Liver Cirrhosis and its Development

FALK SYMPOSIUM 115

Liver Cirrhosis and its Development

Edited by

J. L. Boyer

Liver Center
Section of Digestive Diseases
Yale University School of Medicine
New Haven, CT
USA

H. E. Blum

Medizinische Klinik und Poliklinik
Universitätsklinikum Freiburg
Freiburg
Germany

T. Sauerbruch

Medizinische Klinik
Allgemeine Innere Medizin
Klinikum der Universität
Bonn
Germany

K.-P. Maier

Medizinische Klinik
Fachbereich Gastroenterologie
Städtische Kliniken
Esslingen
Germany

G. A. Stalder

Abteilung Gastroenterologie
Kantonsspital
Basel
Switzerland

Proceedings of the Falk Symposium 115 held in Basel, Switzerland, 22–24 October, 1999 (Part II of the Basel Liver Week 1999; XI International Congress of Liver Diseases)

KLUWER ACADEMIC PUBLISHERS
DORDRECHT / BOSTON / LONDON

Library of Congress Cataloging-in-Publication Data is available.

ISBN 0-7923-8760-0

Published by Kluwer Academic Publishers, BV
P.O. Box 17, 3300 AA Dordrecht, The Netherlands.

Sold and distributed in North, Central and South America
by Kluwer Academic Publishers,
101 Philip Drive, Norwell, MA 02061, USA.

In all other countries, sold and distributed
by Kluwer Academic Publishers, Distribution Center,
P.O. Box 322, 3300 AH Dordrecht, The Netherlands

Printed on acid-free paper

Printed and bound in Great Britain by MPG Books.

Contents

SECTION III: ALCOHOLIC LIVER DISEASE, NASH, DRUGS AND TOXINS

SECTION IV: METABOLIC LIVER DISEASES

List of Principal Contributors

B. R. Bacon
Division of Gastroenterology and Hepatology
Department of Internal Medicine
School of Medicine
Saint Louis University Health Sciences Center
3635 Vista Avenue at Grand Blvd.
St Louis, MO 63110-0250
USA

H. E. Blum
Medizinische Klinik und Poliklinik
Universitätsklinikum Freiburg
Hugstetter Str. 55
D-79106 Freiburg
Germany

J. L. Boyer
Liver Center
Section of Digestive Diseases
1080 LMP
Yale University School of Medicine
333 Cedar Street
New Haven, CT 06520-8019
USA

J. R. Chowdhury
Marion Bessin Liver Research Center
Albert Einstein College of Medicine
1300 Morris Park Avenue
Bronx, NY 10461-1926
USA

H. Denk
Pathologisches Institut
Universität Graz
Auenbruggerplatz 25
A-8036 Graz
Austria

V. J. Desmet
Universitair Ziekenhuis Sint Rafaël
Laboratorium voor Histo- & Cytochemie
Minderbroedersstraat 12
B-3000 Leuven
Belgium

A. M. Di Bisceglie
Department of Internal Medicine
Saint Louis University Health Sciences Center
3635 Vista Ave. at Grand Blvd
PO Box 15250
St. Louis, MO 63110-0250
USA

M. O. Doss
Abteilung für Klinische Biochemie
Fachbereich Humanmedizin
Universität Marburg
Deutschhausstr. 17 1/2
D-35037 Marburg
Germany

G. M. Dusheiko
Royal Free and University College School of Medicine
Centre for Hepatology
Pond Street
Hampstead
London, NW3 2QG
UK

S. Eriksson
Lund University
Department of Medicine
Universitetssjukhuset MAS
SE-205 02 Malmö
Sweden

N. Fausto
Department of Pathology
University of Washington School of Medicine
C-516 Health Science Center
Box 357470
Seattle, WA 98195-7470
USA

P. Ferenci
Klinische Abteilung für Gastroenterologie und Hepatologie
Universitats-Klinik für Innere Medizin IV
Allgem. Krankenhaus der Stadt Wien
Währinger Gürtel 18–20
A-1090 Wien
Austria

C. Ferrari
Laboratorio di Immunologia Virale
Divisione Malattie Infettive
Azienda Ospedaliera di Parma
Via Gramsci 14
I-43100 Parma
Italy

S. L. Friedman
Box 1123, Mount Sinai School of Medicine
1425 Madison Avenue
Room 11-70F
New York, NY 10029-6574
USA

J. L. Gollan
Department of Medicine
Adelaide University
Royal Adelaide Hospital
North Terrace
Adelaide, South Australia 5000
Australia

C. S. Lieber
Alcohol Research and Treatment Center
Liver Disease and Nutrition Section
VA Medical Center (151-2)
130 West Kingsbridge Road
Bronx, NY 10468-3922
USA

K.-P. Maier
Medizinische Klinik
Fachbereich Gastroenterologie
Städtische Kliniken
Hirschlandstr. 97
D-73730 Esslingen
Germany

P. J. Meier-Abt
Abteilung für Klinische Pharmakologie
Medizinische Klinik
Universitätsspital
Rämistr. 100
CH-8091 Zürich
Switzerland

U. A. Meyer
Biozentrum der Universität Basel
Abteilung Pharmakologie/ Neurobiologie
Klingelbergstr. 70
CH-4056 Basel
Switzerland

D. Moradpour
Abteilung Innere Medizin II
Medizinische Universitätsklinik
Hugstetter Str. 55
D-79106 Freiburg
Germany

S. K. Sarin
Department of Gastroenterology
G.B. Pant Hospital
New Delhi 110-002
India

U. Spengler
Medizinische Klinik und Poliklinik
Allgemeine Innere Medizin
Klinikum der Universität
Sigmund-Freud-Str. 25
D-53105 Bonn
Germany

T. Sauerbruch
Medizinische Klinik und Poliklinik
Allgemeine Innere Medizin
Klinikum der Universität
Sigmund-Freud-Str. 25
D-53127 Bonn
Germany

G. A. Stalder
Abteilung Gastroenterologie
Kantonsspital
Petersgraben 4
CH-4031 Basel
Switzerland

J. Stenner
Department of Gastroenterology, Endocrinology and Metabolism
St. George's Hospital Medical School
Cranmer Terrace
London SW17 0RE
UK

W. Stremmel
Abteilung Innere Medizin IV
Universität Heidelberg
Bergheimer Str. 58
D-69115 Heidelberg
Germany

J. H. Teckman
Department of Pediatrics
Washington University
School of Medicine
One Children's Place
St. Louis, MO 63110
USA

H. C. Thomas
Hepatology Section
Department of Medicine A
Imperial College School of Medicine
St Mary's Hospital
London, W2 1PG
UK

M. Trauner
Division of Gastroenterology and Hepatology
Department of Medicine
Karl-Franzens University
Auenbruggerplatz 15
A-8036 Graz
Austria

C. Trepo
INSERM U 271
151 Cours Albert Thomas
F-69003 Lyon Cedex
France

F. von Weizsäcker
Medizinische Klinik und Poliklinik
Universitätsklinikum Freiburg
Hugstetter Str. 55
D-79106 Freiburg
Germany

Introduction

J. L. BOYER

It is a great privilege and honour on behalf of the Scientific organizing committee and the Falk Foundation to introduce the XIth International Congress of Liver Diseases on Liver Cirrhosis and its Development. Although this is the 115th symposium that has been sponsored by the generosity of Herbert Falk and the Falk Foundation over a period that now spans nearly 31 years, this symposium is particularly noteworthy as it is the last of these international congresses of liver diseases to be held in this century. It is fitting, therefore, to first take note of the remarkable progress that has taken place in the field of hepatology during this period, much of which has resulted from discoveries made since the beginning of these congresses.

The presentations in this symposium come from an international faculty of experts who provide us with the very latest concepts concerning the pathogenesis and treatment of chronic liver diseases. These presentations indicate an extraordinary rate of progress in the field of hepatology and are all the more remarkable, given that hepatology as a formal discipline is barely 50 years old. In 1950, the American Association for the Study of Liver Disease was first founded followed shortly by the International Association for the Study of Liver and its regional constituencies. Most of the major landmark discoveries in hepatology in this century have occurred during this period.

Landmark Events in Hepatology in the 20th Century

1. Liver biopsy techniques
2. Liver function tests
3. Identification of hepatitis viruses
4. Effective treatment for chronic liver diseases
5. Liver transplantation
6. Molecular basis for inherited liver disease

Liver biopsy, now taken for granted as a major diagnostic tool, was not generally accepted as a safe procedure until 1958 when Menghini popularized the 'one second' aspiration needle technique. Serum aminotransferases, now routinely used as liver tests to screen for hepatic abnormalities, also came into use only in the late 1950s through the work of LaDue and colleagues. Viral hepatitis, previously thought to result from a catarrh obstruction in the extrahepatic biliary tree, was not recognized as an infectious disease until the middle of this century through pioneering work of Saul Krugman and many others. The discovery of the hepatitis viruses, and the development of tests for their diagnosis, began with Blumberg's Nobel Prize discovery of hepatitis B and are landmark developments that took place only in the past 25 years. Prior to that time, few effective therapies for chronic liver diseases were available other than corticosteroid treatment for autoimmune hepatitis. One of the most remarkable advances has been the development of liver transplantation pioneered by Thomas Starzl, a miraculous accomplishment when viewed from the perspective of many sceptics as recently as the early 1970s. Finally the advent of molecular medicine has led to the identification of specific gene defects in patients with haemochromatosis, Wilson's disease and a number of other inherited liver diseases. Thus, as this century comes to a close and we marvel at the current pace of scientific progress, we have seen far but, like Sir Isaac Newton, we have been standing on the shoulders of giants.

I am sure you will find that this symposium provides an exciting over-view of most of the current major developments in the science and practice of hepatology that are carrying us into the 21st century and the next millennium.

Section I
Cell biology and molecular biology

1
Molecular mechanisms of liver regeneration and hepatocyte apoptosis

N. FAUSTO

The simplest way to conceive the mechanisms that initiate liver regeneration is to assume that at the start of the process, quiescent hepatocytes are propelled into proliferation by the action of a single growth factor. Although compelling, this idea is obviously simplistic and fails to take into account the complexity of gene expression patterns triggered by partial hepatectomy (PH). Recent data from many laboratories, including our own, show instead that liver regeneration after PH is a multistep process and that each step may have its own mediator. Moreover, some of the mediators of the initial steps of regeneration may not function as mitogens. Instead they act by making hepatocytes capable of responding to growth factors (priming effect).

A large number of genes are either newly expressed or show an increase in expression in the regenerating liver. Gene expression during liver regeneration after PH can be divided into a series of stages, starting with the expression of immediate early genes.

IMMEDIATE EARLY GENES

The first phase of gene expression after partial hepatectomy, referred to as the immediate early phase, occurs very rapidly after the operation and lasts approximately 4 h (Fig. 1). The proto-oncogenes c-*fos*, c-*jun* and c-*myc* were the first genes to be identified in this group[1–3]. Subsequent work by Taub and colleagues revealed that as many as 70 genes participate in the immediate early response to partial hepatectomy[4,5]. These genes do not share a common function and include, among others, transcription factors and, tyrosine phosphatases, as well as secreted and intracellular metabolic proteins[6]. It is a difficult and important challenge to determine which among these many genes play essential roles in hepatocyte replication but substantial progress has been made in the identification of such genes[7–9].

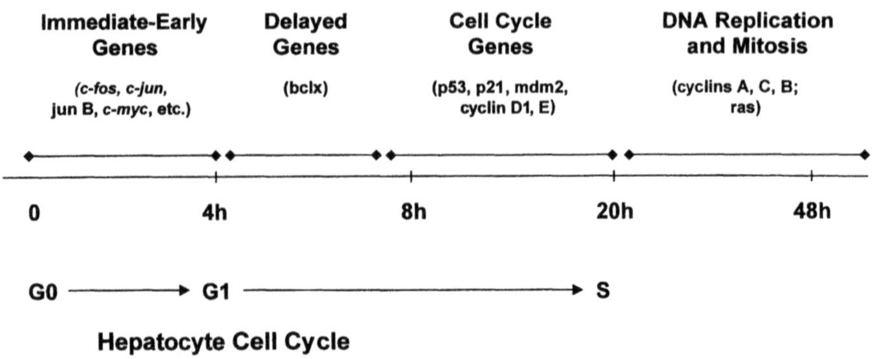

Figure 1 Sequence of gene activation during liver regeneration after partial hepatectomy. The times shown are approximate and represent the timing of events in regenerating rat liver. In mice, DNA replication after partial hepatectomy starts later (around 36 h) and reaches a maximum at 40–44 h after the operation. In both rats and mice the immediate early gene response occurs (approximately) during the first 4 h after partial hepatectomy. At the start of this phase the transcription factors NFκB and STAT3 are activated and hepatocytes are 'primed' by cytokines to fully respond to the growth factors HGF, TGα and EGF.

TRANSCRIPTION FACTOR ACTIVATION AFTER PARTIAL HEPATECTOMY

Transcription factors are proteins which bind specific recognition sites in genes to initiate or enhance their transactivation. Although it was expected that individual transcription factors would bind to single genes, this notion was quickly discarded after the demonstration that a transcription factor can bind and activate multiple genes (target genes). Conversely, it was also demonstrated that single genes bind multiple transcription factors. Thus, transcription factors can propagate signals by activating many different genes while interactions between transcription factors provide another level of regulation for transactivating specific genes.

An important advance in understanding liver regeneration was the finding that the transcription factors NFκB, AP-1, C/EBPβ and STAT3 are activated after partial hepatectomy[10–15]. Activation of these factors does not require protein synthesis, being dependent instead on post-translation mechanisms.

Originally identified in B lymphocytes, NFκB (nuclear factor for the kappa chain of B cells) is found in almost every cell type, including hepatocytes and non-parenchymal cells[11]. In liver cells, it is a heterodimer composed of two protein subunits, referred to as p65 or relA and p50[10,11]. The two subunits are assembled in the cytoplasm but the heterodimer is inactive because an inhibitor, IκB, binds to the p65 subunit. The NFκB heterodimer (p65/p50) free from the IκB inhibitor migrates to the cell nucleus (Fig. 2) where it activates genes involved in inflammation, cell adhesion, stress responses, cell replication and apoptosis. After partial hepatectomy, NFκB is activated very rapidly, within 30 min, if not earlier, after the operation. The activation is transient and is no longer present after 4–5 h[10,11].

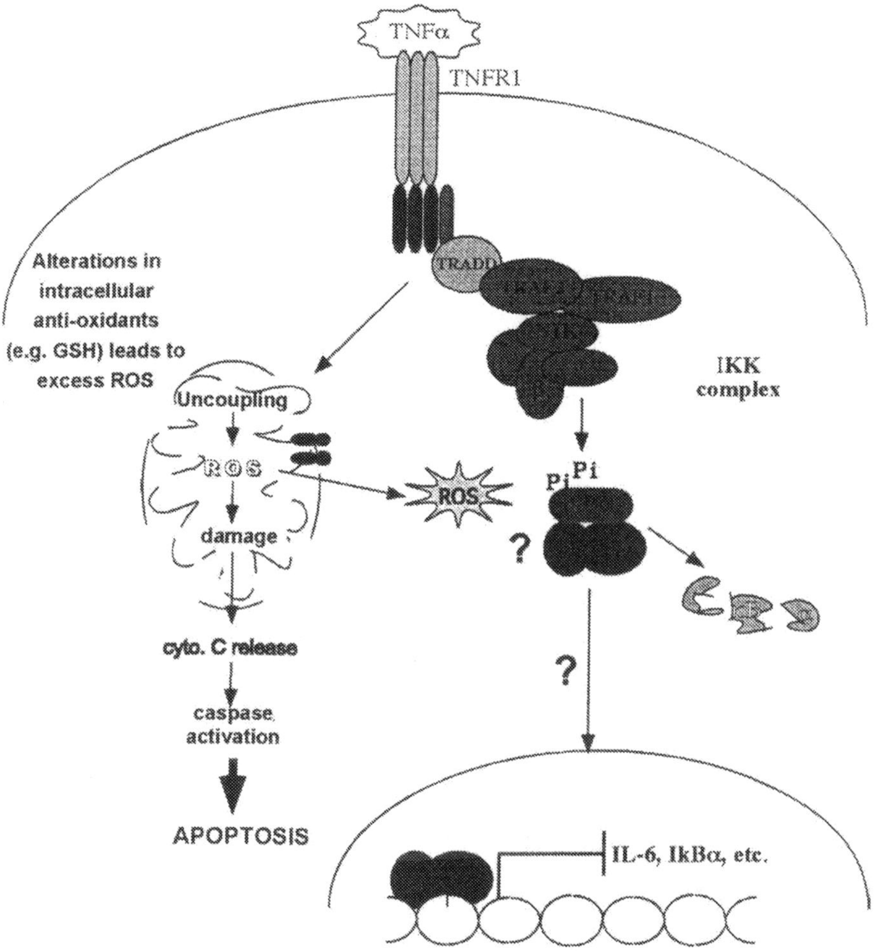

Figure 2 Mechanisms of TNF signalling, NF-κB activation and apoptosis. TNF induces apoptosis in the liver if NFκB activation is blocked or if oxidant stress causes excess production of reactive oxygen species (ROS) that are not captured by cellular antioxidant defences. The figure illustrates excess ROS as a cause of mitochondrial damage, cytochrome C release and caspase activation leading to apoptosis. In this situation TNF functions as an apoptotic rather than a proliferative agent for hepatocytes.

Activation of NFκB involves the phosphorylation of IκB at two critical serine residues. This is followed by the addition of ubiquitin to phosphorylated IκB leading to digestion of phosphorylated, ubiquitinated IκB by the proteasome complex (Fig. 2). The phosphorylation of IκB is controlled by IκB kinases which associate together in a complex. These enzymes are referred to as IKKα (or IKK1) and IKKβ (or IKK2) and appear to respond to different inducible stimuli. While IKKα was found to be required for embryonic development of skin and limbs, the inactivation of IKKβ in knockout mice caused massive liver apoptosis and embryonic lethality[16–18]. Similar effects are also present in mice that lack the p65 (relA) component of NFκB[19]. Thus, the absence of NFκB activity in embryonic development, brought about by either the inactivation of one of its components or the lack of release of the IκB inhibitor preventing the migration of the nucleus of the active NFκB heterodimer, causes liver apoptosis. It has been recently demonstrated that embryonic lethality in RelA knockouts can be eliminated by crossing these animals with mice deficient in TNFR-1 (Rosenfeld et al., Am J Pathol. 2000;156:997–1007). Thus, in the absence of NFκB, TNF functions as an apoptotic agent in liver development. Blockage of NFκB in the regenerating liver by expression of an NFκB superrepressor in an adenovirus vector led to apoptosis after the cells had replicated their DNA[20].

The transcription factor STAT3 is also activated after partial hepatectomy, but the activation is slower than that of NFκB and the mechanism of activation entirely different. STAT3 is detectable in the liver by 1–2 h after partial hepatectomy and the activation lasts for 4–5 h, as determined by gel shift assays[12]. STAT3 is a member of a family of transcription factors known as signal transduction and activators of transcription[21,22]. So far seven mammalian STAT genes have been cloned. STAT3 is activated mainly by IL-6 type cytokines, a family of proteins that includes oncostatin M, leukaemia inhibitory factor (LIF), ciliary neurotrophic factor (CNTF), interleukin-11 (IL-11) and cardiotrophin (CT), all of which use a common gp130 receptor subunit for signal transduction. Binding of IL-6 causes dimerization of the receptor, activation of intracellular tyrosine kinases (JAKs) which phosphorylate gp130 and create docking sites for STAT3 binding. STAT3 is phosphorylated and translocated to the nucleus where it regulates expression of a large number of genes including those involved in inflammation, the acute phase response and proliferation.

LIVER REGENERATION AS A MULTISTEP PROCESS: PRIMING AND CELL CYCLE PROGRESSION

Given the enormous complexity of gene expression in the regenerating liver, it becomes essential to know how the process starts and how the transcription factor and gene activation events are regulated and coordinated. The simplest way to approach these questions is to assume that one or more growth factors can both initiate the process and regulate its progression. To test this hypothesis we have infused growth factors that stimulate hepatocyte replication in primary culture directly into the portal circulation of rats[23]. The infusions were done using osmotic pumps that delivered transforming growth factor α (TGFα), hepatocyte growth factor (HGF) or epidermal growth factor (EGF) with or without insulin for a period of 24 h. DNA synthesis was measured by BrdU incorporation either during the 24 h infusion or for a 48 h period. In all of these experiments no more than 10% of hepatocytes was labelled, a value that is well below the level of hepatocyte replication in the regenerating liver. We found, however, that the same type of infusion in animals with 30% hepatectomies had a much more substantial effect on hepatocyte replication. A 30% hepatectomy by itself has a very small effect on DNA replication but there is absence of a distinct peak of replication at 24 h. Growth factor infusion in these animals restored this peak, and both enhanced and synchronized hepatocyte replication[23]. This, as well as nutritional shift experiments[24], led us to propose that hepatocytes need to be primed to become competent for replication and respond to growth factors. In contrast to cells of proliferative tissues, hepatocytes are resting cells, in the G0 phase of the cell cycle. We hypothesized that gene activation (priming) is required for hepatocytes to go from quiescence to the G1 phase of the cell cycle. In early G1, the cells fully respond to growth factors and can then progress through the cell cycle, overcome the G1 restriction point and undergo DNA replication. Liu et al.[25] used a different approach to show that the response of hepatocytes to growth factors can be greatly enhanced by experimental manipulation. They perfused rat livers with small amounts of collagenase before administration of HGF or TGFα. Collagenase digestion greatly increased the growth factor induced mitogenic response.

The notion that a priming step may be needed for proliferation or more broadly, the view that hepatocyte replication is a multistep process, is not new. Bucher and her colleagues demonstrated in 1970 that the period of time between partial hepatectomy and the peak of DNA replication in rats (22–24 h) can be shortened by stress (such as a sham surgical procedure) and by growth hormone injections[26,27]. These experiments as well as the nutritional modulation experiments conducted by Leduc[28] suggested that primed hepatocytes required less time to undergo DNA replication because the initial phase of the replication process had already taken place. Furthermore, these and the more recent experiments showed that the priming process is reversible and is not sufficient by itself to cause replication (see below).

If hepatocyte replication is a multistep process it follows that agents that initiate liver regeneration should trigger the first phase of gene activation after partial hepatectomy. Because the activation of a transcription factor can increase the transcription of multiple genes, transcription factor activity is a good marker for the initiation events of liver regeneration. Among the transcription factors that are activated after partial hepatectomy we selected NFκB for study. In searching for agents that could trigger NFκB activation as an initiating event for liver regeneration, we found that TNF was a potent NFκB inducer in animals[11].

PROINFLAMMATORY CYTOKINES CAN INITIATE LIVER REGENERATION

TNF is a multifunctional cytokine[29] that signals through 2 distinct receptors, TNFR-1 (p55) and TNFR-2 (p75). In the liver it acts as a mediator of the acute phase response and is a cytotoxic agent in many types of hepatic injury. Nevertheless, Akerman et al.[30] showed that administration of anti-TNF antibodies inhibited liver regeneration after partial hepatectomy in rats, suggesting that TNF may be necessary for hepatocyte proliferation. We approached this problem by studying liver regeneration after partial hepatectomy or CCl_4 injury in knockout mice deficient in either TNFR-1 or TNFR-2[31–33]. Mice lacking functional TNFR-2 showed completely normal DNA replication and gain of liver mass after partial hepatectomy, although activation of AP-1 and C/EBP were delayed[33]. Regeneration after CCl_4 injury was also normal in these animals, indicating that TNFR-2 signaling is not essential for these growth processes. In contrast, lack of signalling through TNFR-1 greatly inhibited DNA replication after partial hepatectomy and caused significant mortality 24–40 h after the operation[32]. In TNFR-1 knockouts activation of NFκB and STAT3 was severely inhibited, while AP-1 activation was decreased. Levels of TNF and IL-6 increase in the blood very quickly after partial hepatectomy in normal animals. In TNFR-1 knockouts TNF also increases, but there is only a very small change in IL-6. A single injection of IL-6 reversed the defect in liver regeneration in TNFR-1 knockouts and restored STAT3 activation. Cressman et al.[34] showed that liver regeneration is impaired in IL-6 knockout mice and that an IL-6 injection corrected the deficits in DNA replication and STAT3 activation after partial hepatectomy and CCl_4 injury.

The work with TNFR-1 and IL-6 knockout mice and with anti-TNF antibodies demonstrates that TNF signalling through TNFR-1 is required for liver regeneration after partial hepatectomy. This signalling pathway follows the sequence TNF $\rightarrow$ TNFR-1 $\rightarrow$ NFκB $\rightarrow$ IL-6 $\rightarrow$ STAT3. The same pathway is also involved in the regeneration of the liver after CCl_4 injury. The regenerative response of TNFR-1 knockout mice after CCl_4 administration was much slower than that of normal animals, but no increased mortality was apparent[31]. Defects were much more severe in IL-6 knockouts injected with CCl_4 (Taub, personal communication). Their livers had a much larger proportion of apoptotic hepatocytes than normal animals, a condition reversed by IL-6 injection. IL-6 has both mitogenic and anti-apoptotic[35] effects on hepatocytes and protects the regenerating liver against ischaemic injury[36].

The observation that TNF and IL-6 are required for liver regeneration is surprising because TNF is a pro-inflammatory cytokine and a mediator of the acute phase response[37]. The proliferative and anti-apoptotic effect of these cytokines takes place only under special conditions, such as those existing after partial hepatectomy. Rai et al.[38] have demonstrated that TNF/IL-6-induced nitric oxide synthase (iNOS) has a cytoprotective role in the regenerating liver. iNOS mRNA increases in the liver before hepatocyte replication and it has been suggested that NO and iNOS may protect the liver from TNF cytotoxicity. Liver regeneration in iNOS knockout mice was severely impaired despite the normal induction of TNF and IL-6 and activation of NFκB and STAT3. Instead of proliferation, cell death predominated in the liver of these knockout mice, demonstrating that NO is required for hepatocyte viability in presence of elevated amounts of TNF and IL-6[38].

TNF PRIMES HEPATOCYTE FOR REPLICATION BUT IS NOT A COMPLETE MITOGEN

TNF injected into rats at relatively high doses induces cell replication in the liver. Replication occurs first in non-parenchymal cells followed a day later by hepatocyte replication. This sequence of cell replication is the opposite of that which takes place after partial hepatectomy (that is, hepatocytes replicate first followed by non-parenchymal cells). The implication of these results is that non-parenchymal cells may release IL-6 or other agents capable of inducing hepatocyte replication[39]. However, when given at low doses to rats or mice, TNF has no effect on hepatocyte replication or apoptosis. We hypothesized that TNF may not have complete mitogenic capacity but functions instead as a priming agent for hepatocytes at the start of liver regeneration. To test this hypothesis we infused rats with growth factors for 24 h and gave the animals a single injection of TNF at the start of the infusion[40]. DNA labelling measured by BrdU incorporation was increased by approximately 4-fold by TNF administration. The cytokine had a stimulatory effect even if given 24 h before the start of the infusion, but the effect was lost if TNF was given 48 h before growth factor infusion. Work with hepatocytes and oval cells in culture demonstrated that TNF stimulates DNA replication in these cells only if they are kept in serum containing medium. TNF had no mitogenic effect for cells maintained in serum free medium in absence of growth factors (Cell Growth Diff. 1999;10:819–28 Kirillova et al.).

In summary, both the animal and cell culture experiments show that TNF primes hepatocytes for proliferation and makes the cells responsive to growth factors (in vivo) or serum (in culture). The TNF priming effect is not specific for any individual growth factor but is equally effective for HGF, TGFα and EGF[40]. Priming of hepatocytes after partial hepatectomy probably involves pathways other than those described here. These may require growth factors rather than cytokines as inducers[41]. For instance, activation of NFκB and STAT3 may not be effective unless the activity of AP-1 and C/EBPβ is enhanced by growth factors. Moreover, increases in protease activity that occur rapidly after partial hepatectomy may cause the release of active HGF and trigger one or more arms of the proliferative cascade.

TNF CAUSES HEPATOCYTE APOPTOSIS THROUGH OXIDATIVE INJURY AND MITOCHONDRIAL DAMAGE

TNF is an initiator of hepatocyte proliferation after partial hepatectomy and CCl_4 injury. However TNF causes apoptosis in many cell types, including hepatocytes. The aims of this work were to determine the conditions under which TNF causes hepatocyte apoptosis instead of proliferation and the mechanisms of TNF-induced apoptosis. Administration of murine TNF (3.3 μg/kg) to mice causes no cell death. However, TNF injection following pretreatment with 800 μg/kg actinomycin D (ActD) caused massive hepatocyte apoptosis within 5–6 h, an effect that was also present in mice that over-express Bcl-2. To study the mechanisms of TNF-induced apoptosis in hepatocytes we used AML-12 cells, a non-transformed, well differentiated murine hepatocyte cell line. Similarly to findings reported with hepatocytes in primary culture, TNF causes apoptosis in AML-12 cells only if given together with a transcriptional blocking agent (ActD in this case). TNF alone can, however, act as an apoptotic agent in thiol-depleted AML-12 cells (treatment with diethylmaleate and buthioninesulfoximine). Treatment with these thiol-depleting agents is associated with a profound inhibition of NFκB transactivation activity in a luciferase assay probably as consequence of oxidation of cysteine 62 in the DNA binding site of the p50 subunit of NFκB. Analysis of carbonyl end-products of lipid peroxidation using napthoic acid hydrazide (NAH) as a reagent showed that these products were removed rapidly from cells treated with TNF alone but were detectable for longer periods of time in TNF+ActD treated cells.

Based on these data, we hypothesized that TNF causes oxidative stress and changes in redox state in hepatocytes and that ActD blocks the induction of reactive oxygen species (ROS) defence/repair mechanisms that protect the cell from apoptosis (Fig. 2). To test this hypothesis we developed multiparametric flow cytometry methods to identify redox-associated changes caused by TNF+ActD prior to nuclear or cellular changes characteristic of apoptosis. The pre-apoptotic phenotype in hepatocytes involved a loss of reduced NAD(P)H (20- to 30-fold decrease in UV-excited 450 nm fluorescence) and concomitant loss of GSH and total reduced thiols (monobromobimane fluorescence). Mitochondrial changes included a reduction in NAO-fluorescence corresponding to loss of cardiolipin from inner mitochondrial membrane, demonstrating oxidative damage in the lipid compartment of mitochondria; decreased mitochondrial potential ($\Delta\Psi_m$) in parallel with a decrease in reduced NAD; and 'uncoupling', indicating loss of proximal electron transport chain integrity (Pierce et al., Am J Pathol. 2000;157:221–36).

Treatment of AML-12 cells with α-lipoate, an agent that prevents GSH decrease, inhibited the loss of cardiolipin, caspase activation and nuclear changes induced by TNF+ActD. Various inhibitors of mitochondrial electron transport blocked the caspase activation and the changes in nuclear morphology caused by TNF+ActD, indicating that the mitochondrial electron transport chain serves as the source of ROS that cause oxidative stress.

We conclude that TNF acts on hepatocytes by increasing ROS through the electron transport chain. It initiates hepatocyte proliferation when ROS are channelled for the activation of NFκB and the excess is dissipated through defence/repair mechanisms. When such mechanisms fail (by a general blockage of transcription or by lack of NFκB activation leading to reduced GSH), structural and functional mitochondrial damage as well as a decrease in reducing equivalents initiate the chain of events that lead to apoptotic cell death.

REFERENCES

1. Thompson NL, Mead JE, Braun L, Goyette M, Shank PR, Fausto N. Sequential protooncogene expression during rat liver regeneration. Cancer Res. 1986;46:3111–17.
2. Alcorn J, Feitelberg S, Brenner D. Transient induction of c-jun during hepatic regeneration. Hepatology. 1990;11:909–15.
3. Morello D, FitzGerald MJ, Babinet C, Fausto N. c-myc, c-fos, and c-jun regulation in the regenerating livers of normal and H-2K/c-myc transgenic mice. Mol Cell Biol. 1990;10:3185–93.
4. Taub R. Expression and function of growth-induced genes during liver regeneration. In: Jirtle RL, ed. Liver Regeneration and Carcinogenesis: Molecular and Cellular Mechanisms. San Diego: Academic Press, Inc., 1995:71–97.
5. Haber AH, Mohn KL, Diamond RH, Taub R. Induction patterns of 70 genes during nine days after hepatectomy define the temporal course of liver regeneration. J Clin Invest. 1993;91:1319–26.
6. Taub R. Transcriptional control of liver regeneration. FASEB J. 1996;10:413–27.
7. Hsu J-C, Bravo R, Taub R. Interactions among LRF-a, JunB, c-Jun, and c-Fos define a regulatory program in the G_1 phase of liver regeneration. Mol Cell Biol. 1992;12:4654–65.
8. Diamond RH, Cressman DE, Laz TM, Abrams CS, Taub R. PRL-1, a unique nuclear protein tyrosine phosphatase, affects cell growth. Mol Cell Biol. 1994;14:3752–62.
9. Peng Y, Du K, Ramirez S, Diamond RH, Taub R. Mitogenic up-regulation of the PRL-1 protein-tyrosine phosphatase gene by Egr-1. Egr-1 activation is an early event in liver regeneration. J Biol Chem. 1999;274(8):4513–20.

10. Tewari M, Dobrzanski P, Mohn KL, Cressman DE, Hsu J-C, Bravo R et al. Rapid induction in regenerating liver of RL/IF-1 (an IκB that inhibits NF-κB, RelB-p50, and c-Rel-p50) and PHF, a novel κB site-binding complex. Mol Cell Biol. 1992; 12:2898–908.
11. FitzGerald M, Webber E, Donovan J, Fausto N. Rapid DNA binding by nuclear factor κB in hepatocytes at the start of liver regeneration. Cell Growth Diff. 1995;6:417–27.
12. Cressman DE, Diamond RH, Taub R. Rapid activation of the Stat3 transcription complex in liver regeneration. Hepatology. 1995;21:1443–9.
13. Diehl AM, Yang SQ. Regenerative changes in C/EBPα C/EBPβ expression modulate binding to the C/EBP site in the c-fos promoter. Hepatology. 1994;19:447–56.
14. Rana B, Xie Y, Mischoulon D, Bucher NL, Farmer SR. The DNA binding activity of C/EBP transcription factor is regulated in the G1 phase of the hepatocyte cell cycle. J Biol Chem. 1995;270:18123–32.
15. Greenbaum LE, Li W, Cressman DE, Peng Y, Ciliberto G, Poli V et al. CCAAT enhancer-binding protein beta is required for normal hepatocyte proliferation in mice after partial hepatectomy. J Clin Invest. 1998;102:996–1007.
16. Takeda K, Takeuchi O, Tsujimura T, Itami S, Adachi O, Kawai T et al. Limb and skin abnormalities in mice lacking IKKalpha. Science. 1999;284:313–16.
17. Hu Y, Baud V, Delhase M, Zhang P, Deerinck T, Ellisman M et al. Abnormal morphogenesis but intact IKK activation in mice lacking the IKKalpha subunit of IkappaB kinase. Science. 1999;284:316–20.
18. Li Q, Van Antwerp D, Mercurio F, Lee KF, Verma IM. Severe liver degeneration in mice lacking the IkappaB kinase 2 gene. Science. 1999;284:321–5.
19. Beg AA, Sha WC, Bronson RT, Ghosh S, Baltimore D. Embryonic lethality and liver degeneration in mice lacking the RelA component of NF-κB. Nature. 1995;376:167–70.
20. Iimuro Y, Nishiura T, Hellerbrand C, Behrns KE, Schoonhoven R, Grisham JW et al. NFkappaB prevents apoptosis and liver dysfunction during liver regeneration (published erratum appears in J Clin Invest. 1998;101:1541). J Clin Invest. 1998;101:802–11.
21. Heinrich PC, Behrmann I, Muller-Newen G, Schaper F, Graeve L. Interleukin-6-type cytokine signalling through the gp130/Jak/STAT pathway. Biochem J. 1998;334:297–314.
22. Darnell JE. Reflections on STAT3, STAT5, and STAT6 as fat STATs. Proc Natl Acad Sci USA. 1996;93:6221–4.
23. Webber EM, Godowski PJ, Fausto N. In vivo response of hepatocytes to growth factors requires an initial priming stimulus. Hepatology. 1994;19:489–97.
24. Mead JE, Braun L, Martin DA, Fausto N. Induction of replicative competence ('priming') in normal liver. Cancer Res. 1990;50:7023–30.
25. Liu M-L, Mars WM, Zarnegar R, Michalopoulos GK. Collagenase pretreatment and the mitogenic effects of hepatocyte growth factor and transforming growth factor-α in adult rat liver. Hepatology. 1994;19:1521–7.
26. Moolten FL, Oakman NJ, Bucher NLR. Accelerated response of hepatic DNA synthesis to partial hepatectomy in rats pretreated with growth hormone or surgical stress. Cancer Res. 1970;30:2353–7.
27. Bucher NLR. Liver regeneration then and now. In: Jirtle RL, ed. Liver Regeneration and Carcinogenesis: Molecular and Cellular Mechanisms. San Diego: Academic Press, 1995:1–25.
28. Leduc EH. Mitotic activity in the liver of the mouse during inanition followed by refeeding with different levels of protein. Am J Anat. 1949;84:397–430.
29. Baker SJ, Reddy EP. Transducers of life and death: TNF receptor superfamily and associated proteins. Oncogene. 1996; 12:1–9.
30. Akerman P, Cote P, Yang SQ, McClain C, Nelson S, Bagby GJ et al. Antibodies to tumor necrosis factor-α inhibit liver regeneration after partial hepatectomy. Am J Physiol. 1992;263:G579–85.
31. Yamada Y, Fausto N. Deficient liver regeneration after carbon tetrachloride injury in mice lacking type 1 but not type 2 tumor necrosis factor receptor. Am J Pathol. 1998;152:1577–89.
32. Yamada Y, Kirillova I, Peschon JJ, Fausto N. Initiation of liver growth by tumor necrosis factor: deficient liver regeneration in mice lacking type I tumor necrosis factor receptor. Proc Natl Acad Sci USA. 1997;94:1441–6.
33. Yamada Y, Webber EM, Kirillova I, Peschon JJ, Fausto N. Analysis of liver regeneration in mice lacking type 1 or type 2 tumor necrosis factor receptor: requirement for type 1 but not type 2 receptor. Hepatology. 1998;28:959–70.

34. Cressman DE, Greenbaum LE, DeAngelis RA, Ciliberto G, Furth EE, Poli V et al. Liver failure and defective hepatocyte regeneration in interleukin-6-deficient mice. Science. 1996;274:1379–83.
35. Sakamoto T, Liu Z, Murase N, Ezure T, Yokomuro S, Poli V et al. Mitosis and apoptosis in the liver of interleukin-6-deficient mice after partial hepatectomy. Hepatology. 1999;29:403–11.
36. Selzner M, Camargo CA, Clavien P-A. Ischemia impairs liver regeneration after major tissue loss in rodents: Protective effects of IL-6. Hepatology. 1999;30:469–75.
37. Xing Z, Richards CD, Braciak T, Thibault V, Gauldie J. Cytokine regulation of hepatic acute phase protein expression. Dordrecht: Kluwer Academic Publishers, 1995.
38. Rai RM, Lee FYJ, Rosen A, Yang SQ, Lin HZ, Koteish A et al. Impaired liver regeneration in inducible nitric oxide synthase-deficient mice. Proc Natl Acad Sci USA. 1998;95:13829–34.
39. Shinozuka H, Ohmura T, Katyal SL, Zedda AI, Ledda-Columbano GM, Columbano A. Possible roles of nonparenchymal cells in hepatocyte proliferation induced by lead nitrate and by tumor necrosis factor α. Hepatology. 1996;23:1572–7.
40. Webber EM, Bruix J, Pierce RH, Fausto N. Tumor necrosis factor primes hepatocytes for DNA replication in the rat. Hepatology. 1998;28:1226–34.
41. Taub R, Greenbaum LE, Peng Y. Transcriptional regulatory signals define cytokine-dependent and -independent pathways in liver regeneration. Semin Liver Dis. 1999;19:117–27.

2
Mechanisms of inflammation

V. J. DESMET

INTRODUCTION

The living organism has developed defence mechanisms against damaging factors that may disturb its homoeostatic equilibrium with the surrounding environment. In addition to passive defence systems (e.g. skin and mucosal barriers), there are active defence mechanisms, of non-specific and specific varieties. Active defence mechanisms are triggered when damage to a tissue is caused by some agent. These mechanisms are operated by cells and soluble factors. The non-specific active defence works via the activation of enzyme systems (such as complement), and/or phagocytosis by neutrophil granulocytes or macrophages, and corresponds to the process of inflammation. The specific active defence is specifically directed against a particular molecule, and corresponds to the immune response. The terms inflammation and immune response are not synonyms, but represent different defence mechanisms which may function separately or jointly.

Inflammation is defined as a response to injury of vascularized tissues, with the purpose of delivering defence materials (blood cells and fluids) to the site of injury[1]. It is, however, nonspecific: it is triggered by virtually any type of injury and varies little with different causal agents. In contrast, the immune response is specifically aimed at certain molecular structures (antigens) which are recognized as foreign. The system works with the specific weapons of antibodies and killer cells. However, both become vastly more powerful with the help of non-specific inflammation. This explains why the immune response often borrows inflammation as one of its effector arms, by inciting the release of inflammatory mediators, a task for which T helper cells are in charge to a large extent. Although inflammation and the immune response can be triggered separately, whenever the immune response is triggered, inflammation follows sooner or later[1].

An example of combined inflammation and immune response is found in liver transplantation. Transplantation initiates both alloantigen-independent and alloantigen-dependent inflammatory responses, both of which are cytokine-dominated processes. The alloantigen-independent factors initiate the response in the transplanted organ. These include mechanical trauma, cold ischaemia and preservation injury, warm ischaemia and reperfusion injury, haemodynamic changes and other factors that occur in the recipient during and after organ transplantation. The actual process of allograft rejection requires other alloantigen-dependent factors produced as a consequence of alloantigen recognition by T cells[2]. Classically, distinction is made between acute and chronic inflammation. Although the terms acute and chronic may appear self-evident, it is important to realize that the biological and clinical concepts of acute and chronic inflammation do not match. In clinical terms, chronic refers to weeks, months or years. However, the biological events run faster. The acute response takes place seconds or minutes after an injury; it is stereotyped because it is virtually immutable: it is the instant reaction to injury of any kind. The chronic or modulated response takes over if the injurious agent is not immediately removed. Its function is to provide a more sophisticated response than phagocytosis by neutrophils alone. It is, therefore, masterminded by an extremely flexible, multipurpose cell : the macrophage[1].

The macrophage can accomplish almost everything the neutrophil can do, albeit more slowly. In addition, if required, it can initiate the immune reaction by summoning lymphocytes; it can activate fibroblasts, induce angiogenesis, clotting and fibrosis; it can scavenge and secrete a variety of proteins; it can cause fever and other general responses. In short, the macrophage is programmed to organize a powerful second line of defence, and this may happen long before the inflammation is considered chronic from a clinical point of view. Acute and chronic inflammation are two overlapping responses, with partially different triggering mechanisms and programmes[1].

GENERAL MECHANISMS OF INFLAMMATION

The inflammatory response involves a great number of mechanisms and mediators, which require long chapters in textbooks to be discussed in detail. One of the best, if not *the* best text on this chapter of general pathology is to be found in *Cell, Tissues and Disease* by G. Majno and I. Joris[1] warmly recommended to the reader.

This overview will shortly summarize the mechanisms of inflammation in general, with somewhat more attention to recent developments in mechanisms of leukocyte emigration (adhesion molecules, cytokines and chemokines).

Acute inflammation

The visible tissular changes during an inflammatory reaction were described by Celsus in the first century BC: rubor (redness), calor (heat), tumor (swelling), dolor (pain). The underlying tissular reaction corresponds to hyperaemia, exudation, infiltration and proliferation in successive phases.

Hyperaemia

Hyperaemia is caused by arteriolar dilatation which is usually preceded by a (very) short phase of vasoconstriction. The latter follows the tissue damage instantly and is caused by nerve stimulation. The ensuing vasodilatation is due to chemical mediators such as histamine and serotonin, released from local tissue mast cells which degranulate as a result of tissue damage. The arteriolar dilatation increases capillary pressure and opens additional capillaries in the microcirculatory network. Although capillary dilatation is minimal the postcapillary venules become distended. Their increased leakiness (see further) results in haemoconcentration caused by fluid exudation. This in turn causes increased resistance, raising the pressure upstream, expansion of the lumen, and slowing down of blood flow. These changes take place within a few minutes.

Exudation

Acute inflammation is associated with increased permeability of the postcapillary venules, whose endothelial cells have the highest density of histamine receptors. The increase in permeability results in vascular leakage, which schematically comprises overlapping phases: an early transient period of increased permeability (less than 1 h); an early prolonged phase of increase in permeability (2–6 hs); and a late prolonged phase of greater leakiness.

The early transient phase of vascular leakage is induced by a group of mediators that are present as preformed molecules in the tissue (e.g. histamine in mast cell granules) or produced within about the first minute (e.g. bradykinin, platelet activating factor (PAF), leukotrienes). It may also be due to mild damage of the vascular endothelium itself, in which case the early transient phase is longer (hours). The early prolonged phase is seen in association with more severe tissular and endothelial damage. The late prolonged phase of vascular leakiness (12–18 hs after challenge) occurs in a focus of inflammation that persists long enough, and appears to be due to the effect of cytokines, which take some time to be produced by the cells involved. The increased vascular permeability is due to endothelial contraction or, in case of direct vascular damage, variable degrees of endothelial destruction. The increased vascular permeability leads to extravasation of fluid and larger molecules (proteins), due to disturbance of the normal circumstances which regulate the normal extravasation of fluid from the capillary network (Starling's law).

Infiltration

As a result of the vasodilatation and slowing down of the bloodstream, leukocytes (neutrophil granulocytes and monocytes) leave the axial blood stream and move towards the vessel wall (margination). This is followed by leukocyte adherence to the endothelial cells with subsequent transmigration into the extravascular space.

The first cells to leave the vessels are neutrophils, followed later by monocytes. Neutrophil granulocytes are short-lived and desintegrate within 24–48 hs, whereas monocytes survive longer in the extravascular space. Once outside the vessels, the extravasated cells move towards the focus of tissue damage and phagocytose the debris of damaged cells and tissue components and, in the case of infections, the invaded bacteria. The processes of leukocyte–endothelial adhesion, diapedesis and extravascular directional movement (chemotaxis) and final phagocytosis are regulated by a large number of inflammatory mediators, including impressive numbers of adhesion molecules, cytokines and chemokines discovered in more recent times. These are shortly reviewed in a subsequent section following the general overview of inflammation.

Proliferation

If the phagocytosing cells succeed in eliminating the causative stimuli, the inflammatory reaction will fade out by lack of generation of additional mediators. With removal of tissue debris by macrophages the tissue returns to its original state when the damage to the local tissue cells and structures was minimal (restitutio ad integrum). This is realized by equilibrated regeneration and proliferation of tissue component cells. In the case of more extensive tissue (especially parenchymal) damage, smaller to larger fractions of the destroyed components may become replaced by connective tissue, due to predominant fibroblast proliferation and new vessel formation (granulation tissue and scar formation).

Chronic inflammation

If the inflammatory reaction does not succeed in eliminating or neutralizing the causative agent tissue damage will persist, with resulting persistence of the inflammatory phenomena. Examples are highly virulent bacteria which persist in spite of the inflammatory defence, or a damaging agent which is continuously renewed, as in the case of repetitive mechanical trauma. In such case, the continuing inflammatory reaction is said to become chronic.

In general, chronic inflammation is preceded by acute inflammation, although the latter may be clinically inapparent. The distinction between acute and chronic inflammation is therefore not so much determined by its chronological duration, as by its all or not successful capability to neutralize or eliminate the causative agent. Chronic inflammation is thus caused by a lack of balance between aggressor and defender. This may be due either to higher intrinsic virulence of the damaging agent, or to a decrease in the defence mechanisms of the host.

The morphology of chronic inflammation differs from the acute inflammatory response in a number of ways. Since neutrophils are short-lived, and monocyte-derived macrophages are more efficient in phagocytosis, chronic inflammation is not dominated by granulocytes, but by mononuclear cells. Furthermore, there is an increasing degree of fibroblast proliferation, resulting from the influence of mediators produced by damaged cells and cytokines secreted by macrophages. In addition, persistence of the causative agent brings with it a higher frequence of involvement of the immune response (although the latter may also be triggered from the very beginning by a variety of pathological stimuli). It follows that lymphocytes and plasma cells, together with macrophages and fibroblasts, are the predominant cell types in the chronic inflammatory infiltrate. Lymphocyte-derived cytokines in turn may stimulate the macrophages, which again respond with secretion of pro-inflammatory cytokines and other mediators, resulting in long-lasting inflammatory reactions with important fibroblastic proliferative component and on-going tissue destruction, as is the case, for example, in chronic rheumatoid arthritis.

Granulomatous inflammation

A special variety of chronic inflammation is granulomatous inflammation. This type is associated with the development of granulomas, which correspond to accumulations (up to a few millimetres) of macrophages, lymphocytes and giant cells. These macrophages are modified by cytokines into a phenotype resembling epithelial cells, hence the term epithelioid cells. Fusion of several epithelioid cells leads to the formation of multinucleated giant cells. The granulomatous type of inflammatory reaction is observed in infections by agents with facultative intracellular life, such as *Mycobacterium tuberculosis*. This microorganism is not digestible by the macrophage after phagocytosis. Granulomatous inflammation also occurs with non-living, indigestible particles, such as silicon crystals and some immune aggregates. Because of the intracellular location of these agents there is no direct tissue damage, and hence no acute inflammatory reaction.

The permanent presence of living or dead indigestible material in the macrophage stimulates the latter to continue to secrete mediators, which summon new macrophages and stimulate others to divide. As a result, an agressive particle or bacillus is retained in loco (sequestration). When the localized and indigestible material corresponds to bacteria or fungi an immune response is usually triggered, directed specifically against the causative agent. Its intracellular location, however, prevents its immediate killing or neutralization. Binding of $CD4^+$-lymphocytes to their cognate antigens results in the production of lymphokines, which attract and activate additional macrophages which differentiate into epithelioid cells. The lymphokines also up-regulate the metabolism of the macrophage containing the bacterium or fungus, enabling it eventually to digest its tough meal. This helpful cytokine storm may come at the price of inducing tissue damage and acute inflammation. In this way, the fight against a virulent bacterium may entail tissue damage. In contrast to the immunological granuloma just described, foreign body granulomas develop around indigestible, but non-antigenic materials (e.g. surgical threads; a thorn).

MECHANISMS OF LEUKOCYTE RECRUITMENT AND CHEMOTAXIS

All free cells, from bacteria to amoeba, have the capacity to move toward a chemical attractant (chemotaxin). This directional movement is termed chemotaxis. Chemotactic agents for leukocytes (leukotaxins) include bacterial chemotaxins (e.g. formyl-methionyl-leucyl-phenylalanine (fMLP), the prototype chemoattractant); chemotaxins derived from complement (the anaphylatoxins C3a, C4a, C5a); chemotaxins secreted by live cells (chemotactic cytokines or chemokines); and chemotaxins (presumably polypeptides) derived from injured tissues, released while the cells are dying[1].

Cytokines and chemokines (originally shown to be derived from activated macrophages, later on from many more cell types) activate the endothelium of the venules in areas of inflammation and also activate the leukocytes flowing with the blood stream through these vessels. Endothelial cells are induced to express adhesion molecules, and leukocytes are stimulated to express surface molecules which act as ligands to adhesion molecules, in homotypic and, mostly, heterotypic interaction.

Adhesion molecules

Adhesion molecules are cell surface glycoproteins involved in cell–cell and cell–matrix communications. According to homology in structure and sequence, cell adhesion molecules are subdivided into four large families: immunoglobulin-related, integrins, selectins and cadherins[3].

Adhesion molecules which belong to the **immunoglobulin superfamily**[4] include intercellular adhesion molecule-1 and -2 and -3 (ICAM-1, ICAM-2, ICAM-3), sheep erythrocyte receptor or CD2, vascular cell adhesion molecule-1 (VCAM-1), platelet endothelial cell adhesion molecule-1 (PECAM-1), neural cell adhesion molecule (NCAM) and the mucosal addressin MadCAM-1.

ICAM-1 (CD54) is one of the best studied adhesion molecules. It is expressed on different cell types and its expression is up-regulated by numerous cytokines. Its ligands are the leukocyte β2-integrins LFA1 and Mac-1. CD2 is expressed on T-lymphocytes and was formerly known as the sheep erythrocyte receptor. It binds to leukocyte function associated antigen-3 (LFA-3). VCAM-1 is induced on endothelial cells by various cytokines, where it mediates the interaction between endothelium and lymphocytes, monocytes and eosinophils[5]. VLA-4, expressed on T-lymphocytes, serves as its ligand. Binding of VLA-4 to VCAM-1 plays a co-stimulatory role in the activation of $CD4^+$ lymphocytes. VCAM-1 is further expressed on a variety of other cell types, including macrophages and dendritic cells. PECAM-1 (CD31) is constitutively expressed on endothelial cells, localized at intercellular junctions. At this site it plays a role in the transmigration of leukocytes, both in vitro and in vivo, since administration of blocking anti-CD31 antibodies prevents leukocyte diapedesis during an exudative inflammatory response[6]. MadCAM-1 is a mucosal addressin, constitutively expressed on high endothelial venules of the intestinal mucosa associated lymphoid tissue (MALT) and is involved in the homing of lymphocytes expressing the homing receptor integrin $\alpha 4\beta 7$.

The integrins are heterodimeric transmembrane proteins, connected to components of the cytoskeleton, that transduce (integrate) signals from the exterior to the interior of the cell. The integrins are subdivided according to their β chain. The β chain is associated with an α chain, of which different types are known. Several α-subunits may associate with different β chains, creating the possibility for several integrin combinations.

The β1-integrins, also called very late activation (VLA) integrins, share a common β1 subunit (CD29), and according to their α-subunit (CD49) serve as receptors for extracellular matrix proteins like collagen, laminin, fibronectin, thrombospondin and vitronectin. In addition, the integrin $\alpha 4\beta 1$ (VLA-4) is involved in the adhesion of various leukocytes to cytokine-activated endothelial cells, and serves as a ligand for VCAM-1. In combination with the β7 chain, the α4 subunit serves as a homing receptor of lymphocytes that binds to MadCAM-1, expressed on the venular endothelium of Peyer's patches and intestinal vessels[7], as mentioned before. The β2 or leukocyte integrins share CD18 as their common β chain, which is associated with either CD11a (in LFA-1), CD11-b (in

Mac-1), or CD11c (in p150,95). LFA-1 is expressed on most leukocytes, Mac-1 predominantly on neutrophil granulocytes, and p150,95 on platelets[5]. One of the characteristic features of integrins is their requirement for activation (conformational change of the α–β chain assembly) before they bind their ligands firmly[8,9].

The members of the selectin family (CD62) are characterized by a lectin-like aminoterminal domain, an epidermal growth factor-like region, a domain resembling some of the complement regulatory proteins, and a short intracytoplasmic region[10]. Selectins are classified according to the cells expressing them, as E-(endothelial), P-(platelet), and L-(leukocyte). These so-called homing receptors are primarily involved in the adhesion of inflammatory cells to vascular endothelium during primary adhesion (tethering), and in the homing of lymphocytes through high endothelial venules. Their ligands are sialylated, fucosylated and sulphated carbohydrates, giving rise to low affinity interactions[11].

Cadherins are calcium-dependent adhesive glycoproteins that frequently have other cadherins as ligands. They have a wide distribution in all tissues, suggesting a role in architectural organization of tissues. Finally, CD44 (hyaluronate receptor) occurs in various isoforms generated by alternative splicing and is widely expressed on a variety of cells. It has a general role in cell–cell and cell–matrix adhesion, including lymphocyte homing.

Chemokines

The attraction of leukocytes to tissues is controlled by chemotactic cytokines, or chemokines, over 40 of which have been identified[12]. They are subdivided into families on the basis of the relative position of their cysteine residues. Two of the four families have been more extensively characterized: the α- and the β-chemokines, which contain four cysteines and are the largest families.

In the α-chemokines, one amino acid separates the first two cysteine residues in the N-terminal portion of the molecule (cysteine–X amino acid–cysteine, or CXC chemokine). In the β-chemokines, the first two cysteine residues are adjacent to each other (cysteine–cysteine, or CC chemokine). Two chemokines do not fit in this grouping: lymphotactin, with only two cysteines, and fractalkine, a membrane-bound glycoprotein with a CXXXC motif, in which the chemokine domain sits on a mucin-like stalk. The CXC chemokines that contain the sequence glutamic acid–leucine–arginine preceding the CXC sequence are chemotactic for neutrophils; those that do not contain this sequence act on lymphocytes. Some of the important human CXC chemokines include IL-8; growth-regulated oncogene (Gro-α, β, γ); platelet factor 4 (PF4); interferon-inducible protein 10 (IP-10), epithelial-cell derived neutrophil activating peptide 78 (ENA-78), and neutrophil activating peptide 2 (NAP-2).

The CC chemokines, in general, do not act on neutrophils, but attract monocytes, eosinophils, basophils, and lymphocytes with variable selectivity. As with the CXC family, the N-terminal amino acids preceding the CC residues of β-chemokines are critical components of the biological activity and leukocyte selectivity of these chemokines[12]. Examples of the human CC family of chemokines include monocyte chemoattractant protein (MCP-1, 2 and 3), macrophage inflammatory protein (MIP-1α, and β), and 'Regulated upon activation normal T-cell expressed and secreted' (RANTES). The CC chemokines are active on a range of cells, predominantly macrophages, lymphocytes and basophils; they have a diversity of action which not only depends on the cell type, but also on the state of activation. For example, RANTES attracts both resting and activated $CD4^+$ T cells, MCP-1 attracts predominantly monocytes, MIP-1α affects activated $CD8^+$ T cells and MIP-1β activated $CD4^+$ T cells[13].

The initial step in chemokine-mediated cellular events involves binding of chemokines to specific cell-surface receptors. The chemokine receptors have a serpentine structure with seven transmembrane domains which is common to all chemokine receptors (and to the receptor for bacterial fMLP, and the receptor for the complement component C5a as well). Chemokine receptors are G-protein coupled cell-surface receptors, that are functionally linked to phospholipases through the G proteins. Receptor activation leads to a cascade of cellular activation, including the generation of inositol triphosphate, the release of intracellular free calcium, and the activation of protein kinase C. The signalling also activ-ates small guanosine triphosphate-binding proteins of the Ras and Rho families; The later are involved in cell motility through actin-dependent processes like membrane ruffling, pseudopod formation, and assembly of focal adhesion complexes[12].

Four human CXC chemokine receptors (CXCR1 – CXCR4); eight human CC chemokine receptors (CCR1–CCR8), and one human CXXXC chemokine receptor (CX3CR1) have been identified[12]. Chemokine receptors are expressed on different types of leukocytes. Some are restricted (e.g. CXCR1 is predominantly restricted to neutrophils), whereas others are more widely expressed (e.g. CCR2 is expressed on monocytes, T cells, natural killer cells, dendritic cells and basophils).

Some chemokine receptors are constitutively expressed, others are inducible, and some constitutive receptors can be down-regulated. Further, the expression of some chemokine receptors is restricted to a state of cell activation and differentiation. For example, CXCR3 is expressed on Th1 type helper lymphocytes, whereas CCR3 is preferentially expressed on activated T helper lymphocytes of the Th2 type. The finding that some chemokine receptors are also expressed on non-haematopoietic cells (including neurons, epithelial and endothelial cells) suggests that the chemokine system has other roles in addition to leukocyte chemotaxis[12].

Chemokines also interact with two types of non-signalling molecules. One is the Duffy antigen receptor for chemokines (DARC) on erythrocytes, which may serve as a sink for chemokines, clearing them from the circulation. The second is a group of heparan sulphate proteoglycans. As chemokines are basic proteins they bind avidly to negatively charged molecules such as heparin and heparan sulphate. Heparan sulphate proteoglycans capture chemokines in the extracellular matrix and on the surface of endothelial cells. This binding may serve to establish a local concentration gradient from the point source of chemokine secretion[12,14].

Chemokines are thought to provide the directional cues for the movement of leukocytes in development, homeostasis, and inflammation. The dramatic increase in the secretion of chemokines during inflammation results in the selective recruitment of leukocytes to inflamed tissue. Chemokines have been detected during inflammation in most organs, where they were identified in many cell types. This suggests that most, if not all, cells can secrete chemokines under appropriate stimulation. Macrophages are potent producers[13,15]. The main stimuli for chemokine production are pro-inflammatory-cytokines such as IL-1 and TNF-α, bacterial products like lipopolysaccharide, and viral infection. In addition, interferon-γ (IFN-γ) and IL-4 which are products of Th1 and Th2 helper lymphocytes, respectively, can induce the production of chemokines. Chemokines often act in concert with other cytokines to cause tissue infiltration, by increasing the circulating pool of a given leucocyte and by up-regulating particular adhesion molecules, as well as by increasing leukocyte responsiveness to a chemokine[12].

Leukocyte–endothelial interactions: recruitment of leukocytes and chemotaxis

The bloodstream slows down in vessels near an inflammatory focus. White blood cells marginate towards the periphery of the vessel, whereas erythrocytes form the central column of the bloodstream. Leukocytes leave the circulation when they recognize and bind to endothelial receptors. This adhesion with endothelium is an important regulatory step in leukocyte recruitment into the tissue. The leukocyte–endothelial interaction is a dynamic process involving several sequential adhesion pathways.

The initial encounter or primary adhesion is a reversible binding: it slows the passing leukocyte by a process of transient tethering to the vessel wall, appearing as rolling or bumping on the endothelium. At this stage, some cells may still disengage and be flushed away by the flow. This leukocyte rolling under flow conditions is usually assured by the selectins. These adhesion molecules are ideal mediators of primary adhesion: they are large molecules that extend above the surrounding glycocalyx; they do not require activation in order to mediate adhesion, and the adhesion they mediate is relatively weak and transient, allowing the leukocyte to come into contact with the endothelium and to subsequently disengage if further strong adhesion is not triggered[16,17]. Under certain conditions, other molecules than relectins may mediate primary adhesion. Under low flow conditions VCAM-1 can mediate both primary and secondary adhesion of lymphocytes[18]. This may particularly apply to the low flow system of hepatic sinusoids[16].

The next step of strong, or secondary, adhesion to the endothelium is assured by the leukocyte integrins. As mentioned, these require activation before they bind their ligands firmly[8]. This activation is provided by a triggering step in the cascade, during which the integrins are functionally activated to bind to their cognate endothelial counter-receptor[19]. Trigger factors include PECAM-1 (CD31)[20] and chemokines[12]. In order to trigger firm adhesion effectively, the proadhesive factors must be available at the vessel wall where they can interact with the circulating leukocytes. As mentioned above, chemokines may be retained on the relevant sites of the endothelium by binding to the proteoglycans present in the endothelial glycocalyx[14]. Thus, activated endothelium can contribute to both the production and the presentation of proadhesive chemokines[16].

Selectivity in leukocyte recruitment to the tissue depends on a number of steps: (1) the type of cytokine(s) activating the endothelium, which may result in the expression of particular sets of adhesion molecules; (2) the type of chemokines involved, since these molecules display some selectivity in their action on various types of leukocytes and subsets of lymphocytes; and (3) the type of endothelial glycocalyx (binding the chemokines), which may vary according to the site and type of bloodvessel and the state of its endothelial activation.

The following step of strong adhesion is mediated by the leukocyte integrins which bind to their respective counter-receptors on the endothelium. These integrins are LFA-1, Mac-1 and VLA-4, binding to the counter-receptors ICAM-1 and VCAM-1. Once firmly adherent to the endothelium, the leukocyte moves to the interendothelial junction, and migrates between the endothelial cells into the extracellular space. The adhesion molecule PECAM-1 (CD31) plays a role in this process of transendothelial migration, or diapedesis[6]. Once outside the vessel, the leukocyte is directed in its amoeboid movements by the gradient in chemoattractants, including the solid gradient of chemokines bound to the heparan sulphate proteoglycans of the extracellular matrix.

Mechanisms of leukocyte recruitment into the liver

There are basically two different anatomical regions for leukocyte infiltration in the liver: the portal tracts and the liver parenchyma. Leukocyte entry via the portal tracts probably occurs through the portal venules, whereas entry into parenchymal territories occurs via the sinusoidal endothelium[7,16,21,22].

Hepatic sinusoidal endothelial cells differ from other microvascular endothelial cells. They do not express P-selectin (CD62-P), since the sinusoidal type of endothelium does not contain Weibel–Palade bodies[23] nor the sialomucin CD34[24,25]. In contrast, they express the CD4 molecule. This characteristic appears to render hepatic sinusoidal endothelium unique among endothelial cells[25]. There is evidence for heterogeneity within the sinusoidal bed, with the possibility of differential regulation of leukocyte recruitment through the centrolobular versus periportal sinusoidal endothelium[26].

Concerning neutrophil infiltration, there appears to exist a significant difference between the liver and most other organs in that, in the liver, those neutrophils which are relevant to hepatocellular injury do not accumulate in postsinusoidal venules, but in the capillary equivalents or sinusoids[27,28]. Despite the expression of adhesion molecules on sinusoidal lining cells, antibodies directed against integrins, selectins or adhesion molecules of the immunoglobulin superfamily do not affect neutrophil sequestration in sinusoids[28]. Immunohistochemical demonstration of increased expression of adhesion molecules at sites of inflammation does not by necessity imply their functional significance[29]. Alternative mechanisms for neutrophil trapping in the sinusoids under inflammatory conditions include swelling of Kupffer cells and endothelial cells, an imbalance between vasoconstrictor (e.g. endothelin-1) and vasodilator (e.g. nitric oxide) formation, and increased stiffness of neutrophils after activation[28].

Lymphocyte recirculation to the non-inflamed liver

The non-inflamed liver has a population of T lymphocytes, located in portal tracts and throughout the parenchyma, presumed to patrol the tissue as part of the process of immune surveillance[30]. Liver associated lymphocytes (LAL)[31] may be recruited into the normal, non-inflamed liver through expression of ICAM-1, ICAM-2, LFA-3, CD44 and, according to some studies, low levels of VCAM-1 on the sinusoidal endothelium[21,32]. The portal vessels and hepatic veins express ICAM-2. In addition, both portal and sinusoidal endothelium express vascular adhesion protein-1 (VAP-1), that may be responsible for the primary adhesion step in non-inflamed liver[7,16,33].

The triggering step to activate the T cell integrins to their endothelial ligands appears to be assured by the chemokines MCP-1 and RANTES[7,16].

Leukocyte recruitment to the inflamed liver via the portal tracts

Recruitment of neutrophils into portal tracts (e.g. in acute cholangitis and cholangiolitis) presumably occurs according to similar mechanisms as in microvessels in other organs, since portal vessels are by and large of the same type.

Concerning lymphocyte migration into portal tracts in case of chronic inflammatory liver disease, the formation of neovessels as demonstrated in chronic viral and autoimmune hepatitis is of significance[34]. The new vessels are found in the centre of dense lymphocytic infiltrates and express PECAM-1 (CD31) and endoglin (a TGF-β-binding molecule found on the surface of human endothelium). This neoangiogenesis in portal tracts is analogous to what happens at other sites of chronic inflammation (e.g. rheumatoid synovium), where vessels of the morphology of high endothelial venules are formed in response to chronic inflammatory stimuli[35]. Such specialized high endothelial venules are likely to facilitate an ongoing influx of lymphocytes to the tissue.

In chronic inflammatory liver disease, the portal vessels can express P-selectin, E-selectin, VCAM-1, and high levels of ICAM-1[16,32]. Moreover, inflammatory cells within inflamed portal tracts synthesize MIP-1a, MIP-1b and RANTES. These chomokines can be detected on portal endothelium where they appear to be retained by proteoglycan binding in the glycocalyx[16]. Thus, portal tract inflammation (in chronic viral infection, autoimmunity and graft rejection) is associated with the expression of adhesion molecules and chemotactic cytokines necessary for the adhesion cascade and transmigration[16]. Moreover, the infiltrating T cells express both LFA-1 and VLA-4[36,37], integrin receptors required for firm endothelial binding.

Of interest is a recent preliminary report of functionally active MAdCAM-1 expression on portal vessel endothelium in a majority of patients with primary sclerosing cholangitis (PSC) or autoimmune hepatitis associated with inflammatory bowel disease (IBD). Large numbers of $\alpha4\beta7$-positive lymphocytes were detected in the serum of these patients, and these gut-derived memory T cells could bind to the MAdCAM-expressing portal endothelium. These findings represent an intriguing immunological link between PSC and IBD[38].

Leukocyte recruitment to the inflamed liver via the sinusoids

According to several studies, E- and P-selectin is only weakly expressed on sinusoidal endothelium during inflammation associated with liver allograft rejection and primary biliary cirrhosis[16,21,22] although a strong expression of E-selectin on sinusoidal endothelium was noted in acute viral hepatitis[32].

The requirements for leukocyte recruitment through sinusoids may differ from those at other vascular sites since blood flow is slow through the sinusoids, and the need for primary, selectin-mediated adhesion is abolished at low flow rates. Lymphocytes may be able to bind to VCAM-1 on the sinusoids directly without the need for prior tethering by selectins[18]. This might explain the lower inducibility of selectins on sinusoidal endothelium[16]. Sinusoidal endothelial ICAM-1 and VCAM-1 is up-regulated in inflammation, allowing for adherence of LFA-1 and VLA-4 positive lymphocytes. Activation of leukocyte integrins by chemokines may be assured by sinusoidal endothelial synthesis and expression of MIP-1α and MIP-1β[16]. Interaction of (cytotoxic) T lymphocytes and hepatocytes is accomplished by several adhesion pathways, including LFA-1 – ICAM-1, CD2 – LFA-3, VLA-4 – VCAM-1 and CD28–B7.

As mentioned before, retention of neutrophils in the sinusoids seems to occur by alternative mechanisms rather than through the expression of adhesion molecules as in postcapillary venules. Strong or even excessive stimulation is required to cause transmigration of neutrophils accumulated in the sinusoids[28]. However, once outside the circulation, neutrophils can attack hepatocytes and cause extensive cell necrosis[27,39]. This suggests that neutrophils are able to use β2-integrins and ICAM-1 for transmigration, in spite of the absence of PECAM-1 (CD31) on sinusoidal endothelium. Chemokine signals that may activate the neutrophil β2-integrins include hepatocellular generation of IL-8 and GRO-α[40,41] and extensive apoptotic cell death of hepatocytes[42].

The last step in neutrophil mediated hepatocellular injury is the adherence of the neutrophil to the hepatocyte. Adherence to a target cell via β2-integrins further activates the neutrophil to generate reactive oxygen species and to release proteolytic enzymes[43]. Cytotoxicity of neutrophils appears to mainly depend on β2-integrins (LFA-1, Mac-1) on the neutrophil and ICAM-1 on the hepatocyte[28]. In alcoholic hepatitis, a co-localization was found between ICAM-1 and TNF-α in the membranes of hepatocytes in contact with Mac-1-positive neutrophils[44].

TYPES OF INFLAMMATORY LIVER DISEASES

Parenchymal liver diseases

Neutrophil-induced liver diseases include alcoholic hepatitis and non-alcoholic steatohepatitis (NASH), hepatic ischaemia reperfusion, endotoxaemia, sepsis, haemorrhagic shock and extensive hepatectomy of cholestatic liver[28]. Macrophage-induced liver disease is found in experimental animal models like the *Propionebacterium acnes*/endotoxin model and the *Corynebacterium parvum* model[28] and in humans the macrophage activation syndrome[45,46]. Lymphocyte-induced liver diseases include viral hepatitis, allograft rejection, late stage alcoholic liver disease and cirrhosis[28].

In several of these conditions, functional studies using, for example, blocking antibodies and neutralizing analogues have shown the involvement of appropriate adhesion molecules on all cell partners involved (leukocytes, endothelial cells and hepatocytes) and in some studies the role of the corresponding CXC or CC chemokines. Several succinct reviews of these studies have been published[13,16,28].

Some of the more recent investigations have focused on the role of P-selectin in reperfusion liver cell injury[47], the expression of adhesion molecules on circulating polymorphonuclear leukocytes during liver transplantation[48], and the influence of Kuppfer cells on endothelial and hepatocellular ICAM-1 expression in rats during endotoxin treatment[49]. Differences in expression of adhesion molecules during alcoholic hepatitis (E-selectin) and later stages of alcoholic liver disease (VLA-4, VCAM-1) have been demonstrated[50], as well as distinct patterns of chemokine expression (IL-8, MCP-1, MIP-1α and MIP-1β in alcoholic hepatitis)[51]. Enhanced MIP-2 and ICAM-1 was found in experimental chronic alcohol-induced liver injury[52].

Expression of adhesion molecules was found on activated hepatic stellate cells[53,54]. Other studies revealed the chemoattractant action of MCP-1 for hepatic stellate cells[55] as well as the production of MCP-1[56,57] and also neutrophil attracting chemokines[58] by the same hepatic stellate cells.

A pivotal role for TARC (thymus and activation regulated chemokine: a C-C chemokine) was demonstrated in bacteria-induced fulminant hepatitis in mice[59], whereas increased generation of fractalkine (CXXXC chemokine) by hepatic stellate cells was shown in liver injury[60].

Diseases of intrahepatic bile ducts

In chronic inflammatory diseases of intrahepatic bile ducts, portal vessels express P-selectin, E-selectin, VCAM-1 and ICAM-1 as in any chronic inflammatory liver disease, and portal inflammatory cells express the chemokines MIP-1α, MIP-1β, MCP-1 and RANTES[16]. Both in vivo and in vitro studies revealed that resting bile duct epithelial cells (BECs) constitutively express high levels of ICAM-1, LFA-3, and HLA-class I, that can be up-regulated under the influence of pro-inflammatory cytokines (IL-1, TNF-α, IFN-γ), which also induce HLA-class II antigen[61]. BECs, stimulated by pro-inflammatory cytokines, can produce the chemokines IL-8 and MCP-1[62], thus promoting the recruitment of neutrophils and lymphocytes in ascending biliary infection and in allograft rejection. In contrast, IFN-γ reduces the secretion of IL-8 and up-regulates the secretion of MCP-1[62]. Cruickshank et al. reported the expression of CD44 on normal and malignant BEC-derived cells[63]. Through this molecule the cells can present chemokines such as MIP-1β[14,64].

Damaged BECs have an increased expression of both IL-6 mRNA and TNF-α mRNA, and express the IL-6 receptor α chain and the TNF receptor[65]. The involvement of these cytokines in BEC pathology is still unclear. BECs in the bile duct lesions of patients with chronic viral hepatitis C express HLA-DR, ICAM-1 and LFA-3[66].

In PBC, ICAM-1 is strongly expressed in about half of the damaged bile ducts, and VCAM-1 in a few of them[67]. Many portal tract lymphocytes express LFA-1, VLA-4, ICAM-1 and VCAM-1, suggesting LFA-1/ICAM-1 and VLA-4/VCAM-1 interactions between damaged BECs and lymphocytes. The same holds true in experimental animal models[68]. The expression of B7 family antigens on BECs has been controversial, but proliferating BECs express B7 antigens in late stage PBC according to one study[67].

The chemokine RANTES, expressed by BECs, may play a role in homing of precursor macrophages and eosinophils near the bile ducts in PBC. These inflammatory cells, in turn, may become activated and express the eosinophil-specific chemokine eotaxin, resulting in recruitment of the well-known eosinophilic infiltrate in PBC[69].

During acute liver allograft rejection, chemotactic activity has been detected in bile; however, the cellular origin and the precise nature of the cytokines was not known[70]. The network of adhesion molecules, cytokines, chemokines and T lymphocyte subsets and their activation and recruitment in allograft rejection was recently reviewed[71].

In PSC, the BECs express HLA class II antigen, and ICAM-1 appears on the cells in later stages of the disease[72]. However, unlike the BECs in PBC, there is no expression of LFA-3, B7-1 (CD80) nor CD95 (Fas)[73]. Bile duct obstruction appears to influence neutrophil chemotaxis, with an enhanced response to IL-8 and f-MLP in obstructive jaundice in rats[74,75]. In biliary atresia in neonates, strong ICAM-1 expression and occasional VCAM-1 staining on BEC cell membranes of both intra- and extrahepatic ductal structures was noted, in contrast with negative immunohistochemical staining for these molecules in control cases with other conditions[76].

In conclusion, it appears that in hepatic inflammatory diseases the liver parenchymal cells are no passive resident cells and remain no innocent bystanders and victims, but actively participate in the inflammatory and immune response by the expression of adhesion molecules and secretion of (chemotactic) cytokines[16,77]. The same applies for intrahepatic bile duct epithelial cells[61,78].

REFERENCES

1. Majno G, Joris I. Cells, Tissues and Disease. Principles of General Pathology. London: Blackwell Science, 1996.
2. Bumgardner GL, Orosz CG. Transplantation and cytokines. Semin Liver Dis. 1999;19:189–204.
3. van den Oord JJ. Adhesion molecules. Hepato-Gastroenterology. 1996;43:1100–2.
4. Williams AF, Barclay AN. The immunoglobulin superfamily – domains for cell surface recognition. Annu Rev Immunol. 1988;6:381–405.
5. Springer TA. Adhesion receptors for the immune system. Nature. 1990;346:425–33.
6. Wakelin MW, Sanz MJ, Albelda SM, Larkin SW, Boughton-Smith N, Williams TJ, Nourshargh S. An anti-platelet-endothelial cell adhesion molecule-1 antibody inhibits leukocyte extravasation from mesenteric microvessels in vivo by blocking the passage through the basement membrane. J Exp Med. 1996;184:229–39.
7. Salmi M, Adams D, Jalkanen S. Cell adhesion and migration. IV. Lymphocyte trafficking in the intestine and liver. Am J Physiol. 1998;274:G1–G6.
8. Hynes RO. Integrins: versatility, modulation, and signaling in cell adhesion. Cell. 1992;69:11–25.
9. Springer TA. Traffic signals for lymphocyte recirculation and leukocyte emigration: the multistep paradigm. Cell. 1994;76:301–14.
10. Bevilacqua MP, Nelson RM. Selectins. J Clin Invest. 1993;91:379–87.
11. Rosen SD. Commentary. Endothelial ligands for L-selectin. From lymphocyte recirculation to allograft rejection. Am J Pathol. 1999;155:1013–20.
12. Luster AD. Chemokines – chemotactic cytokines that mediate inflammation. N Engl J Med. 1998;338:436–45.

13. Thompson K, Wright S, Sheron N. Chemotactic and suppressor cytokine networks. Hepatogastroenterology. 1996;43:15–31.
14. Tanaka Y, Adams D, Hubscher S, Hirano H, Siebenlist V, Show S. T cell adhesion induced by proteoglycan-immobilized cytokine MIP-1b. Nature. 1993;361:79–82.
15. Maher JH. Cytokines: overview. Semin Liver Dis. 1999;19:109–15.
16. Adams DH. Lymphocyte-endothelial cell interactions in hepatic inflammation. Hepatogastroenterology. 1996;43:32–43.
17. Lasky LA. Selectins. Interpreters of cell-specific carbohydrate information during inflammation. Science. 1992;258:964–9.
18. Jones DA, McIntyre LV, Smith CW, Picker LJ. A 2-step adhesion cascade for T cell endothelial-cell interactions under flow conditions. J Clin Invest. 1994;94:2443–50.
19. Adams DH, Shaw S. Leucocyte endothelial interactions and regulation of leucocyte migration. Lancet. 1994;343:831–6.
20. Tanaka Y, Albelda SM, Horgan KJ et al. CD31 expressed on distinctive T cell subsets is a preferential amplifier of b1 integrin-mediated adhesion. J Exp Med. 1992;176:245–53.
21. Steinhoff G, Behrend M, Schrader B, Pichlmayr R. Intercellular immune adhesion molecules in human liver transplants: overview on expression patterns of leucocyte receptor and ligand molecules. Hepatology. 1993;18:440–53.
22. Steinhoff G, Behrend M, Schrader B, Duijvestijn AM, Wonigeit K. Expression patterns of leukocyte adhesion ligand molecules on human liver endothelia. Lack of ELAM-1 and CD62 inducibility on sinusoidal endothelia and distinct distribution of VCAM-1, ICAM-1, ICAM-2 and LFA-3. Am J Pathol. 1993;142:481–8.
23. Wisse E. An ultrastructural characterization of the endothelial cell in the rat liver sinusoid under normal and various experimental conditions as a contribution to the distinction between endothelial and Kupffer cells. J Ultrastruct Res. 1972;38:528–62.
24. Scoazec JY. Adhesion molecules in normal human liver. Hepatogastroenterology. 1996;43:1103–5.
25. Scoazec JY, Feldmann G. The cell adhesion molecules of hepatic sinusoidal endothelial cells. J Hepatol. 1994;20:296–300.
26. Vidal-Vanaclocha F, Rocha MA, Asumendi A, Barbera-Guillem E. Role of periportal and perivenous sinusoidal endothelial cells in hepatic homing of blood and metastatic cancer cells. Semin Liver Dis. 1993;13:60–71.
27. Chosay JG, Essani NA, Dunn CJ, Jaeschke H. Neutrophil margination and extravasation in sinusoids and venules of the liver during endotoxin-induced injury. Am J Physiol. 1997;272 (Gastrointest Liver Physiol 35):G1195–200.
28. Jaeschke H. Cellular adhesion molecules: regulation and functional significance in the pathogenesis of liver disease. Am J Physiol. 1997;273:G602–11.
29. Adams DH, Hübscher SG, Fisher NC, Williams A, Robinson M. Expression of E-selectin and E-selectin ligands in human liver inflammation. Hepatology. 1996;24:533–8.
30. Winnock M, Barcina MG, Lukomska B, Bioulac-Sage P, Balabaud C. Liver associated lymphocytes: role in tumor defense. Semin Liver Dis. 1993;13:81–92.
31. Bioulac-Sage P, Kuiper J, Van Berkel TJC, Balabaud C. Lymphocyte and macrophage populations in the liver. Hepatogastroenterology. 1996;43:4–14.
32. Volpes R, Van den Oord JJ, Desmet VJ. Vascular adhesion molecules in acute and chronic liver inflammation. Hepatology. 1992;15:269–75.
33. McNab G, Reeves JL, Salmi M, Hubscher S, Jalkanen S, Adams DH. Vascular adhesion protein 1 mediates binding of T cells to human hepatic endothelium. Gastroenterology. 1996;110:522–8.
34. Garcia-Monzon C, Sanchez-Madrid F, Garcia-Buey L, Garcia-Arroyo A, Garcia-Sanchez A, Moreno-Otero R. Vascular adhesion molecule expression in viral chronic hepatitis: evidence of neoangiogenesis in portal tracts. Gastroenterology. 1995;108:231–41.
35. Freemont AJ. Functional and biosynthetic changes in endothelial cells of vessels in chronically inflamed tissues: evidence for endothelial control of lymphocyte entry into diseased tissues. J Pathol. 1988;155:225–30.
36. Volpes R, Van den Oord JJ, Desmet VJ. Distribution of the VLA family of integrins in normal and pathological human liver tissue. Gastroenterology. 1991;101:200–6.
37. Steinhoff G, Behrend M, Wonigeit K. Expression of adhesion molecules on lymphocytes/monocytes and hepatocytes in human liver grafts. Hum Immunol. 1990;28:123–7.
38. Grant AJ, Lalor PF, Hübscher SG, Briskin M, Adams DH. MADCAM-1 expression is increased in primary sclerosing cholangitis and supports lymphocyte adhesion to hepatic endothelium: a

mechanism to explain the recruitment of mucosal lymphocytes to the liver in inflammatory bowel disease. Hepatology. 1999;30:232A.
39. Jaeschke H, Farhood A, Smith CW. Neutrophil-induced liver cell injury in endotoxin shock is a CD11b/CD18-dependent mechanism. Am J Physiol. 1991;261 (Gastrointest Liver Physiol 24):G1051–6.
40. Colletti LM, Kunkel SL, Walz A, Burdick MD, Kunkel RG, Wilke CA, Strieter RM. The role of cytokine networks in the local liver injury following hepatic ischemia/reperfusion in the rat. Hepatology. 1996;23:506–14.
41. Thornton AJ, Strieter RM, Lindley I, Baggiolini M, Kunkel SL. Cytokine-induced gene expression of a neutrophil chemotactic factor/IL-8 in human hepatocytes. J Immunol. 1990;144:2609–13.
42. Lawson JA, Fisher MA, Simmons CA, Farhood A, Jaeschke H. Parenchymal cell apoptosis as a signal for sinusoidal sequestration and transendothelial migration of neutrophils in murine models of endotoxin and Fas-antibody-induced liver injury. Hepatology. 1998;28:761–7.
43. Shappell SB, Toman C, Anderson DC, Taylor AA, Entman ML, Smith CW. Mac-1 (CD11b/CD18) mediates adherence-dependent hydrogen peroxyde production by human and canine neutrophils. J Immunol. 1990;144:2702–11.
44. Ohlinger W, Dinges HP, Zatloukal K, Mair S, Gollowitsch F, Denk H. Immunohistochemical detection of tumor necrosis factor-alpha, other cytokines and adhesion molecules in human livers with alcoholic hepatitis. Virchows Archiv A Pathol Anat Histopathol. 1993;423: 169–76.
45. Prieur AM, Stephan JL. Syndrome d'activation du macrophage au cours des maladies rhumatismales chez l'enfant. Rev Rhum (Ed Fr). 1994;6:447–51.
46. Stephan JL, Zeller J, Hubert P, Herbelin C, Dayer JM, Prieur AM. Macrophage activation syndrome and rheumatic diseases in childhood: a report of four new cases. Clin Exp Rheumatol. 1993;11:451–6.
47. Yadav SS, Howell DN, Steeber DA, Harland RC, Tedder TF, Clavien PA. P-selectin mediates reperfusion injury through neutrophil and platelet sequestration in the warm ischemic mouse liver. Hepatology. 1999;29:1494–502.
48. Thiel M, Imendörffer S, Chouker A, Groh J, Briegel J, Anthuber M et al. Expression of adhesion molecules on circulating polymorphonuclear leucocytes during orthotopic liver transplantation. Hepatology. 1998;28:1538–50.
49. Ahmad N, Gardner CR, Yurkow EJ, Laskin DL. Inhibition of macrophages with gadolinium chloride alters intercellular adhesion molecule-1 expression in the liver during acute endotoxemia in rats. Hepatology. 1999;29:728–36.
50. Adams DH, Burra P, Hubscher SG, Elias E, Newman W. Endothelial activation and circulating vascular adhesion molecules in alcoholic liver disease. Hepatology. 1994;19:588–94.
51. Afford SC, Fischer NC, Neil DAH, Fear J, Brun P, Hubscher SG, Adams DH. Distinct patterns of chemokine expression are associated with leukocyte recruitment in alcoholic hepatitis and alcoholic cirrhosis. J Pathol. 1998;186:82–9.
52. Bautista AP. Chronic alcohol intoxication induces hepatic injury through enhanced macrophage inflammatory protein-2 production and intercellular adhesion molecule-1 expression in the liver. Hepatology. 1997;25:335–42.
53. Knittel T, Dinter C, Kobold D, Neubauer K, Mehde M, Eichhorst S, Ramadori G. Expression and regulation of cell adhesion molecules by hepatic stellate cells (HSC) of rat liver. Involvement of HSC in recruitment of inflammatory cells during hepatic tissue repair. Am J Pathol. 1999;154:153–67.
54. Hellerbrand C, Wang SX, Tsukamoto H, Brenner DA, Rippe RA. Expression of intercellular adhesion molecule-1 by activated hepatic stellate cells. Hepatology. 1996;24:670–6.
55. Marra F, Romanelli RG, Giannini C, Failli P, Pastacaldi S, Arrighi MC et al. Monocyte chemotactic protein-1 as a chemoattractant for human hepatic stellate cells. Hepatology. 1999;29:140–8.
56. Sprenger H, Kaufman A, Garn H, Lahme B, Gemsa D, Gressner A. Differential expression of monocyte chemotactic protein-1 (MCP-1) in transforming rat hepatic stellate cells. J Hepatol. 1999;30:88–94.
57. Marra F, De Franco R, Grappone C, Milano S, Pastacaldi S, Pinzani M et al. Increased expression of Monocyte Chemotactic Protein-1 during active hepatic fibrogenesis: correlation with monocyte infiltration. Am J Pathol. 1998;152:423–30.

58. Sprenger H, Kaufmann A, Garn H, Lahme B, Gemsa D, Gressner AM. Induction of neutrophil-attracting chemokines in transforming rat hepatic stellate cells. Gastroenterology. 1997;113:277–85.
59. Yoneyama H, Harada A, Imai T, Baba M, Yoshie O, Zhang Y et al. Pivotal role of TARC, a CC chemokine, in bacteria-induced fulminant hepatic failure in mice. J Clin Invest. 1998;102:1933–41.
60. Efsen E, Caligiuri A, Romanelli RG, Grappone C, De Franco R, Milani S et al. Increased expression of fractalkine, a novel chemokine, during liver injury: role in recruitment and adhesion of leukocytes. J Hepatol. 1999;30 (Suppl 1):89.
61. Reynoso-Paz S, Coppel RL, Mackay IR, Bass NM, Ansari AA, Gershwin ME. The immunobiology of bile and biliary epithelium. Hepatology. 1999;30:351–7.
62. Morland CM, Fear J, McNab G, Joplin R, Adams DH. Promotion of leukocyte transendothelial cell migration by chemokines derived from human biliary epithelial cells in vitro. Proc Assoc Am Phys. 1997;109:1–11.
63. Cruickshank SM, Southgate J, Selby PJ, Trejdosiewicz LK. Expression and cytokine regulation of immune recognition elements by normal human biliary epithelial and established liver cell lines in vitro. J Hepatol. 1998;29:550–8.
64. Tanaka Y, Adams DH, Shaw S. Proteoglycans on endothelial cells present adhesion-inducing cytokines to leukocytes. Immunol Today. 1993;14:111–15.
65. Yasoshima M, Kono N, Sugawara H, Katayanagi K, Harada K, Nakanuma Y. Increased expression of interleukin-6 and tumor necrosis factor-alpha in pathologic biliary epithelial cells: in situ and culture study. Lab Invest. 1998;78:89–100.
66. Mosnier JF, Scoazec JY, Marcellin P, Degott C, Benhamou JP, Feldmann G. Expression of cytokine-dependent immune adhesion molecules by hepatocytes and bile duct cells in chronic hepatitis C. Gastroenterology. 1994;107:1457–68.
67. Yasoshima M, Nakanuma Y, Tsuneyama K, Van de Water J, Gershwin ME. Immunohistochemical analysis of adhesion molecules in the micro-environment of portal tracts in relation to aberrant expression of PDC-E2 and HLA-DR on the bile ducts in primary biliary cirrhosis. J Pathol. 1995;175:319–25.
68. Howell CD, Li J, Chen WR. Role of intercellular adhesion molecule-1 and lymphocyte function-associated antigen-1 during nonsuppurative destructive cholangitis in a mouse graft-versus-host disease model. Hepatology. 1999;29:766–76.
69. Tsuneyama K, Yasoshima M, Hiramatsu K, Harada K, Gershwin ME, Nakanuma Y. A putative role for eotaxin and RANTES in primary biliary cirrhosis: eosinophilic infiltration and damaged bile ducts. Hepatology Res. 1999;16:68–77.
70. Hathaway M, Burnett D, Elias E, Adams DH. Secretion of soluble chemotactic factors, including interleukin-6: a mechanism for the recruitment of CD8-positive T lymphocytes to human liver allografts during rejection. Hepatology. 1993;18:511–18.
71. Vierling JM. Immunology of acute and chronic hepatic allograft rejection. Liver Transplant Surg. 1999;5 (Suppl 1):S1–S20.
72. Bloom S, Fleming K, Chapman R. Adhesion molecule expression in primary sclerosing cholangitis and primary biliary cirrhosis. Gut. 1995;36:604–9.
73. Dienes HP, Lohse AW, Gerken G, Schirmacher P, Gallati H, Lohr HF, Meyer zum Büschenfelde KH. Bile duct epithelia as target cells in primary biliary cirrhosis and primary sclerosing cholangitis. Virchows Archiv. 1997;431:119–24.
74. Yanagitani K, Kubota Y, Tsuji K, Yamamoto S, Amoh Y, Takaoka M et al. Influence of biliary obstruction on neutrophil chemotaxis. J Gastroenterol. 1998;33:536–40.
75. Yamamoto S, Kubota Y, Tsuji K, Yanagitani K, Takaoka M, Kin H et al. Effect of obstructive jaundice on neutrophil chemotactic activity: an in vivo assessment in zymosan-induced peritonitis model in rats. J Gastroenterol Hepatol. 1998;13:405–11.
76. Dillon P, Belchis D, Tracy T, Cilley R, Hafer L, Krummel T. Increased expression of intercellular adhesion molecules in biliary atresia. Am J Pathol. 1994;145:263–7.
77. Volpes R, Van den Oord JJ, Desmet VJ. Can hepatocytes serve as 'activated' immunomodulating cells in the immune response? J Hepatol. 1992;16:228–40.
78. Adams DH. Biliary epithelial cells: innocent victims or active participants in immune-mediated liver disease? J Lab Clin Med. 1996;128:528–30.

3 Mechanisms of hepatic fibrogenesis

S. L. FRIEDMAN

Hepatic fibrosis is a wound healing, or scarring response arising in response to liver damage. This response is an attempt to encapsulate injury, but in doing so liver function is ultimately impaired. The hepatic response to injury represents a paradigm for wound healing in other tissues, including skin, lung and kidney, since it involves many of the same cell types and mediators.

There has been exciting progress in understanding hepatic fibrosis. Advances have occurred in the following areas:

(1) characterization of components of ECM in normal and fibrotic liver;
(2) identification of cellular sources of ECM, especially the establishment of hepatic stellate cells as the major source of ECM in liver fibrosis;
(3) elucidation of key cytokines, their cellular sources, modes of regulation, and pathways of intracellular signaling via membrane receptors;
(4) characterization of key matrix proteases and their inhibitors (MMPs and TIMPs);
(5) identification of apoptotic mediators in stellate cells and exploration of their role in clearance of activated stellate cells during the resolution of liver injury.

EXTRACELLULAR MATRIX (ECM) – THE MICROENVIRONMENT OF HEPATIC FIBROSIS

ECM in the normal and fibrotic liver

Extracellular matrix refers to the array of macromolecules that comprise the scaffolding of normal and fibrotic liver. These macromolecules consist of three main families: collagens, glycoproteins and proteoglycans. The number of collagens identified in liver is rapidly growing, and includes the recent identification of collagen XVIII, which is a precursor to endostatin. Glycoproteins include fibronectin, laminin, merosin, tenascin, nidogen and hyaluronic acid, among others. Proteoglycans include heparan, dermatan sulphates, chondroitin sulphates, perlecan, syndecan, biglycan and decorin. There is remarkable heterogeneity of these matrix macromolecules with respect to their different isoforms, variable combinations within different tissue regions, and changes related to age.

In normal liver, which can be considered as an acinar structure, the subendothelial space of Disse separates the epithelium (hepatocytes) from the sinusoidal endothelium. This space contains a basement membrane-like matrix which, unlike the typical basement membrane, is not electron dense. The hepatic basement membrane is composed of non-fibril-forming collagens including type IV, VI and type XIV, glycoproteins and proteoglycans. This normal subendothelial ECM is critical for maintaining the differentiated functions of resident liver cells, including hepatocytes, stellate cells and sinusoidal endothelium.

In contrast to basement membrane-type matrix, in normal liver the so-called interstitial ECM is largely confined to the capsule, around large vessels, and in the portal areas. It is composed of fibril-forming collagens (e.g. types I and III), together with cellular fibronectin, undulin (collagen XIV), and other glycoconjugates.

As the liver becomes fibrotic, significant changes occur both quantitatively and qualitatively. The total content of collagens and non-collagenous components increases 3- to 5-fold, accompanied by the shift in the type of ECM in subendothelial space from the normal low density basement membrane-like matrix to interstitial type. This 'capillarization' leads to the loss of hepatocyte microvilli and disappearance of endothelial fenestrations.

ECM alterations in hepatic fibrosis – an imbalance between matrix degradation and accumulation

The outcome of fibrogenesis is the conversion of normal low density basement membrane-like matrix to high-density interstitial type matrix. The repertoire of factors responsible for ECM remodelling is rapidly being identified. These include a family of zinc-dependent enzymes matrix-metalloproteinases (MMPs), their inhibitors (tissue inhibitor of metalloproteinases, TIMPs), and several converting enzymes (MT1-MMP, and stromelysin for example). The growing understanding of these factors may ultimately translate into new therapies.

Hepatic stellate cells are the major cellular source of ECM in liver injury

The identification of stellate cells as the key cellular source of extracellular matrix in liver has been a major advance. Hepatocytes were once thought to be the main producer of ECM until the 1980s, when studies using immunohistochemistry, in situ hybridization and cell isolation clearly established the importance of stellate cells. Preferential expression of extracellular matrix genes in stellate cells has been confirmed in mechanistically distinct experiment models of injury, including those induced by carbon tetrachloride, iron overload, and biliary obstruction.

ECM-cell interactions

Changes in the microenvironment of the space of Disse result in phenotypic changes in all resident liver cells. Hepatic stellate cells are activated by the surrounding increase in interstitial matrix. Sinusoidal endothelial cells rapidly deposit cellular fibronectin in very early liver injury, which also contributes to stellate cell activation. In addition, endothelial cells produce type IV collagen, proteoglycans, and factors (eg., urokinase type plasminogen activator) which can activate latent cytokines such as transforming growth factor-β1 (TGFβ1).

General progress in cytokine biology in the past decade has helped elucidate the role played by cytokines in hepatic fibrogenesis. A family of cytokine receptors known as receptor tyrosine kinases are transducers of many key cytokines, including platelet derived growth factor (PDGF), hepatocyte growth factor (HGF), epidermal growth factor (EGF), vascular endothelial growth factor (VEGF) and fibroblast growth factor (FGF).

Integrins are another type of membrane receptor which transduce extracellular signals in liver. Integrins are heterodimeric transmembrane proteins composed of α and β subunits whose ligands are matrix molecules rather than cytokines. In particular integrin ligands contain an Arg-Gly-Asp tripeptide sequence. Several integrins and their downstream effectors have been identified in stellate cells, including $\alpha1\beta1$, $\alpha2\beta1$, $\alpha v\beta1$ and $\alpha6\beta4$.

HEPATIC STELLATE CELL ACTIVATION – THE COMMON PATHWAY LEADING TO HEPATIC FIBROSIS (see Fig. 1)

Hepatic stellate cells, located in subendothelial space of Disse between hepatocytes and sinusoidal endothelial cells, represent one-third of the non-parenchymal population, or about 15% of the total number of resident cells in normal liver. In normal liver they are the principal storage site for retinoids (vitamin A metabolites), which accounts for 40–70% of retinoids in the body.

Following liver injury of any aetiology, stellate cells undergo a process known as activation, which is a transition of quiescent vitamin A-rich cells into proliferative, fibrogenic, and contractile myofibroblasts. Stellate cell activation can be conceptually viewed as a two-stage process, initiation and perpetuation. Initiation refers to early changes in gene expression and phenotype which render the cells responsive to other cytokines and stimuli, while perpetuation results from the effects of these stimuli on maintaining the activated phenotype and generating fibrosis. Initiation is largely due to paracrine stimulation, whereas perpetuation involves autocrine as well as paracrine loops.

Initiation

Stellate cell activation may be initiated by paracrine stimuli from injured neighbouring cells, including hepatocytes, endothelial and Kupffer cells, platelets, as well as infiltrating tumour cells in primary and metastatic cancer.

Hepatocytes promote stellate cell activation by producing lipid peroxides which may be important in many forms of liver fibrosis, especially hepatitis C and iron overload. Moreover, in cirrhotic liver, anti-oxidant levels are commonly depleted, which could amplify the injurious effects of lipid peroxides.

Kupffer cells are another important source of paracrine stimuli driving stellate cell activation. Kupffer cell infiltration occurs just prior to and coincident with the appearance of activated stellate cells. Based on culture studies, Kupffer cells can stimulate matrix synthesis, cell proliferation and release of retinoids by stellate cells.

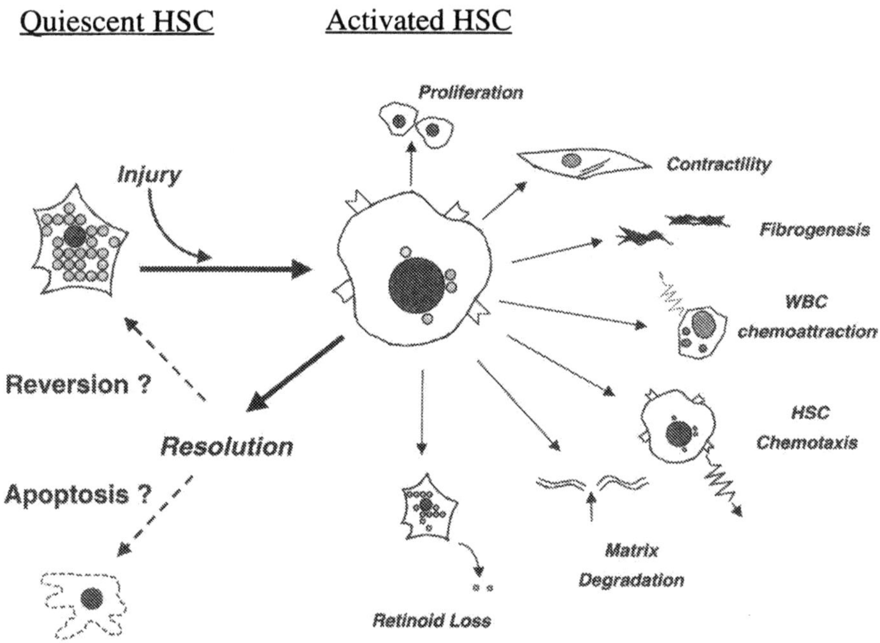

Figure 1 Hepatic stellate cell activation – its features during liver injury and fate during resolution. Following liver injury, hepatic stellate cells undergo activation, transforming from quiescent vitamin A-rich cells into proliferative, fibrogenic and contractile myofibroblasts. The major phenotypic changes after activation include proliferation, contractility, fibrogenesis, WBC chemoattraction, chemotaxis and retinoid loss. The fate of activated stellate cells as liver injury resolves is still unclear but may include reversion to a quiescent phenotype and/or selective clearance by apoptosis. (Reprinted from Dan Li, D and Friedman, SL. Liver fibrogenesis and the role of hepatic stellate cells – new insights and prospects for therapy. J Gastroenterol Hepatol, 1999;14:618–33).

Platelets in injured liver are a potent source of paracrine stimuli by generating multiple potentially important mediators including platelet derived growth factor (PDGF), TGFβ1 and epidermal growth factor (EGF).

Recent interest has been focused on the molecular regulation of gene expression during early stellate cell activation. Several transcription factors have been characterized, including Sp1, c-myb, NFκB, c-jun/AP1, and STAT-1.

Perpetuation

After initiation, activated stellate cells undergo a series of phenotypic changes which collectively lead to the accumulation of extracellular matrix. These changes include: proliferation; contractility; fibrogenesis; chemotaxis; matrix degradation; retinoid loss; cytokine release.

Proliferation

Increased stellate cells, in part due to local proliferation, has been documented in both human and experimental liver injury. Following liver injury, many mitogenic factors and their cognate tyrosine kinase receptors are un-regulated. Of these, PDGF is the best characterized and most potent mitogen towards stellate cells. Up-regulation of PDGF receptor following liver injury enhances the responsiveness to autocrine PDGF, whose expression is also increased. The downstream signalling pathways involves ERK/MAP kinase, phosphoinositol 3 kinase (PI 3-kinase) and STAT-1 (signal transducers and activators of transcription).

Other stellate cell mitogens include endothelin-1 (ET-1) thrombin, FGF, IGF, among others.

Contractility

Contraction by stellate cells may be a major determinant of early and late increases in portal resistance during liver fibrosis. Activated stellate cells impede portal blood flow by both constricting individual sinusoids and by contracting the cirrhotic liver, since the collagenous bands typical of end-stage cirrhosis contain large numbers of these cells.

In addition to ET-1, stellate cells (as well as endothelial and Kupffer cells) also produce nitric oxide (NO), the physiologic antagonist to ET-1. The net contractile activity of stellate cells in vivo reflects the relative strength of these opposing factors. In fact, portal hypertension may reflect diminished NO activity, in addition to increased stimulation by ET-1.

The expression of alpha smooth muscle actin is increased during stellate cell activation. This cytoskeletal filament is a marker of activated cells and may directly participate in their contractility.

Fibrogenesis

Increased fibrogenesis is the most direct way in which the stellate cell contributes to hepatic fibrosis. TGFβ1 is the most potent fibrogenic factor, with lesser fibrogenic activity documented for interleukin-1β, tumor necrosis factor, lipid peroxides and acetaldehyde.

Because of its importance, TGFβ1 regulation has received considerable attention. TGFβ1 is up-regulated in experimental and human hepatic fibrosis. Although sources of this cytokine are multiple, autocrine expression is among the most important. Several mechanisms underlie the increase of TGFβ1 expression by stellate cells during liver injury. The transcription factor Sp1 and a related zinc finger factor Zf9 can transactivate the TGFβ1 promoter, and their combined expression results in synergistic induction. Latent TGFβ1 is activated through increased proteolysis by urokinase-type plasminogen activator (uPA) or tPA. Stellate cell responsiveness to TGFβ1 is also increased during activation by up-regulation of binding to its cognate receptors.

Chemotaxis

Stellate cells may accumulate both through proliferation and via directed migration into regions of injury, or chemotaxis. PDGF and the chemoattractant monocyte chemotactic peptide-1 (MCP-1) have been identified as stellate cell chemoattractants.

Matrix degradation

A greater understanding of matrix degradation in liver is emerging (see above). Quantitative and qualitative changes in the activity of MMPs and their inhibitors play a vital role in extracellular matrix remodeling in liver fibrogenesis. As noted above, the net effect of changes in matrix degradation is the conversion of the low density subendothelial matrix to one rich in interstitial collagens.

Retinoid loss

Activation of stellate cells is accompanied by loss of their characteristic perinuclear retinoid (vitamin A) droplets. Although the intracellular form is largely retinyl esters, when retinol is exported from the cell during activation it is primarily as retinol, suggesting that intracellular hydrolysis of esters occurs prior to export. It is still unknown whether retinoid loss is a requirement for stellate cell activation.

Cytokine release

Autocrine cytokines play vital roles in regulating the activation process of stellate cells. These cytokines include TGFβ1, PDGF, FGF, HGF, PAF and ET-1, among others. Furthermore, stellate cells release neutrophil and monocyte chemoattractants which can amplify inflammation in liver injury.

Anti-inflammatory cytokines produced by stellate cells have also been identified, in particular interleukin-10 (IL-10).

The fate of activated stellate cells during resolution of liver injury

The fate of activated stellate cells as liver injury resolves is under scrutiny. There is now increasing evidence for a role of apoptosis in stellate cell clearance.

Apoptosis may represent one of the central mechanisms modulating fibrosis in vivo. During the resolution of liver injury, there is an increased percentage of apoptotic cells. Interestingly, cells undergoing apoptosis express high levels of TIMP. Activated stellate cells also display an increased susceptibility to apoptotic signals such as soluble Fas ligand and diminished expression of the anti-apoptotic protein bcl-2.

These emerging data raise intriguing questions. What signals in the hepatic microenvironment are responsible for the modulation of apoptosis in stellate cells? The coming years are likely to see rapid growth in our understanding of stellate cell apoptosis as its potential in antifibrotic therapy is explored.

Anti-fibrotic therapies – rationale and specific agents

The paradigm of stellate cell activation provides an important framework to define sites of antifibrotic therapy. These include: cure the primary disease to prevent injury; reduce inflammation or the host response in order to avoid stimulating stellate cell activation; directly down-regulate stellate cell activation; neutralize proliferative, fibrogenic, contractile and/or pro-inflammatory responses of stellate cells; increase the degradation of scar matrix, either by stimulating cells which produce matrix proteases, down-regulating their inhibitors, or by direct administration of matrix proteases.

Cure the primary disease

The most effective way to eliminate hepatic fibrosis is to clear the primary cause of liver disease. This includes abstinence in alcoholic liver disease, removal of excess iron or copper in precirrhotic genetic haemochromatosis or Wilson's disease, clearance of HBV or HCV in chronic viral hepatitis, eradication of organisms in schistosomiasis, or decompression in mechanical bile duct obstruction. Similarly, identification of the pathogenetic mechanisms underlying primary biliary cirrhosis and sclerosing cholangitis could lead to elimination of bile duct injury and periductular fibrosis. Reversal of jejunoileal bypass-related hepatic fibrosis and cessation of methotrexate may also prevent progression to cirrhosis.

Reduce inflammation and immune response

Reduced fibrosis has been reported in some patients treated with α-interferon for HCV presumably through its effect on viral replication and liver injury. The key issue will be whether initial responses to α-interferon in HCV can be maintained over many years, a likely requirement in order to achieve a sustained antifibrotic benefit. A number of agents have anti-inflammatory activity in vitro and in vivo which may eliminate the stimuli to stellate cell activation.

Corticosteroids have been used for decades to treat several types of liver disease. Its activity is solely as an anti-inflammatory agent, with no direct antifibrotic effect on stellate cells.

Efforts to neutralize inflammatory cytokines include an interleukin-1 receptor antagonist, which has shown modest efficacy in rats with dimethylnitrosamine-induced liver injury as well as RGD antagonists, which may limit tumor necrosis factor-related immunologic injury.

Drugs which dampen the allergic response are also under study. Transilast and captopril, an angiotensin converting enzyme inhibitor, have antifibrotic activity attributed to reduced mast cell and eosinophil accumulation. Transilast may also have direct inhibitory effects on stellate cell proliferation and fibrogenesis.

Malotilate is an experimental anti-inflammatory agent. Although reduced fibrogenesis was reported in several experimental models including CCl_4 and dimethylnitrosamine, no clear benefit has been seen in human trials.

An important new approach has used interleukin-12 to modify the host immune response to schistosomiasis rather than the primary infection. IL-12 favours the priming of lymphocytes with a Th1 rather than Th2 cytokine profile. Because Th2 cytokines drive the fibrotic response to this infection, administration of IL-12 markedly reduced the amount of hepatic fibrosis following *S. mansoni* egg inoculation, despite an equal number of worms and eggs in both the control and IL-12 treated groups. These findings could have implications for other human liver diseases where the host response plays an important role, including HCV, primary biliary cirrhosis and autoimmune hepatitis.

Inhibit stellate cell activation

Reducing the transformation of quiescent stellate cells to activated myofibroblasts is a particularly attractive target given its central role in the fibrotic response. The most practical approach is to reduce oxidant stress, which is an important stimulus to activation. Anti-oxidants, including alpha-tocopherol (vitamin E), suppress fibrogenesis in some studies of experimental fibrogenesis, and are currently undergoing limited trials in humans. Phosphatidylcholine, the active ingredient of polyunsaturated lecithin, has been used to protect against fibrosis and cirrhosis in alcohol-fed baboons, presumably through a membrane-stabilizing effect. Encouraging results with this compound have led to ongoing trials in alcoholics.

IL-10 down-regulates inflammation and stellate cell activation which may prove to be useful as a therapeutic, particularly since the agent has already been used in clinical trials for a number of diseases. Induction of IL-10 has been documented during stellate cell activation, leading to reduced collagen secretion and enhanced collagenase gene expression.

Silymarin, a natural flavenoid component of the milk thistle *Silybum marianum* has aroused interest as a potential anti-fibrotic therapy. The compound functions as an antioxidant and may decrease hepatic injury via both cytoprotection and inhibition of Kupffer cell.

The cytokines γ-interferon and hepatocyte growth factor have inhibitory effects on stellate cell activation in animal models of fibrosis.

Neutralize proliferative, fibrogenic, contractile and/or pro-inflammatory responses of stellate cells

Significant advances in growth factor biology will benefit the treatment of hepatic fibrosis through the development of antagonists to cytokines and their receptors. In particular, many proliferative cytokines including PDGF, FGF and TGFβ signal through tyrosine kinase receptors, inhibitors of which are already undergoing clinical trials in other tissues. Because the intracellular signalling pathways for these receptors are well understood, inhibitors to signalling models, including linoleic acid and lipoxygenase inhibitors, are being explored in vivo or in cultured stellate cells. Others include simvastatin, an inhibitor of HMG CoA reductase, pentoxyphylline, which inhibits PDGF receptor signaling, and compounds which elevate intracellular cyclic AMP.

Inhibition of matrix production has been the primary target of most antifibrotic therapies to date. This has been attempted directly by blocking matrix synthesis and processing, or indirectly by inhibiting the activity of TGFβ1, the major fibrogenic cytokine. Inhibitors of collagen synthesis such as HOE 077, which blocks the enzyme prolyl hydroxylase, were among the first antifibrotic compounds tested in liver, but success with this agent has been modest. Colchicine generated excitement at one time because of its apparent efficacy in a small group of patients; however, no confirmation of these results by others has been published. Its presumed mechanism of action was inhibition of collagen secretion, but this has not been established.

TGFβ antagonists are being extensively tested because neutralizing this potent cytokine would have the dual effect of inhibiting matrix production and accelerating its degradation. Concerns that inhibiting TGFβ may alter hepatocellular growth or apoptosis will need to be considered as antagonists reach clinical trials, but in other tissues there is great promise for this approach.

A number of even newer TGFβ antagonists are also being developed and may undergo testing soon. These include soluble receptor antagonists, antisense oligonucleotides and recombinant soluble mannose-6-phosphate. The latter is particularly relevant to hepatic fibrosis because this receptor molecule binds and helps activate TGFβ at the stellate cell surface.

Because endothelin-1 is an important regulator of wound contraction and blood flow regulation mediated by stellate cells, antagonists have been tested as both antifibrotic and portal hypotensive agents. Bosentan, a mixed endothelin A and B receptor antagonist, had antifibrotic activity and reduces stellate cell activation in experimental hepatic fibrosis. This and other endothelin antagonists are under development and could reach clinical testing.

The potential utility of retinoids (vitamin A) as anti-fibrotic therapy has been limited by inadequate knowledge about their regulatory role in stellate cell activation and by toxicity concerns. Although stellate cells export retinoid as they activate, it does not follow that restoration of cellular retinoid will prevent activation. In fact, some retinoids may accelerate fibrosis by augmenting membrane injury as in hypervitaminosis A, or by stimulating the conversion of latent to active TGFβ.

Increase the degradation of scar matrix

This component is very important, because antifibrotic therapy in human liver disease will need to provoke resorption of existing matrix in addition to preventing deposition of new scar. As noted above, TGFβ antagonists have the advantage of stimulating matrix degradation by downregulating TIMPs and increasing net activity of interstitial collagenase. Retinoids may also stimulate matrix degradation but concerns over toxicity limit their utility. Relaxin can directly increase matrix degradation.

THE FUTURE

Our increased understanding of hepatic stellate cell biology over the past decade augurs well for continued progress. Many key questions remain unanswered:

(1) *Is all fibrosis really the same?* We have assumed that the stellate cell responds exactly the same regardless of the type of insult to the liver, yet this may be an oversimplification. There may be subtle, yet important differences in the way the stellate cell behaves in viral vs. alcoholic liver injury, for example, differences which could be exploited therapeutically.

(2) *What distinguishes reversible from irreversible fibrosis?* While it is clear that substantial fibrosis may be reversible, the exact moment at which fibrosis becomes irreversible is not known, either in terms of a histologic marker or a specific change in the matrix composition or content. This remains a key issue, as anti-fibrotic therapies will be most effective if confined to patients with reversible disease.

(3) *What host factors regulate stellate cell activation and fibrosis?* Exciting new data indicate that the host immune phenotype may be an important determinant of the nature of the fibrotic response. It remains uncertain whether

this reflects inherent differences within stellate cells, or responses mediated solely by differences in immune effector cells.

(4) *What is the role of retinoids in driving stellate cell activation?* This is a key unresolved issue which could have therapeutic importance.

(5) *How can stellate cells be targeted for therapies?* Since no genes or receptors are completely unique to stellate cells, any therapy which neutralizes a function of stellate cells must be targeted to avoid unwanted effects on other cells either within or outside the liver.

(6) *Will down-regulating stellate cell activation and hence fibrosis exacerbate the liver injury which the scar is trying to encapsulate?* This remains a fundamental concern of antifibrotic therapy, yet in patients with end-stage liver disease the consequences of scar formation become life-threatening. A reasonable goal of antifibrotic therapy should therefore be the slowing of scar accumulation but not necessarily its total elimination.

BIBLIOGRAPHY

1. Olaso E and Friedman SL. Molecular regulation of hepatic fibrogenesis. J Hepatol. 1998;29:836–47.
2. Ratziu V, Lalazar A, Wong L, Dang Q, Collins C, Shaulian E et al. Zf9, a Kruppel-like transcription factor upregulated in vivo during early hepatic fibrosis. Proc Natl Acad Sci USA. 1998;95:9500–5.
3. Gressner AM. The cell biology of liver fibrogenesis – an imbalance of proliferation, growth arrest, and apoptosis of myofibroblasts. Cell Tiss Res. 1998;292:447–52.
4. Arthur MJ, Mann DA, Iredale JP. Tissue inhibitors of metalloproteinases, hepatic stellate cells and liver fibrosis. J Gastroenterol Hepatol. 1998;13(Suppl):S33–8.
5. Friedman SL. Seminars in medicine of the Beth Israel Hospital, Boston. The cellular basis of hepatic fibrosis. Mechanisms and treatment strategies. N Engl J Med. 1993;328:1828–35.
6. Friedman SL. The virtuosity of hepatic stellate cells. Gastroenterology. 1999;117:1244–6.
7. Li D, Friedman SL. Liver fibrogenesis and the role of hepatic stellate cells: new insights and prospects for therapy. J Gastroenterol Hepatol. 1999;14:618–33.

4
Cellular and molecular mechanisms of cholestasis

M. TRAUNER, P. FICKERT, G. ZOLLNER, R. E. STAUBER, K. ZATLOUKAL, H. DENK and G. J. KREJS

INTRODUCTION*

Recent progress in liver cell and molecular biology has changed our understanding of the pathogenesis of congenital and acquired forms of cholestatic liver diseases. One of the major breakthroughs was the cloning of hepatobiliary transport systems which mediate hepatic uptake and excretion of bile salts and other biliary constituents (e.g. bilirubin)[1,2]. Evidence now exists that decreased or even non-existent expression of hepatobiliary transport proteins in hepatocytes or bile duct epithelial cells (cholangiocytes) may explain impaired transport function resulting in cholestasis[3–13]. This article focuses on molecular alterations of hepatobiliary transport systems and potential mechanisms leading to these changes in cholestasis.

CELLULAR AND MOLECULAR BASIS OF NORMAL BILE SECRETION

Bile is primarily formed at the canalicular level by both bile salt-dependent and -independent mechanisms (canalicular bile, accounting for 75% of daily bile production). Canalicular bile is then further modified along the bile ductules and ducts (ductular/ductal bile, 25% of bile secretion)[14]. Canalicular bile is formed by osmotic filtration of water and electrolytes in response to osmotic gradients generated by active transport systems located at the basolateral and canalicular membrane of hepatocytes. The major determinant of canalicular bile formation is the excretion of bile salts into the canaliculus (bile salt-dependent bile flow).

* Please note that by convention human genes and their products are capitalized, whereas rodent genes and their products are written in lower case throughout this article. Transporter genes are set in *italic* whereas gene products (transporter proteins) are set in normal font.

Other (non-bile salt) organic anions and cations and their conjugates also osmotically influence bile flow. Canalicular excretion of reduced glutathione (GSH) and bicarbonate (HCO_3^-) constitute the major components of the bile salt-independent fraction of bile flow, although the contribution of HCO_3^- occurs mainly at the bile duct level, particularly when stimulated by hormones and regulatory peptides (e.g. secretin and vasoactive intestinal peptide)[15–17]. Normal bile secretion depends on active transmembrane transport systems generating the osmotic gradients for bile flow; an intact cytoskeleton required for the movement of vesicles and bile canalicular contractions; cell contacts sealing off bile canaliculi and maintaining cell polarity; and signal transduction mechanisms regulating and coordinating the various processes involved in bile formation.

Hepatobiliary transport systems

Cloning of hepatobiliary transport systems in rodents and humans has greatly enhanced our understanding of the molecular basis of hepatocellular and cholangiocellular bile formation[1,2,15–18] (for a continuously updated online version see reference 19) (Fig. 1). The hepatocyte is a classical polarized epithelial cell and its basolateral (sinusoidal) and apical (canalicular) plasma membrane domains have distinct features. A basolateral Na^+-dependent Na^+/taurocholate co-transporter (NTCP) is the main uptake system for bile salts[20,21], while an Na^+-independent organic anion transporting protein (OATP) transports not only bile salts, but also a large variety of other (non-bile salt) organic anions (e.g. bromosulphothalein, oestrogen conjugates) and cations (e.g. drugs such as ajmalium)[22,23]. Na^+-dependent bile salt transport via NTCP is driven by a Na^+,K^+-ATPase which generates an inwardly directed Na^+-gradient. Na^+,K^+-ATPase activity depends in turn on the membrane potential generated by a K^+ channel[24]. In contrast to NTCP, OATP functions as a bile salt exchanger with GSH and HCO_3^- [24]. Unlike Na^+-dependent bile salt uptake, Na^+-independent transport of bile salts cannot be attributed to the function of a single transport system[24–26]. In addition to Oatp1[27], a second Oatp2 with uniquely high affinity for the cardiac glycoside digoxin is highly expressed in rat liver[28]. The general importance of the OATP/Oatp family is further emphasized by the recent cloning of a third Oatp3 expressed in the ileum and in cholangiocytes[29,30]. Recently, a novel liver-specific organic anion transporter (LST-1) also belonging to the OATP family was identified in human and rodent liver[31,32]. Basolateral bile salt transport systems are essential for bile formation since the majority (approximately 95%) of bile salts excreted by the liver is reabsorbed on each pass through the intestine (mainly in the terminal ileum) and returned to the liver (enterohepatic circulation)[14]. Little is known about intracellular transport of bile salts from the basolateral to the canalicular membrane. Bile salts appear to be retained in the cytosol by specific bile salt binding proteins such as 3α-hydroxysteroid dehydrogenase, which prevent their efflux from the liver and are required for their rapid excretion by the canalicular transporter[24].

Canalicular bile secretion is the rate-limiting step of bile formation[33]. The canalicular membrane contains both adenosine triphosphate (ATP)-dependent and ATP-independent transport systems[1,2,18,33]. ATP-dependent transport systems (also known as ATP-binding cassette (ABC) proteins) transport biliary constituents

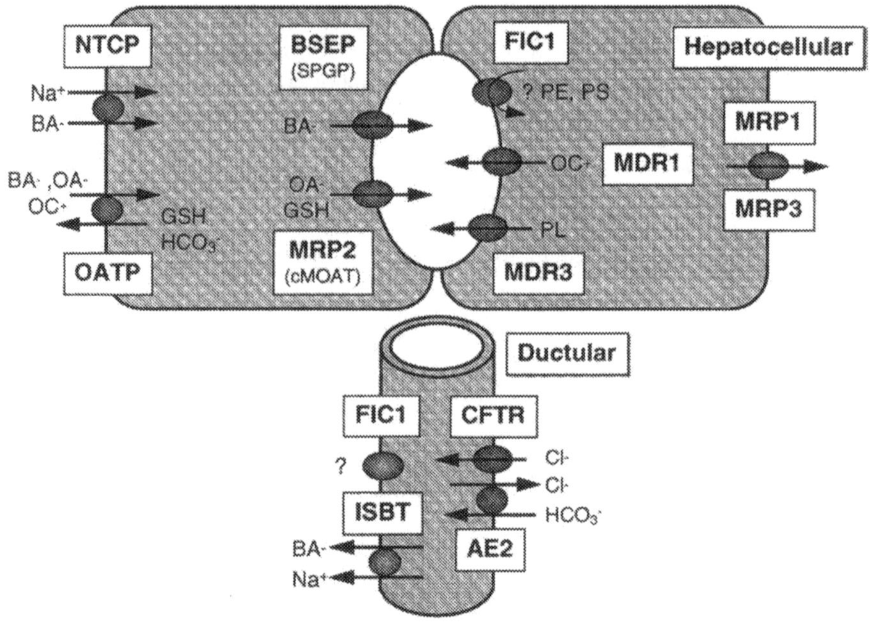

Figure 1 Hepatobiliary transport systems in human liver. A Na^+/taurocholate cotransporter (NTCP) at the basolateral membrane of hepatocytes mediates hepatic bile salt (BA^-) uptake, while a Na^+-independent organic anion transporting polypeptide (OATP) also transports (non-bile salt) organic anions (OA^-) and cations (OC^+). Recently, another liver-specific organic anion transporter (LST-1) has been identified (not shown). Bile salts are excreted into bile via a canalicular bile salt export pump (BSEP) which is the 'sister of P-glycoprotein' (SPGP), while reduced glutathione (GSH) and (non-bile salt) organic anions (e.g., conjugated bilirubin) are excreted via a canalicular conjugate export pump (MRP2, also known as canalicular multispecific organic anion transporter, cMOAT). Other multidrug resistance-associated protein (MRP) isoforms such as MRP1 and 3 are located on the (baso)lateral membrane where they may serve as a compensatory overflow system under cholestatic conditions. In addition, the canalicular membrane contains a multidrug export pump (MDR1), a phospholipid export pump (MDR3). A P-type ATPase (FICl) is a putative aminophospholipid (PE, phosphatidylethanolamine; PS, phosphatidylserine) transporter (from the outer to the inner leaflet of the cell membrane), but may also play a direct or indirect role for canalicular bile salt excretion. Bile duct epithelial cells (cholangiocytes) contain a Cl^- -channel which is the cystic fibrosis transmembrane regulator (CFTR) driving HCO_3^- excretion via a chloride/bicarbonate (Cl^-/HCO_3^-) anion exchanger (AE2). AE2 is also expressed at the canalicular membrane (not shown). In addition, cholangiocytes contain the ileal sodium-dependent bile salt transporter (ISBT) for reabsorption and cholehepatic cycling of bile salts, as well as FICl (which might also play a role in bile salt reabsorption).

against steep concentration gradients across the canalicular membrane (often in the range of 100- to 1000-fold). Most canalicular ABC proteins belong to the multidrug resistance protein (MDR) or multidrug resistance-associated protein (MRP) gene superfamily[33]. A multidrug export pump (MDR1) excretes hydrophobic cationic compounds (e.g. anticancer drugs, calcium channel blockers, cyclosporin A, various other drugs)[34–36], while a phospholipid export pump (MDR3) acts as a phospholipid flippase/translocase[37–39]. A conjugate export pump (MRP2)[40–43], functionally also known as the canalicular multispecific organic anion transporter (cMOAT), mediates the canalicular excretion of a broad range of organic anions, most of which are amphiphilic anionic conjugates with glutathione, glucuronate and sulphate formed by phase II conjugation in the hepatocyte (e.g. bilirubin diglucuronide)[44]. Canalicular excretion of GSH also appears to be mediated through MRP2[45]. Other MRP isoforms such as MRP1 and MRP3 are located on the basolateral membrane[46] where they may serve as a compensatory overflow system under cholestatic conditions with impaired canalicular (MRP2) excretory function[47]. A bile salt export pump (BSEP) which is the sister of P-glycoprotein (SPGP) excretes monovalent bile salts[48,49]. Recently, a P-type ATPase (FIC1; mutated in familial intrahepatic cholestasis) belonging to a family of aminophospholipid transporters[50,51] has also been localized to the canalicular membrane[52] and the bile duct epithelium[53]. The detailed function of FIC1 is unclear, but may involve the transfer of aminophospholipids (e.g. phosphatidylserine, phosphatidylethanolamine) from the outer to the inner leaflet of the canalicular membrane bilayer[50–52]. Mutations of this gene result in variants of familial intrahepatic cholestasis (see below), suggesting that it must play an important direct or indirect role in bile salt excretion[51]. Strong expression of FIC1 in extrahepatic tissues such as pancreas, small intestine and kidney suggests a more general role in the regulation of secretory processes (e.g. by maintaining membrane asymmetry required for the function of embedded transport systems and/or fusion of vesicles targeting these transport proteins to the canalicular membrane) and may explain some of the extrahepatic features (in addition to cholestasis) associated with these syndromes (e.g. pancreatitis, diarrhoea, nephrolithiasis; see below)[50,51].

In addition to these ATP-dependent transport systems, the canalicular membrane also contains ATP-independent transport systems. Canalicular bicarbonate secretion is mediated via the Cl^-/HCO_3^- exchanger belonging to a family of anion exchangers (AE1–3). AE2 is encountered in various tissues, including the liver and secretory epithelia, and plays a major role in mediating hepatic Cl^-/HCO_3^- exchange. The AE2 protein is localized to both bile canaliculi and bile ducts[54]. In addition to AE2, large but not small bile duct epithelial cells (cholangiocytes) contain several other transport systems for their secretory and absorptive functions[15–17,55], including a Cl^- channel which is the cystic fibrosis transmembrane regulator (CFTR)[56,57]. Interestingly, the ileal sodium-dependent bile salt transporter (ISBT) has also been identified on the apical domain of large but not small cholangiocytes[58,59], where together with a recently identified new organic anion transporter subtype (Oatp3)[29,30] it may be involved in the reabsorption and cholehepatic shunting of bile salts. Cholangiocytes also contain aquaporin-1 (AQP1) water channels which facilitate water transport down osmotic gradients[60,61]. In contrast to bile ducts, osmotic flow of water into the bile canaliculus occurs primarily through semipermeable tight junctions and by diffusion via the lipid bilayer across hepatocyte membranes[62,63].

Role of vesicular trafficking, cytoskeleton and cell contacts in normal bile secretion

In addition to hepatobiliary transport proteins mediating active transmembrane transport of biliary constituents, normal bile secretion also heavily depends on transcellular movement of vesicles (vesicular trafficking), as well as an intact cytoskeleton and cell contacts. Vesicular trafficking serves the blood-to-bile transport of exogenous substances (derived from receptor-mediated or fluid-phase endocytosis) following the transcytotic pathway from the sinusoidal membrane to the bile canaliculus[64–66]. Proteins destined for secretion or insertion in the plasma membrane are synthesized in the endoplasmatic reticulum, processed in the Golgi apparatus, and transported to the sinusoidal membrane. Current evidence suggests that many canalicular membrane proteins are first delivered to the basolateral membrane, before they are then selectively retrieved and delivered by recruitment of transcytotic vesicular pathways to the canalicular (apical) pole[64–66]. More recently, a direct Golgi to apical membrane exocytotic pathway has been identified for canalicular ABC transporters (e.g. MDR1, MRP2, BSEP)[67,68]. In addition to vesicular targeting to the canaliculus, there must also be brisk endocytotic retrieval of canalicular membrane material to prevent massive increases in surface area[65], although little is known about the potential mechanisms involved. Insertion and retrieval of membrane transporters into/from the sinusoidal and canalicular membrane is a dynamic process regulating the number of transport proteins in the plasma membrane. This may be especially important for handling sudden increases in the hepatic flux of biliary constituents under physiologic and pathologic conditions. Vesicular trafficking is regulated by various hormones as well as acute changes in cell volume and intracellular pH[64,69].

The cytoskeleton of the hepatocyte, like that of other epithelial cells, is composed of three components: microtubules, microfilaments and intermediate filaments[70–73]. Microtubules consist of polymerized heterodimers of α- and β-tubulins and are the principal cytoskeletal element along which vesicles travel. Two classes of microtubule motors move vesicles along the microtubular network: kinesin translocates vesicles as a (+) end-directed motor, whereas cytoplasmic dynein acts as a (–) end-directed motor[73,74]. Microtubules play a major role in endocytosis, transcytosis, and exocytosis of vesicles (vesicular trafficking) to the basolateral and apical (bile canalicular) surface. Microfilaments consist of actin and are distributed along the cytoplasmic face of the plasma membrane. They are especially abundant around the bile canaliculus, where they form a contractile system which provides tone to the canaliculus and facilitates bile flow from pericentral to periportal regions through active contractions of the canalicular membrane[70,75,76]. Tight junction permeability may also be influenced by microfilaments interacting with tight junction proteins[70–73]. The motor molecule myosin interacts with actin (analogous to the microtubule motors interacting with tubulin) and may facilitate vesicle movement to the cell membrane surface after the vesicles have reached the end of the microtubules underneath the plasma membrane[74]. Microfilaments may also play an important role as a barrier regulating the fusion of vesicles at the plasma membrane. Thus, insertion of bile salt transporters such as Ntcp into the plasma membrane depends on an intact microfilament system[77]. Intermediate filaments of hepatocytes are composed of cytokeratin 8/18 heteropolymers[78]. A pericanalicular keratin sheath forms a supportive network around the bile canaliculus and is essential for the structural integrity of the bile canaliculus and for normal bile secretion[79]. In addition to mechanical roles in the maintenance of hepatocyte integrity, keratins also appear to be important for protection from non-mechanical cell stresses (e.g. exposure to drugs, toxins)[78].

Cell contacts such as tight junctions seal off the bile canaliculus and create a barrier between sinusoidal blood and canalicular bile. Furthermore, they maintain cell polarity by defining the border of the apical and (baso)lateral membrane surfaces[80,81]. Several tight-junction-specific proteins have been identified (e.g. zonula occludens 1 and 2, occludin) which form the molecular basis of this seal[81]. While tight junctions are impermeable for biliary constituents, they are semipermeable for water and small electrolytes, allowing them to follow osmotic gradients. Gap junctions provide intercellular communication between individual hepatocytes through migration of calcium waves and other second messengers. Several studies have implicated hormones (e.g. vasopressin, glucagon at the hepatocellular level; secretin, vasoactive intestinal peptide at the cholangiocellular level) in the regulation of bile secretion. These hormones activate intracellular second messenger systems and signal transduction cascades (e.g. adenosine 3′,5′-cyclic monophosphate, protein kinase C, phosphoinositide 3-kinase, calcium) which in turn modulate transporter function, vesicle movement, canalicular contractions and tight junction permeability[82,83].

CELLULAR AND MOLECULAR MECHANISMS OF CHOLESTASIS

Cholestasis may result either from a functional defect in bile formation at the level of the hepatocyte (hepatocellular cholestasis) or from an impairment in bile secretion and flow at the level of bile ductules or ducts (ductular/ductal cholestasis)[84]. Molecular probes for hepatobiliary transport systems in experimental and clinical forms of cholestasis have demonstrated decreased or even non-existent expression of transporter proteins (Fig. 2), which may explain the impairment of transport functions with subsequent reduction in bile flow and the development of cholestasis[3–13]. Other mechanisms which may also contribute to cholestasis include changes in membrane fluidity altering the function of embedded transport proteins and enzymes; disruption of the cytoskeleton and vesicle transport which normally determine the hepatocyte's secretory polarity and target transport proteins to the basolateral and canalicular membrane; defects in tight junctional structures that lead to dissipation of osmotic gradients via leaky paracellular pathways; impairment of signal transduction pathways that normally coordinate cell functions in the hepatic lobule via gap junctions and stimulate bile canalicular contractions[3,66,70,80,85,86] (Fig. 2). While these general concepts had already been recognized by the late 1970s[87], only recent advances in molecular and cell biology have permitted exploration of these potential mechanisms in more detail.

Hepatocellular alterations

Insights from experimental animal models of cholestasis

Several experimental models of cholestasis have been developed to study the mechanisms of human cholestatic liver diseases including inflammation-induced cholestasis (endotoxin (lipopolysaccharide, LPS)-treated rats), oral contraceptive-induced cholestasis/cholestasis of pregnancy (ethinylestradiol (EE)-treated rats), and extrahepatic biliary obstruction (common bile duct

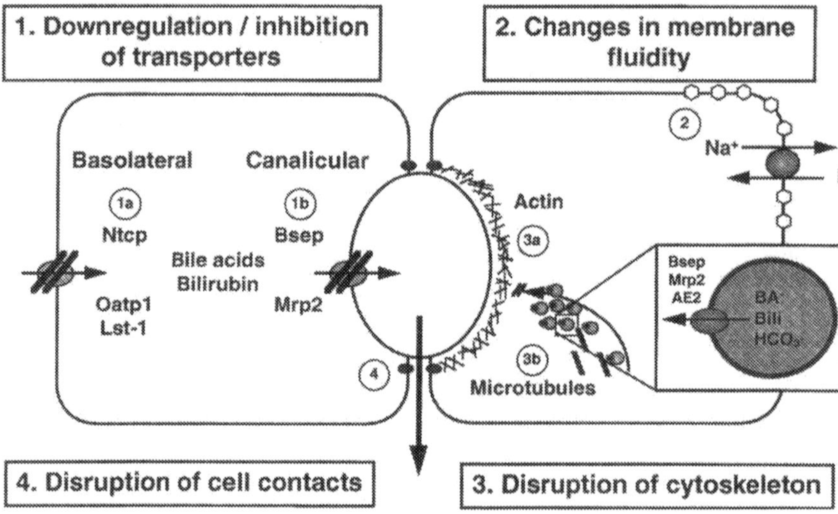

Figure 2 Hepatocellular alterations in experimental cholestasis. Cholestasis may result from (1) down-regulation and inhibition of transport systems (normally mediating vectorial transport of biliary constituents such as bile acids and bilirubin); (2) decreased membrane fluidity with subsequent reduction in the activity of the embedded transporters or enzymes such as Na^+,K^+-ATPase (normally maintaining the membrane potential and driving Na^+-dependent bile acid uptake); (3) disruption of cytoskeletal elements such as (3a) pericanalicular actin microfilaments (resulting in impaired bile canalicular contractions normally mediating the forward flow of bile from pericentral to periportal regions of the hepatic lobule) and (3b) microtubules (resulting in impaired movement of vesicles targeting transport proteins (insert) to the canalicular membrane) or (4) disruption of cell contacts such as tight junctions (normally sealing off the bile canaliculus) resulting in leaky junctions with the regurgitation of bile into the plasma (large arrow).

ligation (CBDL)[8,9,88]. Administration of LPS, EE, or CBDL to rats results in a marked reduction of mRNA and protein levels of the basolateral Na^+/taurocholate co-transporter (Ntcp) and organic anion transporting proteins (Oatp1, 1st-1), as well as the canalicular conjugate export pump (mrp2) and, to a lesser extent, the bile salt export pump (Bsep)[32,89–98]. Decreased expression of these transporters may explain impaired hepatocellular uptake and canalicular excretion of bile salts and other (non-bile salt) organic anions (e.g. bilirubin diglucuronide) in cholestasis (Fig. 2). Expression of the canalicular bile salt export pump Bsep initially decreases and partially recovers with prolonged cholestasis[96,98]. Thus, Bsep is more stably expressed than the other transporters (Ntcp, Oatp1, and mrp2)[98] and may continue to excrete bile salts into bile even under cholestatic conditions[99]. This response, together with the down-regulation of Ntcp, would tend to reduce the hepatocellular retention of bile salts and the degree of bile salt-mediated liver injury. Since canalicular transport represents the rate limiting step in bile secretion, alterations of canalicular transporter expression are considered the primary events, while alterations of basolateral transport systems may be secondary[10,100]. However, this concept is challenged by findings in estrogen-induced cholestasis and mouse models of cholestasis (e.g., mdr2 (rodent homologue of human MDR3) (-/-) and a mouse model of erythropoietic protoporphyria), where massive down-regulation of the basolateral bile salt transporter Ntcp appears to be an early event leading to the retention of bile salts[101-103]. In contrast to the down-regulation of these transporters, expression of the multidrug export pump (Mdr1) at the canalicular membrane and isoforms of the multidrug-resistance-associated protein (Mrp1 and 3) at the (baso)lateral membrane increases following cholestatic injury[47,96,97,104]. Up-regulation of these transport systems in cholestasis could be a compensatory mechanism that prevents further accumulation of potentially toxic biliary constituents within cholestatic hepatocytes.

Although much information has been gathered on the molecular alterations of hepatobiliary transport systems at the mRNA and protein levels, only limited information is currently available regarding the transcriptional and/or post-transcriptional/post-translational mechanisms and potential mediators leading to these events[10]. Evidence so far suggests that cytokines, bile salts and hormones could be potential modulators of transporter expression during cholestasis[10]. Such effects could be mediated by changes in the rate of gene transcription regulated by the promoter region of each gene, post-transcriptional changes (affecting mRNA processing, stability, and translational efficiency), as well as post-translational mechanisms (impaired intracellular sorting/targeting of transport proteins to the membrane, impaired protein activation by (de-) phosphorylation/(de-)glycosylation)[10].

Recent findings suggest that the down-regulation of transporter gene expression may occur to large extent at the transcriptional level[89,94], and that the reduction in gene transcription may be due to alterations in the quantity or function of nuclear transcription factors binding to the promoter region and regulating the transcriptional activity of these genes[94]. Administration of LPS in vivo and cytokines in vitro (e.g., TNF-α, IL-1β) reduces the activity of liver-specific transcription factors normally regulating the *Ntcp* promoter (e.g., hepatocyte nuclear factor 1 (HNF1) and a retinoid X receptor (RXR): retinoic acid receptor (RAR) heterodimer, formerly known as footprint B binding protein), thus providing a molecular mechanism for decreased *Ntcp* gene transcription in a rat model of inflammation-induced cholestasis[94,105,106].

Hepatic steady state mRNA levels of basolateral bile salt transporter Ntcp are inversely related to serum bile salt levels in rats subjected to CBDL and choledochocaval fistulas, suggesting that bile salts may suppress *Ntcp* gene expression[107]. Similarly, hepatic levels of human NTCP also correlate inversely with the levels of bile salts and bilirubin[108]. Bile salts suppress *Ntcp* gene promoter activity in vitro[109], similar to the negative feedback inhibition of cholesterol-7α-hydroxylase (a key enzyme for bile salt synthesis) by bile salts[110]. The *Ntcp* promoter contains a sequence homologous to a putative bile acid response element (BARE) recently described in the cholesterol-7α-hydroxylase promoter[111]. In addition, bile salts have been identified as natural ligands for the farsenoid X receptor (FXR)[112-117] which also down-regulates cholesterol-7α-hydroxylase, thus providing a molecular mechanism for negative feedback inhibition of cholesterol-7α-hydroxylase by bile salts[118-120]. Theoretically, down-regulation of *Ntcp* gene expression by elevated intrahepatic bile salt levels in cholestasis could be secondary to interaction of bile salts with BARE or the nuclear bile salt receptor RXR:FXR competing for co-factors with the retinoic acid receptor RXR:RAR[105,120].

Ganguly et al.[121] have shown that hormones such as prolactin and growth hormone up-regulate *Ntcp* expression via signal transducer and activator of transcription (STAT) 5 binding to two closely spaced consensus sites within the *Ntcp* promoter. Theoretically, reduced Ntcp levels in oestrogen-induced cholestasis could be explained in part by the effects of oestrogen on the pituitary growth hormone secretory pattern (disruption of the pulsatile secretory pattern)[101], possibly resulting in decreased stimulation of constitutive *Ntcp* gene expression by growth hormone. In addition, the *Ntcp* promoter contains a steroid hormone response element which could also result in down-regulation of *Ntcp* gene expression by estrogen[111].

Potential interactions between proinflammatory cytokines, bile salts, and hormones in regulating hepatobiliary transporter expression remain to be explored. Similar to *Ntcp*, the *mrp2* promoter is also regulated by HNF1 and RXR:RAR, which may explain their coupled down-regulation by cytokines and bile salts in cholestasis[105,122]. In particular, the *mrp2* promoter contains several glucocorticoid-response elements[122], which (in addition to anti-inflammatory and immunosuppressive effects) may explain up-regulation of mrp2 expression by glucocorticoids[123] and previous observations on the beneficial effects of corticosteroids in the treatment of cholestatic jaundice (corticosteroid whitewash)[88]. In contrast to Ntcp and mrp2, mdr1b expression is stimulated by TNF-α via activation of the inflammation-inducible nuclear transcription factor nuclear factor-κB (NF-κB), consistent with the presence of a functional NF-κB response element in the *mdr1b* promoter[124,125].

In addition to these transcriptional events, post-transcriptional and/or post-translational mechanisms such as enhanced protein degradation, transporter redistribution, direct protein modifications (e.g. (de-) phosphorylation, (de-) glycosylation), or direct cis-/trans-inhibition of transport systems by cholestatic agents (e.g. drugs) may also play an important role in the pathogenesis of cholestasis. The canalicular localization of Bsep and mrp2 becomes irregular and fuzzy, with a less well defined canalicular membrane, indicating a general disturbance of ATP-binding cassette proteins at the canalicular membrane in cholestasis[96–98,126,127]. This finding could be explained by impaired targeting or increased retrieval of transport systems in cholestasis (see below). Since the half-life of most hepatic transport proteins is probably on the order of several days, post-transcriptional/post-translational effects may be early events while transcriptional mechanisms may maintain alterations of transporter expression and function during cholestasis. For example, in LPS-induced cholestasis, retrieval of mrp2 from the canalicular membrane appears to be an early event (first 6 h after LPS)[126], whereas down-regulation of mrp2 mRNA may be a later event (occurring beyond 12 h after LPS)[96–98,126]. Furthermore, precholestatic or mild cholestatic conditions may affect transporter expression primarily at the post-transcriptional/post-translational level, while more severe cholestatic injury may result in alterations at the transcriptional level[102]. These findings suggest a complex hierarchy of events resulting in reduced transporter expression and function, depending on severity and duration of the cholestatic injury.

Besides down-regulation of transport systems, cholestasis may also result from altered membrane fluidity with subsequent reduction in the activity of the embedded transporters or enzymes such as Na^+-K^+-ATPase (which maintains the membrane potential and normally drives sodium dependent bile salt uptake; Fig. 2). Alterations of membrane fluidity may be particularly important in oestrogen-induced cholestasis[101], since oestrogen (via modulation of pituitary growth hormone secretion; see above) may increase hepatic low-density lipoprotein receptor expression, resulting in increased cholesterol incorporation into the cell membrane with decreased membrane lipid fluidity and Na^+, K^+-ATPase activity[101]. However, the correlation of restoration of normal fluidity (e.g., by S-adenosyl-L-methionine) and the correction of bile flow has been poor, and the role of alterations in membrane fluidity in the pathogenesis of cholestasis remains controversial[101,128].

Cholestasis is associated with profound alterations of the cytoskeleton of hepatocytes, including disruption of the microtubular system and actin microfilament network, as well as increases in cytokeratin intermediate filaments[70] (Fig. 2). Altered function of different components of the cytoskeleton may lead to cholestasis by interference with transcellular transport processes of biliary constituents or carrier proteins, increased tight junctional permeability, and impaired contraction of bile canaliculi[76,85]. Under baseline conditions, disruption of microtubules (e.g., by colchicine) does not cause cholestasis, but bile flow rapidly decreases under conditions with increased bile salt flux[129], since the vesicular pathway is an important way of rapidly adapting the number of transport proteins in the canalicular membrane. Cholestatic concentrations of hydrophobic bile salts such as chenodeoxycholate inhibit microtubular motors such as kinesin and dynein *in vitro*[130], which could be a critical factor in the impairment of vesicle movement during cholestasis. Accumulation of vesicles within the pericanalicular region of the hepatocyte is a characteristic morphological finding in many forms of cholestatic liver injury[84]. Impaired vesicular trafficking of transport proteins to the canalicular membrane will result in a decreased number of functional transporters in the canalicular membrane and thus contribute to cholestasis[131]. Ursodeoxycholic acid (UDCA) partially restores defective vesicular exocytosis in cholestatic livers[132]. Microfilament disrupting agents (e.g. phalloidin, cytochalasin D, norethandrolone, chlorpromazine) impair canalicular contractility, cause loss of microvilli, and disrupt tight junctions, resulting in cholestasis[70]. Certain forms of hereditary cholestasis (North American Indian childhood cirrhosis) are associated with increased pericanalicular microfilaments resembling phalloidin toxicity[133]. Although phalloidin does not directly affect the function of canalicular export pumps[134], it destabilizes the canalicular membrane with subsequent loss of canalicular membrane proteins through membrane invaginations[127]. Very little is known about the role of the cytokeratin (CK) intermediate filament network[135]. Obstructive cholestasis and feeding of hydrophobic (but not of hydrophilic) bile salts induce hepatic CK 8/18 expression with an increased density of the pericanalicular CK sheath[136–138] which may help hepatocytes to resist increased mechanical and toxic stress during cholestasis. Transgenic mice with disrupted CK 8/18 network due to ectopic CK 14 expression[139] and CK 8 (–/–) mice[140] show decreased bile flow and bile salt excretion, suggesting that CK intermediate filaments could have a role in bile secretion, although the detailed mechanisms have not been described[78]. Thus, it is reasonable to speculate, that CK intermediate filaments could also be primary targets in cholestasis.

Disruption of cell contacts such as tight junctions (which normally seal off the bile canaliculus) results in leaky junctions with the regurgitation of bile into plasma and reduction of the osmotic gradients in the bile canaliculi that normally constitute the driving force for bile secretion (Fig. 2)[80]. The hepatic localization and expression of tight junction-associated protein such as zonula occludens 1 and occludin are altered by CBDL, EE, bacterial toxins and LPS, resulting in leaky junctions[141–146]. Gap junction proteins such as connexins disappear rapidly after CBDL, resulting in a decline in the migration of calcium waves between individual hepatocytes that normally coordinate cell functions in the hepatic lobule and stimulate bile canalicular contractions[147]. Alterations of second messenger and signal transduction systems (e.g., cAMP-mediated intracellular signalling, protein kinase C, calcium, phosphoinositide 3-kinase) regulating various steps in bile formation (e.g. transporter activity, vesicular trafficking, tight junction permeability) may also contribute to cholestasis[3,82,83].

Further studies in human cholestatic liver diseases will have to show the extent to which these experimental findings in rodents (mostly rats) can be applied to humans.

Hereditary cholestasis syndromes

Mutations of transporter genes can result in hereditary cholestasis[3–6,10,12] (for a continuously updated online version see reference 148) (Fig. 3). Generally,

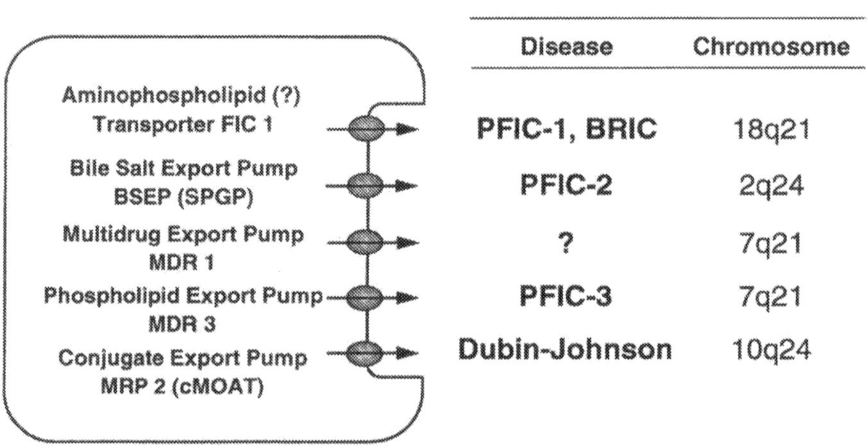

Figure 3 Hereditary defects of hepatocellular transport systems. Mutations of transporter genes can cause congenital cholestasis or hyperbilirubinemia. PFIC, progressive familial intrahepatic cholestasis; BRIC, benign recurrent intrahepatic cholestasis. Chromosomal localizations of cholestatic/ hyperbilirubinemic syndromes are given on the right. Mutations of the putative aminophospholipid transporter FICl result in PFIC-1 (Byler Disease) or BRIC (Summerskill-Walshe syndrome), depending on the severity of the mutation. PFIC-2 (Byler syndrome) is caused by mutations in the *BSEP* gene. No mutations of MDR1 have been described so far. PFIC-3 is caused by mutations of the *MDR3*-gene. Dubin–Johnson syndrome is caused by mutations of the *MRP2* gene.

these mutations cause defects in protein production, processing, regulation (of transport function), or channel/pore function[149]. Most of these mutations are nonsense (single base) or frameshift (deletion/insertion) mutations with introduction of a premature stop codon resulting in a truncated or even completely absent protein, while missense mutations result in a malfunctioning protein which is still expressed (or even overexpressed) with residual function. Progressive familial intrahepatic cholestasis (PFIC) is a severe type of cholestatic liver disease in infants and children which is inherited in an autosomal recessive fashion[150,151].

Four types (PFIC 1–4) have been identified: PFIC-1 (also known as Byler disease) is characterized by low γ-glutamyl transpeptidase (γ-GT) serum levels, elevated serum bile salts, normal serum cholesterol and low biliary bile salt levels. This form of PFIC has been mapped to chromosome 18q21-22[152]. Benign recurrent intrahepatic cholestasis (BRIC), a recurrent cholestatic disorder in children or adults (also known as Summerskill–Walshe syndrome), has also been mapped to chromosome 18q21-22[153], indicating that there may be a familial cholestasis gene that is responsible for both PFIC-1 and BRIC. Recently, a gene encoding a P-type ATPase (*FIC*1) likely to be involved in hepatic bile salt excretion and/or the enterohepatic circulation of bile salts and mutated in both PFIC-1 and BRIC has been described[50]. The mutations were found in different regions of the *FIC*1 gene, possibly explaining the different phenotypic appearances of PFIC-1 and BRIC. In contrast to PFIC-1, BRIC is characterized by recurrent episodes of cholestasis which do not progress to liver cirrhosis. Extrahepatic manifestations in both diseases (e.g. diarrhoea, bile salt malabsorption, pancreatitis, nephrolithiasis) may be explained by the extrahepatic expression of FIC1 and can persist after liver transplantation in patients with PFIC-1[51]. Recently it has become clear that these two diseases may overlap considerably; BRIC and PFIC-1 may represent the extreme ends of a whole spectrum of cholestatic syndromes.

A second type, PFIC-2, is similar phenotypically to PFIC-1, but is different genetically since the gene locus is on chromosome 2q24[154]. PFIC-2 is caused by mutations in the *BSEP/SPGP* gene[99] resulting in a defective or even completely absent canalicular bile salt export pump (BSEP) in the liver of these patients[155]. Extrahepatic manifestations are typically absent and the defect is restricted to the liver.

In contrast to PFIC-1 and PFIC-2, the third subtype, PFIC-3, is characterized by high γ-GT serum levels, as well as bile duct proliferation and inflammatory infiltrates in portal areas. This type of cholestasis is caused by mutations of the *MDR3*-gene encoding the canalicular phospholipid export pump and resulting in a marked reduction of biliary phospholipid (phosphatidylcholine) levels[156,157]. Since phospholipids in bile normally protect bile duct epithelial cells from bile salt toxicity by the formation of mixed micelles, the marked reduction or even absence of biliary phospholipids may explain bile duct injury in these patients. UDCA may benefit some patients with PFIC-3 with a partial or incomplete defect by exerting its protective effect from the biliary lumen, presumably by counteracting the toxic effects of other (more hydrophobic) bile salts in bile[158]. The pathophysiological consequences and potential therapeutic approaches were originally discovered in mdr2 (rodent homologue of human MDR3) (–/–) knockout mice and stimulated the research that led to the discovery of a human equivalent for this defect[38,159–166]. PFIC-3 provides an important link between a hepatocellular (canalicular) transport defect and the development of cholangiopathies. Many human neonatal and adult cholangiopathies/cholestatic syndromes now are reevaluated for possible MDR3 defects[159]. Notably, patients with primary biliary cirrhosis (PBC) have normal MDR3 -mRNA levels[167] suggesting that decreased *MDR3*-gene expression is not involved in the pathogenesis of this vanishing bile duct syndrome. Furthermore, bile analysis from patients with acquired destructive cholangiopathies (e.g. PBC and primary sclerosing cholangitis), drug-induced cholestasis, and several forms of idiopathic cholestasis has not revealed a pathological bile salt/phospholipid ratio (indicating a defect in biliary phospholipid excretion)[164]. The only exception was total parenteral nutrition-induced cholestasis[165], although the molecular basis for defective phospholipid excretion in this condition remains to be clarified[164–166]. A fourth subtype (PFIC-4) is caused by hereditary bile acid synthesis defects and is not a transporter defect[11,166].

Dubin–Johnson syndrome is caused by mutations of the human *MRP2* gene encoding a (bilirubin) conjugate export pump[168–179]. This syndrome is characterized by abnormal biliary excretion of various endogenous and exogenous substances (e.g. bilirubin diglucuronide, bromosulphophthalein conjugates, oral cholecystographic agents) which are normally excreted by MRP2[180,181]. Although patients with Dubin–Johnson syndrome are usually hyperbilirubinemic rather than cholestatic, this is yet another important example of how a mutation of a hepatocellular transporter gene can impair bile excretory function[182].

What could be the role of hereditary transporter defects for adult cholestatic liver diseases? Homozygotes or compound heterozygotes (carrying two different mutations of the same gene) are already cholestatic under baseline conditions depending on the severity of the underlying mutation. Most mutations identified so far cause severe cholestatic liver disease early on in life. Although these syndromes offer interesting new insights into biliary physiology and pathophysiology, they are exceedingly rare and of limited clinical relevance for liver disease in adults. However, a larger number of still-to-be-identified defects may be incomplete or mild, and may not become evident until later in life (e.g. when challenged with a cholestatic agent). Heterozygotes are unremarkable under normal conditions, since they have a second normal copy of the gene, but they may also have an increased suceptibility to cholestatic injury (e.g. drugs and sex hormones). Interestingly, some heterozygous mothers of PFIC-3 patients had recurrent episodes of cholestasis during pregnancy as a result of a transient decompensation of their heterozygous state due to female sex hormones and their metabolites[157,183]. Therefore, hereditary transporter mutations may also predetermine the individual susceptibility to cholestatic liver injury and may explain the broad clinical spectrum of cholestatic liver diseases.

Acquired cholestatic liver diseases

Very little is so far known about alterations of hepatobiliary transport systems in acquired cholestatic liver disease in humans (Fig. 4). Messenger RNA levels of the basolateral bile salt transporter NTCP are decreased in patients with extra-

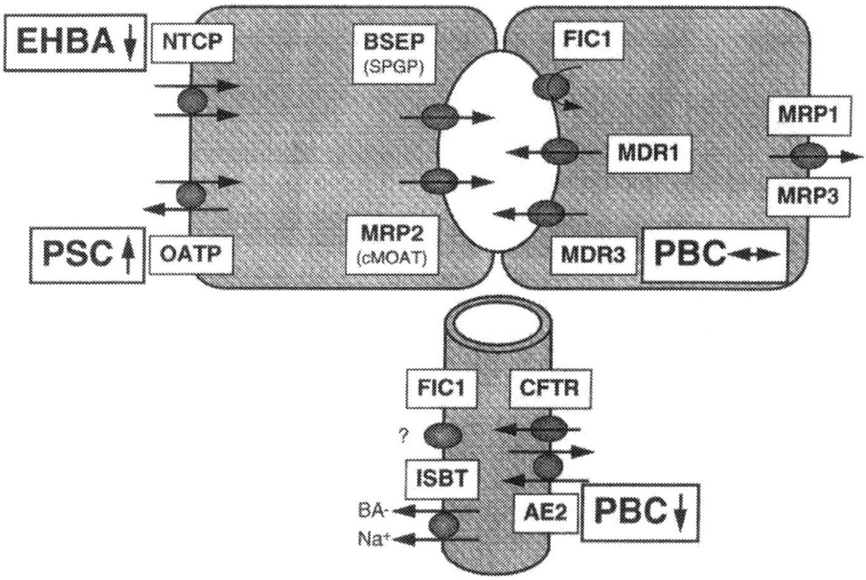

Figure 4 Alterations of hepatobiliary transport systems in acquired forms of cholestatic liver diseases. NTCP mRNA levels are decreased in children with extrahepatic biliary atresia (EHBA), while OATP mRNA levels are increased in patients with primary sclerosing cholangitis (PSC). MDR3 mRNA levels remain unchanged in patients with primary biliary cirrhosis (PBC), while AE2 expression is reduced in both hepatocytes (not shown) and cholangiocytes in these patients. Only data published as full papers (refs 23, 108, 167, 186, 187) have been considered in this figure.

hepatic biliary atresia and subsequently increase if complete biliary drainage is achieved by portoenterostomy (Kasai procedure)[108]. In contrast to the down-regulation of NTCP, the expression of the canalicular bile salt export pump BSEP is not reduced in these patients[184]. On the other hand, MDR1 and MDR3 - mRNA levels are increased in patients with obstructive cholestasis[185]. These findings resemble those obtained in the CBDL rat model of obstructive cholestasis (see above). Expression of the Cl^-/HCO_3^- anion exchanger isoform AE2 is reduced in livers from patients with PBC[186,187]. Since Cl^-/HCO_3^- exchange activity contributes to secretion of both canalicular and ductular bile, decreased hepatic expression of AE2 could lead to impaired bile flow. Up-regulation of AE2 mRNA and protein levels as well as improved HCO_3^- secretion (in response to the cholangiocyte secretagogue secretin) has been reported in PBC patients treated with UDCA, indicating that improvement of hepatobiliary excretory function under UDCA treatment could in part be mediated by stimulation of gene expression of defective hepatobiliary transport systems[186–188]. UDCA might also increase the number of transport proteins contained in the canalicular membrane by stimulating vesicular exocytosis and targeting of transporters to the canalicular membrane[132,189] (see above). Future studies should determine whether UDCA also stimulates the expression of hepatobiliary transport systems for canalicular excretion of bile salts and conjugated bilirubin (e.g. BSEP,

MRP2). OATP mRNA expression is up-regulated in patients with cholestasis due to primary sclerosing cholangitis[23]. This up-regulation might minimize the accumulation of potentially toxic compounds by transporting these substances out of the hepatocytes into portal venous plasma, since the exchange mechanism for bile salts by OATP may be reversed under cholestatic conditions[23]. However, expression of OATP is already extremely low in normal human liver[22,31] and these finding need to be reevaluated in the light of the recently identified liver-specific organic anion transporter LST-1 (see above). In a preliminary report, MRP2 mRNA was found to be reduced in patients with advanced PBC[190]. However, only a very small number of patients, mainly with cirrhotic PBC stage IV, was studied, and down-regulation of MRP2 in these patients could be a non-specific finding secondary to cirrhosis.

The expression of hepatobiliary transport systems has not yet been studied systematically in adult cholestatic liver diseases, mainly due to the limitations resulting from the small amount of liver tissue available from percutaneous biopsies. Quantitative, competitive RT-PCR using homologous internal RNA standards (with mutated restriction enzyme sites) permits the simultaneous and accurate quantification of mRNA expression of a whole panel of hepatobiliary transport systems utilizing only very small amounts of RNA as isolated from routine percutaneous liver biopsies[191]. Applying this technique to liver biopsies from patients with acute icteric cholestasis (mostly cholestatic alcoholic hepatitis), NTCP mRNA levels were found to be significantly decreased, while BSEP mRNA expression was only slightly reduced. Interestingly, no changes were seen at the RNA level for the bilirubin conjugate export pump MRP2, despite the presence of pronounced cholestasis and jaundice. RNA levels of MRP3 (basolateral MRP isoform), MDR1 (multidrug export pump), MDR3 (phospholipid flippase), FIC1 (a transporter affected in hereditary cholestasis), and GAPDH (housekeeping gene) also remained unchanged. These findings suggest that regulation of hepatocellular transport systems in human cholestatic liver disease can occur at the RNA level (as observed for NTCP), consistent with previous findings in experimental animal models of cholestasis (see above). However, the observed mRNA changes are moderate compared to those seen in experimental animal models of cholestasis. Furthermore, conserved mRNA levels of MRP2 in severely cholestatic and jaundiced patients suggest that post-translational mechanisms directly affecting protein function may also play an important role in the pathogenesis of human cholestatic liver disease.

Cholangiocellular alterations

The bile duct epithelium has become a new frontier in hepatobiliary research[15]. Although they contribute to only 3–5% of the total liver cell mass, cholangiocytes play an important role in normal bile secretion[16,17,55] (see above) and may become a primary target for the cholestatic injury in various genetic, immune-mediated, infectious and drug-induced cholangiopathies[16,55,192,193].

Defects in cholangiocellular transport systems such as mutations of the *CFTR* gene (encoding a chloride channel) in cystic fibrosis[149,192] and decreased expression of the Cl^-/HCO_3^- exchanger AE2 in PBC[186,187] may also cause or contribute to cholestasis (Fig. 5). Understanding the molecular basis of the morphological and functional heterogeneity of the intrahepatic bile duct

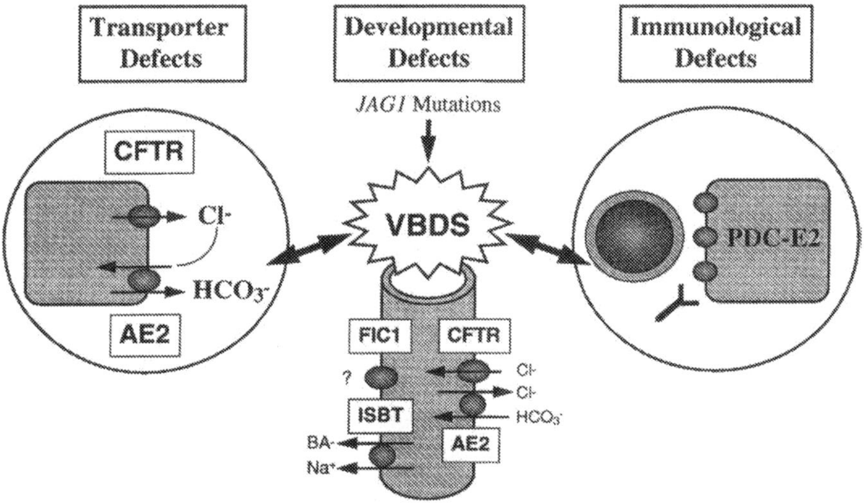

Figure 5 Cholangiocellular alterations in cholestasis. Defects in cholangiocellular transport systems such as mutations of the *CFTR* gene encoding a chloride channel in cystic fibrosis and decreased expression of the Cl^-/HCO_3^- exchanger AE2 in PBC may cause cholestasis. Transport systems for intestinal reabsorption of bile acids such as the ileal sodium-dependent bile salt transporter ISBT and the putative aminophospholipid transporter FICl have also been identified in cholangiocytes, and these transport systems may also undergo pronounced changes in cholestasis. Mutations of the *JAG1* gene (encoding a ligand for the Notch receptor signaling pathway which plays a critical role in the determination of cell fate during development) result in Alagille syndrome, characterized by cholestasis due to ductopenia in combination with multiple extrahepatic abnormalities. Finally immunological abnormalities such as aberrant expression of the E2 subunit of the pyruvate dehydrogenase complex (PDC-E2) or related antigens in the apical region of intrahepatic bile ducts is one of the earliest immunological abnormalities in primary biliary cirrhosis. This antigen is recognized by antimitochondrial antibodies and specific T cells, resulting in the destruction of small interlobular bile ducts. VBDS, vanishing bile duct syndrome.

epithelium[15–17,55–57] may be a key to a better understanding of the segmental character of the vanishing bile duct syndromes (VBDS). Mutations of the human *ISBT* gene cause primary bile salt malabsorption in the ileum[194], but further studies will have to investigate the role of cholangiocyte ISBT/isbt in cholestasis. Proliferation of cholangiocytes during obstructive cholestasis (rat CBDL model) may at least in part be induced by bile salts retained during cholestasis[195] and results in increased expression (and possibly) function of cholangiocyte isbt[103,196,197]. Since the relative stability of hepatocellular Bsep expression during cholestasis enables some bile salts to continue to be excreted into bile, increased expression and functional capacity of cholangiocyte isbt could facilitate the return of bile salts to the systemic circulation. Urinary excretion of bile salts then provides an overflow pathway by partially reducing the bile salt pool that accumulates in the systemic circulation. Therefore, recent studies have focused on renal expression of hepatobiliary transporters such as isbt and mrp2, which are also expressed in the apical membrane of kidney proximal tubules[198–202]. In contrast to hepatic down-regulation of mrp2 and up-regulation of isbt, renal mrp2 is up-regulated while isbt in the kidney is down-regulated[197]. These reciprocal changes in liver and kidney expression of both mrp2 and isbt may help the renal elimination of biliary constituents (e.g. bile salts) during cholestasis and suggest organ-specific differences in their gene regulation. On the other hand, increased isbt activity due to bile duct proliferation has also been implicated in the intrahepatic bile salt recirculation, contributing to intrahepatic retention of bile salts and, by spillover, to increased systemic bile salt concentrations in cholestasis[103]. Enhanced secretin-stimulated ductal secretion in obstructive cholestasis (rat CBDL model), as reflected in increased secretin receptor gene expression, secretin-induced cAMP synthesis, Cl^-/HCO_3^- exchanger activity and apical insertion of AQP1 water channels[17,60,61], could also account for the well-known clinical observation of white bile that occurs during prolonged obstruction of bile ducts. FIC1 is also highly expressed at the level of the bile duct epithelium but its physiological role is unknown and bile duct damage is remarkably absent in patients with PFIC-1 and BRIC[50,51].

Major progress has been made in understanding the molecular genetic basis of VBDS. Mutations of the *JAG1* gene result in Alagille syndrome[202–205], characterized by cholestasis due to ductopenia in combination with multiple extrahepatic abnormalities (heart, skeletal, ocular, facial, renal, and pancreatic abnormalities). *JAG1* normally encodes a ligand for the Notch receptor signalling pathway which in turn plays a critical role in the determination of cell fate during differentiation and development, explaining the widespread phenotypic appearances of Alagille syndrome[206].

Immunological abnormalities such as aberrant expression of the E2 subunit of the pyruvate dehydrogenase complex or related antigens in the apical region of intrahepatic bile ducts are one of the earliest immunological abnormalities in PBC. This antigen is recognized by antimitochondrial antibodies and specific T cells, resulting in the destruction of small interlobular bile ducts[207]. Finally the bile duct epithelium is not just an innocent bystander, but actively produces cytokines, chemokines and adhesion molecules and thus actively contributes to immune-mediated injury[207].

SUMMARY AND OUTLOOK

Hereditary mutations of transporter genes, exposure to cholestatic injury through drugs, hormones, proinflammatory cytokines, and biliary obstruction, or the combination of both hereditary and exogenous cholestatic factors result in decreased or even non-existent expression of hepatobiliary transport systems (Fig. 6). These molecular changes may explain impaired hepatic uptake and excretion of bile salts and other organic anions in cholestasis. It is conceivable that some of these hepatobiliary transport systems and their alterations in cholestatic liver diseases may become the target of specific therapeutic interventions in the near future. Some drugs already used to treat cholestatic liver diseases and their complications such as pruritus (e.g. UDCA, phenobarbital) may act via stimulation and restoration of defective hepatobiliary transporter expression and function[208–211]. Increasing information on the molecular regula-

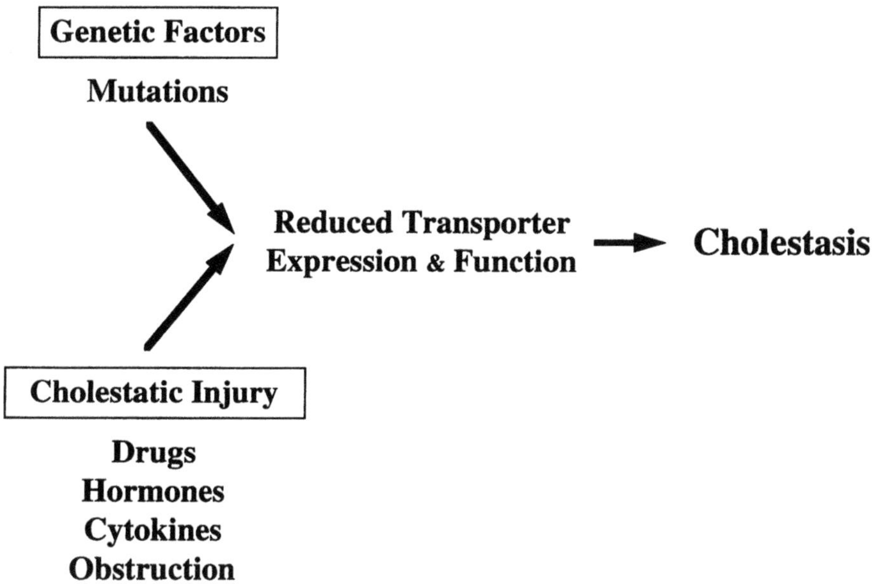

Figure 6 Molecular mechanisms of cholestasis. Genetic factors such as mutations of hepatobiliary transporter genes, exposure to cholestatic injury such as drugs, hormones, proinflammatory cytokines, and biliary obstruction, or a combination of both hereditary and acquired factors, may result in decreased or even non-existent expression of hepatobiliary transport systems, which may explain impaired transport function causing cholestasis.

tion of hepatobiliary transport systems in cholestasis should lead to the identification of novel drugs for the treatment of cholestatic liver diseases. Finally, gene therapy and hepatocyte transplantation may be a feasible approach to the correction of hereditary transporter defects[3,212].

ACKNOWLEDGEMENT

This work was supported by the Jubilaeumsfonds of the Austrian National Bank and the Joseph Skoda Prize of the Austrian Society of Internal Medicine.

REFERENCES

1. Müller M, Jansen PLM. Molecular aspects of hepatobiliary transport. Am J Physiol. 1997;272:G1285–1303.
2. Müller M, Jansen PLM. The secretory function of the liver: new aspects of hepatobiliary transport. J Hepatol. 1998;28:344–54.
3. Trauner M, Meier PJ, Boyer JL. Molecular pathogenesis of cholestasis. N Eng J Med. 1998;339:1217–27.

4. Arias IM. New genetics of inheritable jaundice and cholestatic liver disease. Lancet. 1998;352:82–3.
5. Arrese M, Ananthanarayanan M, Suchy FJ. Hepatobiliary transport: molecular mechanisms of development and cholestasis. Pediatric Res. 1998;44:141–7.
6. Jansen PL, Mueller MM. Progressive familial intrahepatic cholestasis types 1,2, and 3. Gut. 1998;42:766–7.
7. Koopen NR, Mueller M, Vonk RJ, Zimniak P, Kuipers F. Molecular mechanisms of cholestasis: causes and consequences of impaired bile formation. Biochem Biophys Acta. 1998;1408:1–17.
8. Trauner M. Molecular alterations of canalicular transport systems in experimental models of cholestasis: possible functional correlations. Yale J Biol Med. 1997;70:365–78.
9. Gartung C, Matern S. Molecular regulation of sinusoidal liver bile acid transporters during cholestasis. Yale J Biol Med. 1997;70:355–63.
10. Trauner M, Meier PJ, Boyer JL. Molecular regulation of hepatocellular transport systems in cholestasis. J Hepatol. 1999;31:165–78.
11. Balistreri WF. Inborn errors of bile acid synthesis and transport. Novel forms of metabolic liver disease. Gastroenterol Clin N Am. 1999;28:145–72.
12. Shneider BL. Genetic cholestatic syndromes. J Pediatr Gastr Nutr. 1999;28:124–31.
13. Trauner M, Boyer JL. Cholestatic syndromes. Curr Opin Gastroenterol. 1999;15:217–28.
14. Boyer JL, Nathanson MH. Bile formation. In: Schiff ER, Sorrell MF, Maddrey WC, eds. Schiff's Diseases of the Liver, 8th edition. Philadelphia: Lippincott-Raven Publishers, 1999: pp. 119–46.
15. Boyer JL. Bile duct epithelium: frontiers in transport physiology. Am J Physiol. 1996;270:G1–5.
16. Strazzabosco M. New insights into cholangiocyte physiology. J Hepatol. 1997;27:945–52.
17. Baiocchi L, LeSage G, Glaser S, Alpini G. Regulation of cholangiocyte bile secretion. J Hepatol. 1999;31:179–91.
18. Oude Elferink RPJ, Meijer DKF, Kuipers F, Jansen PLM, Groen AK, Groothuis GMM. Hepatobiliary secretion of organic compounds; molecular mechanisms of membrane transport. Biochim Biophys Acta. 1995;1241:215–68.
19. Müller M, Jansen PLM. The transporter page. http://www.med.rug.nl/mdl/tab3.htm
20. Hagenbuch B, Meier PJ. Molecular cloning, chromosomal localization, and functional characterization of a human Na^+/bile acid cotransporter. J Clin Invest. 1994;93:1326–31.
21. Hagenbuch B, Stieger B, Foguet M, Luebbert H, Meier PJ. Expression cloning and characterization of the hepatocyte Na^+/bile acid cotransport system. Proc Natl Acad Sci USA. 1991;88:10629–33.
22. Kullak-Ublick GA, Hagenbuch B, Stieger B, Schteingart CD, Hofmann AF, Wolkoff AW, Meier PJ. Molecular and functional characterization of an organic anion transporting polypeptide cloned from human liver. Gastroenterology. 1995;109:1274–82.
23. Kullak-Ublick GA, Beuers U, Fahney C, Hagenbuch B, Meier PJ, Paumgartner G. Identification and functional characterization of the promoter region of the human organic anion transporting polypeptide gene. Hepatology. 1997;26:991–7.
24. Meier PJ. Molecular mechanisms of hepatic bile salt transport from sinusoidal blood into bile. Am J Physiol. 1995;269:G801–12.
25. Meier PJ, Eckhardt U, Schroeder A, Hagenbuch B, Stieger B. Substrate specificity of sinusoidal bile acid and organic anion uptake systems in rat and human liver. Hepatology. 1997;26:1667–77.
26. Kullak-Ublick GA. Regulation of organic anion and drug transporters of the sinusoidal membrane. J Hepatol. 1999;31:563–73.
27. Jacquemin E, Hagenbuch B, Stieger B, Wolkoff AW, Meier PJ. Expression cloning of a rat liver Na^+-independent organic anion transporter. Proc Natl Acad Sci USA. 1994;91:133–7.
28. Noe B, Hagenbuch B, Stieger B, Meier PJ. Isolation of a multispecific organic anion and cardiac glycoside transporter from rat brain. Proc Natl Acad Sci USA. 1997;94:10346–50.
29. Abe T, Kakyo M, Sakagami H, Tokui T, Nishio T, Tanemoto M et al. Molecular characterization and tissue distribution of a new organic anion transporter subtype (oatp3) that transports thyroid hormones and taurocholate and comparison with oatp2. J Biol Chem. 1998;273:22395–401.
30. Walters HC, Craddock AL, Dawson PA. Identification of a novel rat ileal organic anion transporter. Hepatology. 1998;28:386A.

31. Abe T, Kakyo M, Tokui T, Nakagomi R, Nishio T, Nakai D et al. Identification of a novel gene family encoding human liver-specific organic anion transporter LST-1. J Biol Chem. 1999;274:17159–63.
32. Kakyo M, Unno M, Tokui T, Nakagomi R, Nishio T, Iwasashi H et al. Molecular characterization and functional regulation of a novel rat liver-specific organic anion transporter rlst-1. Gastroenterology. 1999;117:770–75.
33. Keppler D, Arias IM. Introduction: transport across the hepatocyte canalicular membrane. FASEB J. 1997;11:15–8.
34. Ueda K, Clark DP, Chen CJ, Roninson IB, Gottesman MM, Pastan I. The human multidrug resistance (mdrl) gene. cDNA cloning and transcription initiation. J Biol Chem. 1987;262:505–8.
35. Gottesman MM, Pastan I. Biochemistry of multidrug resistance mediated by the multidrug transporter. Annu Rev Biochem. 1993;62:385–427.
36. Silverman JA, Thorgeirson SS. Regulation and function of the multidrug resistance genes in liver. In: Boyer JL, Ockner RK, eds. Progress in Liver Disease. Volume 13. Philadelphia: WB Saunders, 1995: pp. 101–23.
37. van der Bliek AM, Kooiman PM, Schneider C, Borst PA. Sequence of mdr3 cDNA encoding a human P-glycoprotein. Gene. 1988;71:401–11.
38. Smit JJM, Schinkel AH, Oude Elferink RPJ, Groen AK, Wagenaar E, Van Deemter L et al. Homozygous disruption of the murine *mdr2* P-glycoprotein gene leads to complete absence of phospholipids from bile and to liver disease. Cell. 1993;75:451–62.
39. Ruetz S, Gros P. Phosphatidylcholine translocase: a physiological role for the mdr2 gene. Cell. 1994;77:1071–81.
40. Büchler M, König J, Brom M, Kartenbeck J, Spring H, Horie T, Keppler D. cDNA cloning of the hepatocyte canalicular isoform of the multidrug resistance protein, cMrp, reveals a novel conjugate export pump deficient in hyperbilirubinemic mutant rats. J Biol Chem. 1996;271:15091–8.
41. Taniguchi M, Wada M, Kohno K, Nakamura T, Kawabe T, Kawakami M et al. A human canalicular multispecific organic anion transporter (cMOAT) gene is overexpressed in cisplatin-resistant human cancer cell lines with decreased drug accumulation. Cancer Res. 1996;56:4124–9.
42. Paulusma CC, Bosma PJ, Zaman GJR, Bakker CTM, Otter M, Scheffer GL et al. Congenital jaundice in rats with a mutation in a multidrug resistance-associated protein gene. Science. 1996;271:1126–28.
43. Ito K, Suzuki H, Hirohashi T, Kume K, Shimizu T, Sugiyama Y. Molecular cloning of canalicular multispecific organic anion transporter defective in EHBR. Am J Physiol. 1997;272:G16–22.
44. Oude Elferink RPJ, Jansen PLM. The role of the canalicular multispecific organic anion transporter in the disposal of endo- and xenobiotics. Pharmacol Ther. 1994;64:77–97.
45. Paulusma CC, van Geer MA, Evers R, Heijn M, Ottenhoff R, Borst P, Oude Elferink RPJ. The canalicular multispecific organic anion transporter (cMOAT/MRP2) mediates low-afinity transport of reduced glutathione. Biochem J. 1999;338:393–401.
46. Koenig J, Rost D, Cui Y, Keppler D. Characterization of the human multidrug resistance protein isoform MRP3 localized to the basolateral hepatocyte membrane. Hepatology. 1999;29:1156–63.
47. Hirohashi T, Suzuki H, Ito K, Ogawa K, Kume K, Shimizu T, Sugiyama Y. Hepatic expression of multidrug resistance-associated protein-like proteins maintained in Eisai hyperbilirubinemic rats. Mol Pharmacol. 1998;53:1068–75.
48. Gerloff T, Stieger B, Hagenbuch B, Madon J, Landmann L, Roth J et al. The sister of P-glycoprotein represents the canalicular bile salt export pump of mammalian liver. J Biol Chem. 1998;273:10046–50.
49. Strautnieks SS, Bull LN, Knisely AS, Kocoshis SA, Dahl N, Arnell H et al. A gene encoding a liver-specific ABC transporter is mutated in progressive familial intrahepatic cholestasis. Nature Genet. 1998;20:233–38.
50. Bull LN, van Eijk MJT, Pawlikowska L, DeYoung JA, Juijn JA, Liao M et al. A gene encoding a P-type ATPase mutated in two forms of hereditary cholestasis. Nature Genet. 1998;18:219–24.
51. Oude Elferink RPJ, Van Berge Henegouwen GP. Cracking the genetic code for benign recurrent and progressive familial intrahepatic cholestasis. J Hepatol. 1998;29:317–20.

52. Ujhazy P, Ortiz DF, Misra S, Li S, Arias IW. ATP-dependent aminophospholipid translocase activity in rat canalicular membrane vesicles and its relationship to FIC1 (Abstract). Hepatology. 1999;30:462A.
53. Mutero JA, Bull LN, Pawlikowska L, Freimer NB, Scharschmidt BF, Lomri N. Cloning and tissue distribution of the rat homologue of the human gene involved in familial intrahepatic cholestasis type 1. Hepatology. 1998;28:530A.
54. Martinez-Anso E, Castillo JE, Diez J, Medina JF, Prieo J. Immunohistochemical detection of chloride/bicarbonate anion exchangers in human liver. Hepatology. 1994;19:1400–6.
55. Strazzabosco M. Transport systems in cholangiocytes: their role in bile formation and cholestasis. Yale J Biol Med. 1997;70:427–34.
56. Cohn JA, Strong TV, Piccioto MR, Nairn AC, Collins FS, Fitz JG. Localization of the cystic fibrosis transmembrane conductance regulator in human bile duct epithelial cels. Gastroenterology. 1993;105:1857–64.
57. Alpini G, Ulrich C, Roberts S, Phillips JO, Podila PV, Colegio O et al. Molecular and functional heterogeneity of cholangiocytes from rat liver after bile duct ligation. Am J Physiol. 1997;272:G289–97.
58. Alpini G, Glaser SS, Rodgers R, Phinizy JL, Robertson WE, Lasater J et al. Functional expression of the apical Na^+-dependent bile acid transporter in large but not small rat cholangiocytes. Gastroenterology. 1997;113:1734–40.
59. Lazaridis KN, Pham L, Tietz P, Marinelli RA, deGroen PC, Levine S et al. Rat cholangiocytes absorb bile acids at their apical domain via the ileal sodium-dependent bile acid transporter. J Clin Invest. 1997;100:2714–21.
60. Marinelli RA, Pham L, Agre P, LaRusso NF. Secretin promotes osmotic water transport in rat cholangiocytes by increasing aquaporin-1 water channels in plasma membrane. Evidence for a secretin-induced vesicular translocation of aquaporin-1. J Biol Chem. 1997;272:12984–8.
61. Marinelli RA, Tietz PS, Pham LD, Rueckert L, Agre P, LaRusso NF. Secretin induces the apical insertion of aquaporin-1 water channels in rat cholangiocytes. Am J Physiol. 1999;276:G280–6.
62. Yano M, Marinelli RA, Roberts SK, Balan V, Pham L, Tarara JE et al. Rat hepatocytes transport water mainly via a non-channel pathway. J Biol Chem. 1996;271:6702–7.
63. Marinelli RA, LaRusso NF. Aquaporin water channels in liver: their significance in bile formation. Hepatology. 1997;26:1081–4.
64. Nathanson MH, Boyer JL. Vesicular trafficking in the hepatocyte. In: Arias IM, Boyer JL, Fausto N, Jakoby WB, Schachter DA, Shafritz DA, eds. The Liver: Biology and Pathobiology. 3rd edn. New York: Raven Press, 1994: pp. 33–44.
65. Crawford JM. Role of vesicle-mediated transport pathways in hepatocellular bile secretion. Semin Liver Dis. 1996;16:169–89.
66. Stieger B, Landmann L. Effects of cholestasis on membrane flow and surface polarity in hepatocytes. J Hepatol. 1996;24:128–34.
67. Sai Y, Nies AT, Arias IM. Bile acid secretion and direct targeting of mdr1-green fluorescent protein from golgi to the canalicular membrane in polarized WIF-B cells. J Cell Sci. 1999;112:4535–45.
68. Misra S, Ujhazy P, Gatmaitan Z, Varticovski L, Arias IM. The role of phosphoinositide 3-kinase in taurocholate-induced trafficking of ATP-dependent canalicular transporters in rat liver. J Biol Chem. 1998;273:26638–44.
69. Kubitz R, D'Urso D, Keppler, Haeussinger D. Osmodependent dynamic localization of the multidrug resistance protein 2 in the rat hepatocyte canalicular membrane. Gastroenterology. 1997;113:1438–42.
70. Phillips MJ, Poucell S, Oda M. Biology of disease: mechanisms of cholestasis. Lab Invest. 1986;54:593–608.
71. Feldmann G. The cytoskeleton of the hepatocyte. Structure and functions. J Hepatol. 1989;8:380–6.
72. Phillips MJ. Biology and pathobiology of actin in the liver. In: Arias IM, Boyer JL, Fausto N, Jakoby WB, Schachter DA, Shafritz DA, eds. The Liver: Biology and Pathobiology. 3rd edn. New York: Raven Press, 1994: pp. 19–32.
73. Satir P. Motor molecules of the cytoskeleton. In: In: Arias IM, Boyer JL, Fausto N, Jakoby WB, Schachter DA, Shafritz DA, eds. The Liver: Biology and Pathobiology. 3rd edn. New York: Raven Press, 1994: pp. 45–52.

74. McNiven MA, Marlowe KJ. Contributions of molecular motor enzymes to vesicle-based protein transport in gastrointestinal epithelial cells. Gastroenterology. 1999;116: 438–51.
75. Tsukada N, Ackerley CA, Phillips MJ. The structure and organization of the bile canalicular cytoskeleton with special reference to actin and actin-binding proteins. Hepatology. 1995;21:1106–13.
76. Watkins JB, Klaasen CD. Mechanisms of drug-induced cholestasis. In: Cameron RG, Feuer G, de la Iglesia FA, editors. Drug-Induced Hepatotoxicity. Berlin, Springer-Verlag, 1996: pp. 155–83.
77. Dranoff JA, McClure M, Burgstahler AD, Denson LA, Crawford AR, Crawford JM et al. Short-term regulation of bile acid uptake by microfilament-dependent translocation of rat ntcp to the plasma membrane. Hepatology. 1999;30:223–9.
78. Omary MB, Ku NO. Intermediate filament proteins of the liver: emerging disease associations and functions. Hepatology. 1997;25:1043–8.
79. Kawahara H, Cadrin M, Perry G, Autilio-Gambetti L, Swierenga SHH, Metuzals J et al. Role of cytokeratin intermediate filaments in transhepatic transport and bile secretion. Hepatology. 1990;11:435–48.
80. Anderson JM. Leaky junctions and cholestasis: a tight correlation. Gastroenterology. 1996;110:1662–74.
81. Mitic LL, Anderson JM. Molecular architecture of tight junctions. Annu Rev Physiol. 1998;60:121–4.
82. Nathanson MH, Schlosser SF. Calcium signaling mechanisms in liver in health and disease. In: Boyer JL, Ockner RK, ed. Progress in Liver Disease. Philadelphia: WB Saunders Company, 1996: pp. 1–27.
83. Bouscarel B, Kroll SD, Fromm H. Signal transduction and hepatocellular bile acid transport: cross talk between bile acids and second messengers. Gastroenterology. 1999;117:433–52.
84. Erlinger S. What is cholestasis in 1985? J Hepatol. 1985;1:687–93.
85. Reichen J, Simon FR. Cholestasis. In: Arias IM, Boyer JL, Fausto N, Jakoby WB, Schachter DA, Shafritz DA, eds. The Liver: Biology and Pathobiology, 3rd edn. New York: Raven Press, 1994: pp. 1105–24.
86. Landmann L. Cholestasis-induced alterations of the trans- and paracellular pathways in rat hepatocytes. Histochemistry. 1995;103:3–9.
87. Popper H. Cholestasis: the future of a past and present riddle. Hepatology. 1981;1:187–91.
88. Trauner M, Fickert P, Stauber RE. Inflammation-induced cholestasis. J Gastroenterol Hepatol. 1999;14:946–59.
89. Gartung C, Ananthanarayanan M, Rahman MA, Schuele S, Nundy S, Soroka CS et al. Down-regulation of expression and function of the rat liver Na^+/bile acid cotransporter in extrahepatic cholestasis. Gastroenterology. 1996;110:199–209.
90. Green RM, Beier D, Gollan JL. Regulation of hepatocyte bile salt transporters by endotoxin and inflammatory cytokines in rodents. Gastroenterology. 1996;111:193–8.
91. Moseley RH, Wang W, Takeda H, Lown K, Shick L, Ananthanarayanan M, Suchy FJ. Effect of endotoxin on bile acid transport in rat liver: a potential model for sepsis-associated cholestasis. Am J Physiol. 1996;271:G137–46.
92. Simon FR, Fortune J, Iwahashi M, Gartung C, Wolkoff A, Sutherland E. Ethinyl estradiol cholestasis involves alterations in expression of liver sinusoidal transporters. Am J Physiol. 1997;271:G1043–52.
93. Trauner M, Gartung C, Schlosser SF, Boyer JL. Role of nitric oxide in the transcriptional regulation of bile acid transporters in endotoxin-induced cholestasis (Abstract). Gastroenterology. 1996;110:A1349.
94. Trauner M, Arrese M, Lee H, Boyer JL, Karpen SJ. Endotoxin downregulates rat hepatic *ntcp* gene expression via decreased activity of critical transcription factors. J Clin Invest. 1998;101:2092–100.
95. Dumont M, Jacquemin E, D'Hont C, Descout C, Cresteil D, Haouzi D et al. Expression of the liver Na^+-independent organic anion transporting polypeptide (oatp-1) in rats with bile duct ligation. J Hepatol. 1997;27:1051–6.
96. Vos TA, Hooiveld GJEJ, Koning H, Childs S, Meijer DKF, Moshage H et al. Up-regulation of the multidrug resistance genes, mrp1 and mdr1b, and down-regulation of the organic anion transporter, mrp2, and the bile salt transporter, spgp, in endotoxemic rat liver. Hepatology. 1998;28:1637–44.

97. Trauner M, Arrese M, Soroka CJ, Ananthanarayanan M, Koeppel TA, Schlosser SF et al. The rat canalicular conjugate export pump (Mrp2) is down-regulated in intrahepatic and obstructive cholestasis. Gastroenterology. 1997;113:255–64.
98. Lee JM, Trauner M, Soroka CJ, Stieger B, Meier PJ, Boyer JL. The molecular expression of the bile salt export pump, sister of P-glycoprotein, is selectively preserved in cholestatic liver injury. Gastroentrology. 1999, in press.
99. Buscher HP, Miltenberger C, MacNelly S, Gerok W. The histoautoradiographic localization of taurocholate in rat liver after bile duct ligation. Evidence for ongoing secretion and reabsorption processes. J Hepatol. 1989;8:181–91.
100. Bolder U, Ton-Nu HT, Schteingart CD, Frick E, Hofmann AF. Hepatocyte transport of bile acids and organic anions in endotoxemic rats: impaired uptake and secretion. Gastroenterology. 1997;112:214–25.
101. Simon FR. The role of sex hormones and hepatic plasma membranes in the pathogenesis of cholestasis. In: Reyes HB, Leuschner U, Arias IM, eds. Pregnancy, Sex Hormones and the Liver. Dordrecht: Kluwer Academic Publishers, 1996: pp. 51–9.
102. Koopen NR, Wolters H, Voshol P, Stieger B, Vonk RJ, Meier PJ et al. Decreased Na^+-dependent taurocholate uptake and low expression of the sinusoidal Na^+-taurocholate cotransporting protein (Ntcp) in livers of mdr2 P-glycoprotein-deficient mice. J Hepatol. 1999;30:14–21.
103. Meerman L, Koopen NR, Bloks V, van Goor H, Havinga R, Wolthers BG et al. Biliary fibrosis associated with altered bile composition in a mouse model of erythropoietic protoporphyria. Gastroenterology. 1999;117:696–705.
104. Schrenk D, Gant TW, Preisegger KH, Silverman JA, Marino PA, Thorgeirsson SS. Induction of multidrug resistance gene expression during cholestasis in rats and nonhuman primates. Hepatology. 1993;17:854–60.
105. Denson LA, Auld KL, Schiek DS, McClure MH, Mangelsdorf DJ, Karpen SJ. The gene promoters for two critical hepatobiliary transporters, *Ntcp* and *Mrp2*, are coordinately induced by retinoids and suppressed by IL-1b and bile acids via RXR:RAR response elements (Abstract). Hepatology. 1999;30:305A.
106. Denson LA, McClure MH, Karpen SJ. Identification of a novel negative-acting cytokine response element in the rat liver sodium-dependent bile acid cotransporter gene promoter (Abstract). Gastroenterology. 1998;114:A1232.
107. Gartung C, Schuele S, Schlosser SF, Boyer JL. Expression of the rat liver Na^+/taurocholate cotransporter is regulated in vivo by retention of biliary constituents but not their depletion. Hepatology. 1997;25:284–90.
108. Shneider BL, Fox VL, Schwarz KB, Watson CL, Ananthanarayanan M, Thevananther S et al. Hepatic basolateral sodium-dependent-bile acid transporter expression in two unusual cases of hypercholanemia and in extrahepatic biliary atresia. Hepatology. 1997;25:1176–83.
109. Karpen SJ, Ananthanarayanan M, Potselueva T, Suchy FJ. Bile acids suppress the rat liver Na^+-dependent bile acid cotransporter promoter (Abstract). Hepatology. 1995;22:318A.
110. Chiang JYL, Stroup D. Identification and characterization of a putative bile acid-responsive element in cholesterol 7α-hydrohylase gene promoter. J Biol Chem. 1994;269:17502–7.
111. Karpen SJ, Sun AQ, Kudish B, Hagenbuch B, Meier PJ, Ananthanarayanan M, Suchy FJ. Multiple factors regulate the rat liver basolateral sodium-dependent bile acid cotransporter promoter. J Biol Chem. 1996;271:15211–21.
112. Mangelsdorf DJ, Evans RM. The RXR heterodimers and orphan receptors. Cell. 1995;83:841–50.
113. Mangelsdorf DJ, Thumel C, Beato M, Herrlich P, Schuetz G, Umesono K et al. The nuclear receptor superfamily: the second decade. Cell. 1995;83:835–9.
114. Blumberg B, Evans RM. Orphan nuclear receptors – new ligands and new possibilities. Genes Dev. 1998;12:3149–55.
115. Kliewer SA, Lehmann JM, Willson TM. Orphan nuclear receptors: shifting endocrinology into reverse. Science. 1999;284:757–60.
116. Carlberg C, Polly P. The nuclear receptor superfamily. Retinoids. 1999;15:71–4.
117. Russell DW. Nuclear orphan receptors control cholesterol catabolism. Cell. 1999;97:539–42.
118. Makishima M, Okamoto AY, Repa JJ, Tu H, Learned RM, Luk A et al. Identification of a nuclear receptor for bile acids. Science. 1999;284:1362–5.

119. Parks DJ, Blanchard SG, Bledsoe RK, Chandra G, Consler TG, Kliewer SA et al. Bile acids: natural ligands for an orphan nuclear receptor. Science. 1999;284:1365–8.
120. Karpen SJ. Bile acids go nuclear. Hepatology. 1999;30:1107–9.
121. Ganguly TC, O'Brien ML, Karpen SJ, Hyde JF, Suchy FJ, Vore M. Regulation of the rat liver sodium-dependent bile acid cotransporter gene by prolactin. Mediation of transcriptional activation by Stat5. J Clin Invest. 1997;15:2906–14.
122. Kauffmann HM, Schrenk D. Sequence analysis and functional characterization of the 5′-flanking region of the rat multidrug resistance protein 2 (mrp2) gene. Biochem Biophys Res Commun. 1998;245:325–31.
123. Demeule M, Jodoin J, Neaulieu E, Brossard M, Beliveau R. Dexamethasone modulation of multidrug transporters in normal tissues. FEBS Lett. 1999;442:208–14.
124. Zhou G, Kuo MT. NF-kappaB-mediated induction of mdr1b expression by insulin in rat hepatoma cells. J Biol Chem. 1997;272:15174–83.
125. Ros JE, Geuken M, Schuetz J, Koning H, Kuipers F, Manns MP et al. TNF-α mediated upregulation of the multidrug resistance gene mdr1b but not of mrp1 in rat hepatocytes is dependent on NF-κB activation (Abstract). Hepatology. 1999;30:462A.
126. Kubitz R, Wettstein M, Warskulat U, Haeussinger D. Regulation of the multidrug resistance protein 2 in the rat liver by lipopolysaccharide and dexamethasone. Gastroenterology. 1999;116:401–10.
127. Rost D, Kartenbeck J, Keppler D. Changes in the localization of the rat canalicular conjugate export pump mrp2 in phalloidin-induced cholestasis. Hepatology. 1999;29:814–21.
128. Reyes H, Simon F. Intrahepatic cholestasis of pregnancy: an estrogen-related disease. Semin Liver Dis. 1993;13:289–301.
129. Dubin M, Maruice M, Feldman G, Erlinger S. Influence of colchicine and phaloidin on bile secretion and hepatic ultrastructure in the rat: possible interaction between microtubules and microfilaments. Gastroenterology. 1980;79:646–54.
130. Marks DL, La Russo NF, McNiven MA. Isolation of the microtubule-vesicle motor kinesin from rat liver: selective inhibition by cholestatic bile acids. Gastroenterology. 1995;108:824–33.
131. Boyer JL, Soroka CJ. Vesicle targeting to the apicaldomain regulates bile excretory function in isolated rat hepatocyte couplets. Gastroenterology. 1996;109:1600–11.
132. Beuers U, Nathanson MH, Isales CM, Boyer JL. Tauroursodeoxycholic acid stimulates hepatocellular exocytosis and mobilizes extracellular Ca^{++} mechanisms defective in cholestasis. J Clin Invest. 1993;92:2984–93.
133. Weber AM, Tuchweber B, Yousef I, Brochu P, Turgeon C, Gabbiani G et al. Severe familial cholestasis in North American Indian children: a clinical model of microfilament dysfunction. Gastroenterology. 1981;81:653–62.
134. St-Pierre MV, Dufour JF, Arias IM. Disruption of actin organization by cytochalasin D does not impair biliary secretion of organic anions in the rat. Hepatology. 1997;25:970–5.
135. Van Eyken P, Desmet VJ. Cytokeratins and the liver. Liver. 1993;13:113–22.
136. Fickert P, Trauner M, Fuchsbichler A, Zatloukal K, Denk H. Cholestasis and bile acid feeding induce cytoheratin 8/18 expression and Mallory body formation in mice (Abstract). Hepatology. 1999;30:464A.
137. Ohta M, Marceau N, French SW. Pathologic changes in the cytokeratin pericanalicular sheath in experimental cholestasis and alcoholic fatty liver. Lab Invest. 1988;59:60–74.
138. Song JY, Van Noorden CJF, Frederiks WM. Alterations of hepatocellular intermediate filaments during extrahepatic cholestasis in rat liver. Virchows Arch. 1997;430:253–60.
139. Albers KM, Davis FE, Perrone TN, Lee EY, Liu Y, Vore M. Expression of an epidermal keratin protein in liver of transgenic mice causes structural and functional abnormalities. J Cell Biol. 1995;128:157–69.
140. Loranger A, Duclos S, Grenler A, Price J, Wilson-Heiner M, Baribault H, Marceau N. Simple epithelium keratins are required for maintenance of hepatocyte integrity. Am J Pathol. 197;151:1673–83.
141. Anderson JM, Glade JL, Stevenson BR, Boyer JL, Mooseker MS. Hepatic immunohistochemical localization of the tight junction protein ZO-1 in rat models of cholestasis. Am J Pathol. 1989;134:1055–62.
142. Fallon MB, Mennone A, Anderson JM. Altered expression and localization of the tight junction protein ZO-1 after common bile duct ligation. Am J Physiol. 1993;264:C1439–447.

143. Fallon MB, Brecher AR, Balda MS, Matter K, Anderson JM. Altered hepatic localization and expression of occludin after common bile duct ligation. Am J Physiol. 1995;269:C1057–62.
144. Rahner C, Stieger B, Landmann L. Structure-function correlation of tight junctional impairment following intrahepatic and extrahepatic cholestasis in rat liver. Gastroenterology. 1996;110:1564–78.
145. Kawaguchi T, Sakisaka S, Sata M, Mori M, Tanikawa K. Different lobular distributions of altered hepatocyte tight junctions in rat models of intrahepatic and extrahepatic cholestasis. Hepatology. 1999;29:205–16.
146. Lora L, Mazzon E, Martines D, Fries W, Muraca M, Martin A et al. Hepatocyte tight-junctional permeability is increased in rat experimental colitis. Gastroenterology. 1997;113:1347–54.
147. Fallon MB, Nathanson MH, Mennone A, Saez JC, Burgstahler AD, Anderson JM. Altered expression and function of hepatocyte gap junctions after common bile duct ligation in the rat. Am J Physiol. 1995;268:C1186–94.
148. Müller M, Jansen PLM. The cholestasis page. http://www.med.rug.nl/mdl/table1.htm
149. Welsh MI. The path of discovery in understanding the biology of cystic fibrosis and approaches to therapy. Am J Gastroenterol. 1994;89(Suppl):S97–105.
150. Sela-Herman S, Bull L, Lomri N, Rahmaoui C, Luther TT, Hammermann P et al. In search of a gene for hereditary cholestasis. Biochem Mol Med. 1996;59:98–103.
151. Bull LN, Carlton VEH, Stricker NL, Baharloo S, DeYoung JA, Freimer NB et al. Genetic and morphological findings in progressive familial intrahepatic cholestasis (Byler disease [PFIC-1] and Byler syndrome): evidence for heterogeneity. Hepatology. 1997;26:155–64.
152. Carlton VEH, Knisely AS, Freimer AB. Mapping a locus for progressive familial intrahepatic cholstasis (Byler disease) to 18q21-q22, intrahepatic cholestasis region. Hum Mol Genet. 1995;4:1049–53.
153. Houwen RHJ, Baharloo S, Blankenship K, Raeymaekers P, Juyn J, Sandkuijl LA, Freimer NB. Genome screening by searching for shared segments: mapping a gene for benign recurrent intrahepatic cholestasis. Nature Genet. 1994;8:380–6.
154. Strautnieks SS, Kagalwalla AF, Tanner MS, Knisely AS, Ball L, Freimer N et al. Identification of a locus for progressive familial intrahepatic cholestasis PFIC2 on chromosome 2q24. Am J Hum Genet. 1997;61:630–3.
155. Jansen PLM, Strautnieks SS, Jacquemin E, Hadchouel M, Sokal EM, Hooivield GJEJ et al. Hepatocanalicular bile salt export pump deficiency in patients with progressive familial intrahepatic cholestasis. Gastroenterology. 1999;117:1370–9.
156. Deleuze JF, Jacquemin E, Dubuisson C, Cresteil D, Dumont M, Erlinger S et al. Defect of multidrug resistance 3 gene expression in a subtype of progressive familial intrahepatic cholestasis. Hepatology. 1996;23:904–8.
157. de Vree JML, Jacquemin E, Sturm E, Cresteil D, Bosma PJ, Aten J et al. Mutations in the MDR3 gene cause progressive familial intrahepatic cholestasis. Proc Natl Acad Sci USA. 1998;95:282–7.
158. Jacquemin E, Hermans D, Myara A, Habes D, Debray D, Hadchouel M et al. Ursodeoxycholic acid therapy in pediatric patients with progressive familial intrahepatic cholestasis. Hepatology. 1997;25:519–23.
159. Borst P, Schinkel AH. What have we learnt thus far from mice with disrupted P-glycoprotein genes? Eur J Cancer. 1996;32A:985–90.
160. Mauad TH, van Nieuwkerk CMJ, Dingemans KP, Smit JJM, Schinkel AH, Notenboom RGE et al. Mice with homozygous disruption of the mdr2 P-glycoprotein gene. A novel animal model for studies of nonsuppurative inflammatory cholangitis and hepatocancerogenesis. Am J Pathol. 1994;145:1237–45.
161. Oude Elferink RPJ, Ottenhoff R, van Wijland M, Smit JJM, Schinkel AH. Regulation of biliary lipid secretion by mdr2 P-glycoprotein in the mouse. J Clin Invest. 1995;95:31–8.
162. Van Nieuwkerk CMJ, Oude Elferink RPJ, Groen AK, Ottenhoff R, Tytgat GNJ, Dingemans KP et al. Efects of urodeoxycholate and cholate feeding on liver disease in FVB mice with a disrupted *mdr2* P-glycoprotein gene. Gastroenterology. 1996;111:165–71.
163. Smith AJ, de Vree JML, Ottenhoff R, Oude Elferink RPJ, Schinkel AH, Borst P. Hepatocyte-specific expression of the human MDR3 P-glycoprotein restores the biliary phosphatidylcholine excretion absent in mdr2 (–/–) mice. Hepatology. 1998;28:530–6.
164. De Vree JML. Defects in hepatobiliary lipid transport. Genetics and therapy of progressive familial intrahepatic cholestasis (Dissertation). Amsterdam: University of Amsterdam, 1999.

165. De Vree JML, Romijn JA, Mok KS, Mathus-Vliegen LMH, Stoutenbeek CP, Ostrow JD et al. Lack of enteral nutrition during critical illness is associated with profound decrements in biliary lipid concentrations. Am J Clin Nutr. 1999;70:70–7.
166. Oude Elferink RPJ, Groen AK. The mechanism of biliary lipid secretion and its defects. Gastroenterology Clin N Am. 1999;28:59–74.
167. Dumoulin FL, Reichel C, Sauerbruch T, Spengler U. Semiquantitation of intrahepatic MDR3 mRNA levels by reverse transcription/competitive polymerase chain reaction. J Hepatol. 1997;26:852–6.
168. Kartenbeck J, Leuschner U, Mayer R, Keppler D. Absence of the canalicular isoform of the MRP gene encoded conjugate export pump from the hepatocytes in Dubin–Johnson syndrome. Hepatology. 1996;23:1061–6.
169. Paulusma CC, Kool M, Bosma PJ, Scheffer GL, terBorg F, Scheper RJ et al. A mutation in the human canalicular multispecific organic anion transporter gene causes the Dubin–Johnson syndrome. Hepatology. 1997;25:1539–42.
170. Wada M, Toh S, Taniguchi K, Nakamura T, Uchiumi T, Kohno K et al. Mutations in the canalicular multispecific organic anion transporter (*cMOAT*) gene, a novel ABC transporter, in patients with hyperbilirubinemia II/Dubin Johnson syndrome. Hum Mol Genet. 1998;7:203–7.
171. Kagawa T, Sato M, Hosoi K, Uchiyama J, Nishizaki Y, Watanabe N et al. Absence of R1066X mutation in six Japanese patients with Dubin–Johnson syndrome. Biochem Mol Biol Int. 1999;47:639–44.
172. Kajihara S, Hisatomi A, Mizuta T, Hara T, Ozaki I, Wada I, Yamamoto K. A splice mutation in the human canalicular multispecific organic anion transporter gene causes Dubin–Johnson syndrome. Biochem Biophys Res Commun. 1998;18:454–7.
173. Toh S, Wada M, Uchiumi T, Inokuchi A, Makino Y, Horie Y et al. Genomic structure of the canalicular multispecific organic anion-transporter gene (*MRP2/cMOAT*) and mutations in the ATP-binding-cassette region in Dubin–Johnson syndrome. Am J Hum Genet. 1999;64:739–46.
174. Tsujii H, Koenig J, Rost D, Stoeckel B, Leuschner U, Keppler D. Exon-intron organization of the human multidrug-resistance protein 2 (*MRP2*) gene mutated in Dubin–Johnson syndrome. Gastroenterology. 1999;117:653–60.
175. Paulusma CC, Oude Elferink RP. The canalicular multispecific organic anion transporter and conjugated hyperbilirubinemia in rat and man. J Mol Med. 1997;75:420–8.
176. Keppler D, Koenig J. Hepatic canalicular membrane 5: expression and localization of the conjugate export pump encoded by the *MRP2* (*cMRP/cMOAT*) gene in liver. FASEB J. 1997;11:509–16.
177. Keppler D, Kartenbeck J. The canalicular conjugate export pump encoded by the cmrp/cmoat gene. In: Boyer JL, Ockner RK, eds. Progress in Liver Disease. Vol. 14. Philadelphia: WB Saunders, 1996: pp. 55–67.
178. Iyanagi T, Emi Y, Ikushiro S. Biochemical and molecular aspects of genetic disorders of bilirubin metabolism. Biochim Biophys Acta. 1998;1407:173–84.
179. Konig J, Nies AT, Cui Y, Leier I, Keppler D. Conjugate export pumps of the multidrug resistance protein (MRP) family: localization, substrate specificity, and MRP2-mediated drug resistance. Biochim Biophys Acta. 1999;1461:377–94.
180. Roy Chowdhury J, Roy Chowdhury N, Wolkoff AW, Arias IM. Heme and bile pigment metabolism. In Arias IM, Boyer JL, Fausto N, Lakoby WB, Schachter DA, Shafritz DA, eds. The Liver: Biology and Pathobiology, 3rd edn. New York: Raven Press, 1994: pp. 471–504.
181. Nowicki MJ, Poley JR. The hereditary hyperbilirubinemias. Baillières Clin Gastroenterol. 1998;12:355–57.
182. Douglas JG, Beckett GJ, Percy-Roob IW, Finlayson ND. Bile salt transport in the Dubin–Johnson syndrome. Gut. 1980;21:890–3.
183. Jacquemin E, Cresteil D, Manouvrier S, Boute O. Hadchouel M. Heterozygous non-sense mutation of the *MDR3*-gene in familial intrahepatic cholestasis of pregnancy. Lancet. 1999;353:210–11.
184. Kogan D, Ananthanarayanan M, Emre S, Suchy FJ, Shneider BL. The bile salt export pump (BSEP/SPGP) is not down-regulated in human cholestasis associated with extrahepatic biliary atresia (EHBA). Hepatology. 1999;30:468A.
185. Nozawa S, Miyazaki M, Tou HI, Nakagawa KN, Ambiru S, Shimizu H. Human MDR1 and MDR3 gene expression in the liver with obstructive jaundice (Abstract). Gastroenterology. 1997;112:A1349.

186. Prieto J, Qian C, Garcia N, Diez J, Medina JF. Abnormal expression of anion exchanger genes in primary biliary cirrhosis. Gastroenterology. 1993;105:572–8.
187. Medina JF, Martinez-Anso E, Vazquez JJ, Prieto J. Decreased anion exchanger 2 immunoreactivity in the liver of patients with primary biliary cirrhosis. Hepatology. 1997;25:12–17.
188. Prieto J, Garcia N, Marti-Climent JM, Penuelas I, Richter JA, Medina JF. Assessment of biliary bicarbonate secretion in humans by positron emission tomography. Gastroenterology. 1999;117:167–72.
189. Beuers U, Throckmorton DC, Anderson MS, Isales CM, Thasler W, Kullack-Ublick GA et al. Tauroursodeoxycholic acid activates protein kinase C in isolated rat hepatocytes. Gastroenterology. 1996;110:1553–63.
190. Oswald M, Kullak-Ublick GA, Beuers U, Paumgartner G. Expression of the hepatocyte canalicular multidrug rsistance associated protein 2 (MRP2) in primary biliary cirrhosis (Abstract). Hepatology. 1998;28:544A.
191. Zollner G, Zenz R, Fickert P, Kenner L, Stauber RE, Denk H et al. Quantification of hepatobiliary transporter expression in liver biopsies from patients with cholestasis (Abstract). Hepatology. 1999;30:467A.
192. Welsh MJ, Smith AE. Molecular mechanisms of CFTR chloride channel dysfunction in cystic fibrosis. Cell. 1993;73:1251–4.
193. Roberts SK, Ludwig J, LaRusso NF. The pathobiology of biliary epithelia. Gastroenterology. 1997;112:269–79.
194. Oelkers P, Kirby LC, Heubi JE, Dawson PA. Primary bile acid malabsorption caused by mutations in the ileal sodium-dependent bile acid transporter gene (SLC10A2). J Clin Invest. 1997;15:1880–7.
195. Alpini G, Glaser S, Ueno Y, Rodgers R, Phinizy JL, Francis H et al. Bile acid feeding induces cholangiocyte proliferation and secretion; evidence for bile acid-regulated ductal secretion. Gastroenterology. 1999;116:179–86.
196. Elsing C, Fitscher BA, Boker C, Kramer W, Stengelin S, Stremmerl W. Expression of a bile acid transporter in biliary epithelial cells from normal and cholestatic rat livers. Eur J Med Res. 1999;27:165–8.
197. Lee JM, Azzaroli F, Gigliozzi A, Mennone A, Boyer JL. Adaptive regulation of the ileal sodium-dependent bile salt transporter (Isbt) and the multispecific organic anion transporter (Mrp2) in kidney and cholangiocytes in chronic cholestasis – alternative pathways for bile salt excretion (Abstract). Hepatology. 1999;30:417A.
198. Christie DM, Dawson PA, Thevananther S, Shneider BL. Comparative analysis of the ontogeny of a sodium-dependent bile acid transporter in rat kidney and ileum. Am J Physiol. 1996;271:G377–85.
199. Schaub TP, Kartenbeck J, Koenig J, Vogel O, Witzgall R, Kriz W, Keppler D. Expression of the conjugate export pump encoded by the mrp2 gene in the apical membrane of kidney proximal tubules. J Am Soc Nephrol. 1997;8:1213–21
200. Schaub TP, Kartenbeck J, Koenig J, Spring H, Dorsam J, Staehler G et al. Expression of the MRP2 gene-encoded conjugate export pump in human kidney proximal tubules and renal cell carcinoma. J Am Soc Nephrol. 1999;10:1159–69.
201. Belinsky MG, Kruh GD. MOAT-E (ARA) is a full length MRP/cMOAT subfamily transporter expressed in kidney and liver. Br J Cancer. 1999;80:1342–9.
202. Craddock AL, Love MW, Daniel RW, Kirby LC, Walters HC, Wong MH, Dawson PA. Expression and transport properties of the human ileal and renal sodium-dependent bile acid transporter. Am J Physiol. 1998;274:G157–69.
203. Li L, Krantz ID, Deng Y, Genin A, Banta AB, Collins CC et al. Alagille syndrome is caused by mutations in human Jaggedl, which encodes a ligand for Notch l. Nature Genet. 1997;16:243–51.
204. Oda T, Elkahloun AG, Pike BL, Okajima K, Krantz ID, Genin A et al. Mutations in the human *Jagged1* gene are responsible for Alagille syndrome. Nature Genet. 1997;16:235–42.
205. Crosnier C, Driancourt C, Raynaud N, Shorne-Pollet S, Pollet N, Bernard O et al. Mutations in *JAGGED1* gene are predominantly sporadic in Alagille syndrome. Gastroenterology. 1999;116:1141–8.
206. Spinner NA. Alagille syndrome and the notch signaling pathway: new insights into human development. Gastroenterology. 1999;116:1257–60.
207. Reynoso-Paz S, Coppel RL, Mackay IR, Bass NM, Ansari AA, Gershwin ME. The immunobiology of bile and biliary epithelium. Hepatology. 1999;30:351–7.

208. Trauner M, Graziadei IW. Mechanisms of action and therapeutic applications of ursodeoxycholic acid in chronic liver diseases. Aliment Pharmacol Ther. 1999;13:979–95.
209. Kauffmann HM, Keppler D, Gant TW, Schrenk D. Induction of hepatic *mrp2 (cmrp/cmoat)* gene expression in nonhuman primates treated with rifampicin and tamoxifen. Arch Toxicol. 1998;72:763–8.
210. Kim RB, Leake B, Cvetkovic M, Roden MM, Nadeau J, Walubo A, Wilkinson GR. Modulation by drugs of human hepatic sodium-dependent bile acid transporter (sodium taurocholate cotransporting polypeptide) activity. J Pharmacol Exp Ther. 1999;291:1204–9.
211. Green RM, Hoda F, Ward K. Effect of dexamethasone and rifampin on the gene expression of hepatic bile salt transporters (Abstract). Hepatology. 1999;30:468A.
212. Gupta S, Gorla GR, Irani AN. Hepatocyte transplantation: emerging insights into mechanisms of liver repopulation and their relevance to potential therapies. J Hepatol. 1999;30:162–70.

Section II
Chronic viral hepatitis

5
Hepatitis B and D: virology and diagnosis

F. von WEIZSÄCKER and H. E. BLUM

With an estimated 350 million chronic carriers worldwide, hepatitis B virus (HBV) infection still represents a major health care problem. The spectrum of disease includes the asymptomatic carrier status, acute and fulminant hepatitis as well as chronic hepatitis which may eventually progress to liver cirrhosis and hepatocellular carcinoma[1]. Superinfection or co-infection with the hepatitis delta virus (HDV) may result in a more severe clinical course[2]. Treatment of chronic HBV infection is still unsatisfactory. At present, interferon alpha and lamivudine are the only therapeutic options[3]. A better understanding of basic virological aspects as well as virus–host interactions are a prerequisite for the development of urgently needed new therapeutic strategies. In the following, new aspects in virology as well as diagnosis of hepatitis B and D will be discussed.

STRUCTURE AND REPLICATION STRATEGY

HBV[4] is a small DNA virus that belongs to the family of hepadnaviruses which includes the woodchuck hepatitis virus (WHV), ground squirrel hepatitis virus (GSHV), Peking duck hepatitis B virus (DHBV) and heron hepatitis B virus (HHBV). More recently, endogenous hepadnaviruses were also identified in woolly monkeys[5] and orang utans[6]. The HBV genome consists of a partially double-stranded DNA molecule of about 3200 nucleotides. The genetic organization of the viral genome and the viral proteins are known in great detail. The viral envelope ist made up of hepatitis B virus surface antigen (HBsAg) which exists in three different forms (small, middle and large HBsAg). The nucleocapsid is made up of the hepatitis B core antigen (HBcAg) that is encoded by the core gene. The structure of the HBV nucleocapsids has been elucidated by electron cryomicroscopy[7] as well as crystallography[8]. It is a highly symmetric icosahedral shell formed by core protein dimers. The pre-core/core gene codes for a protein that is processed by amino- and carboxyterminal truncation yielding hepatitis B e antigen (HBeAg) that indicates high level viral replication. The viral genome further encodes for a polymerase/ reverse transcriptase and a small protein with transactivating properties[9], termed X-antigen (HBxAg). Studies in the woodchuck model revealed that the X protein is essential for establishing persistent viral infection[10,11]. Upon entry into the target cell the partially double-stranded HBV genome is converted into covalently closed circular (ccc) DNA, which resides in the nucleus and serves as template for RNA synthesis. This DNA species has a long half-life (presumably several months or more) and plays an important role in viral persistence. Different from all other animal DNA viruses hepadnaviral replication is not semi-conservative but is asymmetrical, with the reverse transcription of a RNA intermediate into minus strand DNA and subsequent plus strand synthesis within viral nucleocapsids. HBV replication, therefore, has molecular characteristics of retroviruses rendering them sensitive to strategies aimed at blocking reverse transcription.

HDV[12] is a defective RNA virus which is only capable of synthesizing infectious particles in the presence of HBV. It has a diameter of 36 nm and, similar to HBV, consists of an outer envelope composed of HBsAg. The nucleocapsid contains the hepatitis delta antigen (HDAg) and the single-stranded viral RNA genome. At 1679 nucleotides, the HDV genome is by far the smallest of all known animal viruses. Through extensive base pairing it is predicted to form a rodlike structure involving about 70% of the genome. HDV replicates via a 'rolling circle' mechanism. This process involves RNA-directed RNA synthesis using a host polymerase as well as HDV-ribozyme-mediated RNA processing. The viral genome codes for one 195 amino acid protein, the 'small' HDAg. As a RNA chaperone which stabilizes HDV RNA and facilitates ribozyme action, the small HDAg plays an important role in HDV replication. Some HDV RNAs undergo RNA editing and thus allow for the synthesis of a carboxy-terminally extended HDAg, the 215 amino acid 'large' HDAg. This protein acts as a dominant repressor of viral replication and is required for particle assembly.

VIRUS–HOST INTERACTIONS

The first important virus–host interaction in the viral life cycle is the specific attachment to the target cell and virus internalization. Due to the lack of readily available infection models, the search for the HBV receptor(s) has long been unsuccessful. Studies in the DHBV system have now established that carboxypeptidase D (CPD) mediates binding and internalization of DHBV[13,14]. However, in non-permissive cells that have been reconstituted with duck CPD the viral life cycle is not complete, i.e., the virus is taken up but replication is not initiated. Thus, is appears likely that co-receptors are required to complete the import of the viral genome into the nucleus. Glycine decarboxylase has recently been identified as one such co-receptor candidate[15]. Since human CPD has been cloned, similar reconstitution experiments can be expected for HBV in the near future. Cellular proteins also play an important role in virus replication and assembly. Thus, activation of in vitro translated DHBV polymerase requires the presence of cellular chaperones including Hsp 90, p23 and probably other cellular proteins as well[4]. This process resembles the chaperone-mediated activation of steroid receptors. Hsp 70, which co-purifies with virions, and calnexin seem to play an essential role in chaperoning viral enveloping and export[4,16].

Finally, the HBxAg was shown to transactivate a large number of cellular genes and has been incriminated in hepatocarcinogenesis. Its precise molecular function, however, has still not been fully clarified[9].

VIRAL QUASISPECIES, VIRAL MUTANTS

Due to the lack of proofreading ability of the HBV reverse transcriptase/polymerase mutations can occur during viral replication. The mutation rate of HBV is estimated as 1 nucleotide per 10 000 bases and year of infection. This mutation rate is 10–1000 times lower than that of RNA viruses but about 100 times higher than that of other DNA viruses due to the asymmetrical replication strategy of HBV. Over time a mixed population of genetically similar, but not identical viral genomes, termed viral quasispecies, evolves in the infected individual. HBV mutants can accumulate and become clinically significant. Prominent examples include escape mutants occurring during antiviral therapy with lamivudine or escape mutants within the a-determinant of the surface protein which have been associated with diagnostic and vaccine escape[17,18]. Diagnostic escape is defined as active HBV replication in the presence of anti-HBs antibodies with HBsAg not being detectable by commonly used commercial assays. A vaccine escape is referred to as productive HBV infection despite successful active or passive immunization. A recent study in chimpanzees, however, challenged the current view that mutants in the a-determinant result from antibody-mediated immune pressure, since commercially available standard vaccines elicited protective immunity against a prototype HBsAg variant[19]. Further experiments in animal models of HBV infection are clearly needed to resolve this issue.

HDV displays a marked sequence heterogeneity with up to 28% diverging nucleotides among different genotypes[20]. Also viral quasispecies are found in infected individuals. A precise correlation between HDV, genotypes and molecular or clinical consequences has not yet been established. Analogous to HBV and the hepatitis C virus (HCV), it seems very likely, however, that genetic factors play an important role in the biology, clinical course and efficacy of treatment of HDV infection.

NEW ANIMAL MODELS

Animal models of HBV/HDV infection are of paramount importance to analyse the viral life cycle and evaluate new antiviral strategies. HBV transgenic mice[21–23] have yielded important insights into the virology and immune-pathogenesis of HBV infection. Mice cannot be naturally infected with HBV, however, and transgenic mice fail to produce sizable amounts of ccc DNA, a hallmark of HBV replication and persistence. Surrogate models of HBV infection, such as woodchucks and ducks have contributed substantially to our understanding of the virology of HBV but the immunological characterization of these animals has only recently begun. Tree shrews can be infected with HBV[24,25] and HCV[26], but reproducible long-term studies in these animals are still lacking. In the search for new animal models, transplantation of infectible hepatocytes to immunocompromised mice has recently been evaluated. Thus, human HBV-infected liver tissue was transplanted into lethally irradiated mice, radioprotected with SCID mouse bone marrow cells[27]. In this model a peak of viraemia was observed between days 18 and 25 thus leaving ample room for the evaluation of antiviral drugs. In another approach, woodchuck hepatocytes were transplanted into the regenerating liver of uPA/RAG-2 mice. In these mice the transgene (urokinase-type plasminogen activator, UPA) is toxic to hepatocytes and individual cells that have deleted the transgene can repopulate the whole liver[28]. An elegant study by Petersen et al. showed that transplanted normal adult woodchuck hepatocytes proliferated and reconstituted up to 90% of the uPA/RAG-2 mouse liver[29]. In this model, persistent experimental WHV infection could be established. Efforts to adapt this system for human hepatocyte xenotransplantation are currently under way. Both systems would also allow to address specific immunological questions, for example via T-cell transfer.

DIAGNOSIS

The diagnosis of HBV infection includes past history, physical examination, clinical chemistry (ALT, AST, GGT, bilirubin), virological and imaging analyses (e.g. abdominal ultrasound, duplex sonography, computer tomography) and in some patients histopathology. Virological analyses should be performed in the context of the diagnostic hierarchy mentioned above. HBsAg positivity establishes the diagnosis of HBV infection and is the screening test of choice[2]. Other serological HBV markers (HBeAg, anti-HBe) are not useful as screening tests but are important for the indication to and follow-up of patients receiving antiviral therapy as well as for scientific studies. Apart from the serological detection of viral antigens and antibodies, molecular hybridization analyses, PCR amplification or branched DNA (bDNA) assays allow the direct demonstration of HBV DNA. It is important to note, however, that low levels of HBV DNA can persist for decades in patients who have clinically and serologically recovered from HBV infection[30]. In clinical practice, therefore, HBV DNA analysis should only be performed in special situations such as monitoring of therapy, scientific studies on viral mutants or screening for HBV infection in immunocompromized patients.

The specific diagnosis of HDV infection is based on the detection of antibodies against HDAg (anti-HDAg), either as anti-HDV IgM or anti-HDV IgG, in serum concomitantly with markers of HBV infection[2]. HDAg can be detected in infected liver cells by immunohistochemistry. HDV RNA can be detected by PCR amplification or molecular hybridization analyses. Clinically, these analyses are not important, however, and should be restricted to special situations as outlined above.

SUMMARY AND PERSPECTIVES

HBV and HDV are structurally and genetically well defined. Serological and molecular analyses allow their specific and sensitive detection. Main topics of current research activities include the characterization of membrane proteins responsible for viral attachment and uptake, virus–host interactions during viral replication and morphogenesis and the search for new antiviral strategies. Novel small animal models for HBV/HDV infection that have recently been developed will provide important tools to address these issues.

REFERENCES

1. Wright TL, Lau JY. Clinical aspects of hepatitis B virus infection. Lancet. 1993;342:1340–4.
2. Blum HE, Wieland S, Walter E, von Weizsäcker F, Offensperger W-B, Moradpour D. Natural course of HBV infection. In: (Koshy R and Caselmann WH, eds.) Hepatitis B Virus. London: Imperial College Press, 1998: pp. 75–92.
3. Hoofnagle JH. Therapy of viral hepatitis. Digestion. 1998;59:563–78.
4. Nassal M. Hepatitis B virus replication: novel roles for virus host interactions. Intervirology. 1999;42:100–16.
5. Lanford RE, Chavez D, Brasky KM, Burns RBr, Rico-Hesse R. Isolation of a hepadnavirus from the woolly monkey, a New World primate. Proc Natl Acad Sci USA. 1998;95:5757–61.
6. Warren KS, Heeney JL, Swan RA, Heriyanto, Verschoor EJ. A new group of hepadnaviruses naturally infecting orangutans (Pongo pygmaeus). J Virol 1999;73:7860–65.
7. Crowther RA, Kiselev NA, Bottcher B, Berriman JA, Borisova GP, Ose V, Pumpens P. Three-dimensional structure of hepatitis B virus core particles determined by electron cryomicroscopy. Cell. 1994;77:943–50.
8. Wynne SA, Crowther RA, Leslie AG. The crystal structure of the human hepatitis B virus capsid. Mol Cell. 1999;3:771–80.
9. Andrisani OM, Barnabas S. The transcriptional function of the hepatitis B virus X protein and its role in hepatocarcinogenesis. Int J Oncol. 1999;15:373–9.
10. Chen HS, Kaneko S, Girones R, Anderson RW, Hornbuckle WE, Tennant BC et al. The woodchuck hepatitis virus X gene is important for establishment of virus infection in woodchucks. J Virol. 1993;67:1218–26.
11. Zoulim F, Saputelli J, Seeger C. Woodchuck hepatitis virus X protein is required for viral infection in vivo. J Virol. 1994;68:2026–30.
12. Taylor JM. Hepatitis delta virus. Intervirology. 1999;42:173–8.
13. Breiner KM, Urban S, Schaller H. Carboxypeptidase D (gp180), a Golgi resident protein, functions in the attachment and entry of avian hepatitis B viruses. J Virol. 1998;72:8098–104.
14. Tong S, Li J, Wands JR. Carboxypeptidase D is an avian hepatitis B virus receptor. J Virol. 1999;73:8696–702.
15. Li J, Tong S, Wands JR. Identification and expression of glycine decarboxylase (p120) as a duck hepatitis B virus pre S envelope binding protein. J Biol Chem. 1999;274:27658–65.
16. Prange R, Werr M, Loffler-Mary H. Chaperones involved in hepatitis B virus morphogenesis. Biol Chem. 1999;380:305–14.
17. Carman WF. The clinical significance of surface antigen variants of hepatitis B virus. J Viral Hepatol. 1997;1:11–20.
18. Chen WN, Oon CJ. Human hepatitis B virus mutants: significance of molecular changes. FEBS Lett. 1999;453:237–42.
19. Ogata N, Cote PJ, Zanetti AR, Miller RH, Shapiro M, Gerin J, Purcell RH. Licensed recombinant hepatitis B vaccines protect chimpanzees against infection with the prototype surface gene mutant of hepatitis B virus. Hepatology. 1999;30:779–86.
20. Wu JC, Huang IA, Huang YH, Chen JY, Sheen IJ. Mixed genotypes infection with hepatitis D virus. J Med Virol. 1999;57:64–7.
21. Chisari FV. Hepatitis B virus transgenic mice: models of viral immunobiology and pathogenesis. Curr Top Microbiol Immunol. 1996;206:149–73.
22. Chisari FV. Hepatitis B virus transgenic mice: insights into the virus and the disease. Hepatology. 1995;22:1316–25.
23. Larkin J, Clayton M, Sun B, Perchonock CE, Morgan JL, Siracusa LD et al. Hepatitis B virus transgenic mouse model of chronic liver disease. Nature Med. 1999;5:907–12.

24. Yan RQ, Su JJ, Huang DR, Gan YC, Yang C, Huang GH. Human hepatitis B virus and hepatocellular carcinoma I. Experimental infection of tree shrews with hepatitis B virus. J Cancer Res Clin Oncol. 1996;122:283–8.
25. Walter E, Keist R, Niederöst B, Pult I, Blum HE. Hepatitis B virus infection of Tupaia hepatocytes in vitro and in vivo. Hepatology. 1996;24:1–5.
26. Xie ZC, Riezu-Boj JI, Lasarte JJ, Guillen J, Su JH, Civeira MP, Prieto J. Transmission of hepatitis C virus infection to tree shrews. Virology. 1998;244:513–20.
27. Ilan E, Burakova T, Dagan S, Nussbaum O, Lubin I, Eren R et al. The hepatitis B virus trimera mouse: a model for human HBV infection and evaluation of anti HBV therapeutic agents. Hepatology. 1999;29:553–62.
28. Sandgren EP, Palmiter RD, Heckel JL, Daugherty CC, Brinster RL, Degen JL. Complete hepatic regeneration after somatic deletion of an albumin plasminogen activator transgene. Cell. 1991;66:245–56.
29. Petersen J, Dandri M, Gupta S, Rogler CE. Liver repopulation with xenogenic hepatocytes in B and T cell deficient mice leads to chronic hepadnavirus infection and clonal growth of hepatocellular carcinoma. Proc Natl Acad Sci USA. 1998;95:310–15.
30. Rehermann B, Ferrari C, Pasquinelli C, Chisari FV. The hepatitis B virus persists for decades after patients' recovery from acute viral hepatitis despite active maintenance of a cytotoxic T lymphocyte response. Nature Med. 1996;2:1104–8.

6
Liver damage and control of HBV infection: role of the cell-mediated immune response

A. PENNA, C. BONI, A. CAVALLI, C. CAVALLO, G. MISSALE, M. MALPELI, M. PILLI, J. UGGERI, S. URBANI and C. FERRARI

Since viruses are intracellular parasites, anti-viral cytotoxic T-lymphocytes (CTL) are believed to play a major role in eradication of infection by virtue of their capacity to identify and kill virus-infected cells through recognition of viral peptides displayed in association with HLA class I molecules on the surface of the cells[1]. Therefore, in infections with non-cytopathic viruses, such as HBV, immunopathology has been considered to be the result of a lytic mechanism of protection that leads to termination of infection when it is efficient, or to a chronic inflammation of the liver when it is weak. According to these concepts, acute self-limited hepatitis B can be viewed as the result of a coordinate activity of cellular and humoral anti-viral responses leading to control of infection, through CTL-mediated destruction of infected cells and antibody-mediated neutralization of free circulating viral particles responsible for liver cells reinfection. Chronic hepatitis B was interpreted as a condition of CTL activity capable of maintaining liver damage and inflammation but insufficient to cause complete elimination of infected cells. A lack of CTL activity was considered the hallmark of the asymptomatic HBV carrier state.

GENERAL FEATURES OF THE PROTECTIVE HBV-SPECIFIC T-CELL RESPONSE

During the acute phase of HBV infection the CTL response is generally polyclonal and multispecific since multiple epitopes located within different structural and non-structural HBV antigens are recognized simultaneously by individual patients[2–6], making unlikely the possibility that viral mutations within CTL epitopes can allow viral escape from immune surveillance. Similarly, a vigorous HLA class II restricted peripheral blood T-cell response to HBcAg and

HBeAg is detectable in virtually all patients during the symptomatic phase of acute self-limited hepatitis B[7,8] and it is directed against several epitopes, a few of which are strongly immunodominant and widely recognized by patients with different HLA backgrounds[9]. It is of note that the appearance of a strong T-cell response to nucleocapsid antigens in the peripheral blood is temporally associated in most patients with clearance of serum HBV envelope antigens, suggesting that an optimal development of CD4-mediated responses is required to supplement CTL and B-cell mediated events to fully control the infection. Indeed, HBV nucleocapsid-specific $CD4^+$ T-cells are probably essential for optimal activation of HBV-specific $CD8^+$ CTL, as suggested by the observation that both kinetics and vigour of the CD4 response in acute HBV infection parallels those of HLA class I-restricted CTL[2,5,7,8]. Moreover, HBcAg-specific helper T-cells could facilitate viral clearance by a direct cooperation with HBV envelope-specific B-cells, through a mechanism of 'intermolecular' help[10], leading to amplification of the virus-neutralizing anti-envelope antibody response. Finally, HBV-specific helper and CTL have been shown to be still present in an activated state several years after recovery from acute hepatitis as a likely result of a continuous stimulation by minute amounts of persisting virus detectable only by PCR[11,12]. Therefore, resolution of disease does not imply complete eradication of infection but more likely reflects the capacity of anti-viral T cells to keep HBV infection under tight and persistent control.

MECHANISMS OF ELIMINATION OF INTRACELLULAR VIRUS IN ACUTE HBV-INFECTED INDIVIDUALS

The notion that the lytic activity of the CTL is the most important mechanism of elimination of intracellular virus is difficult, however, to reconcile with the evidence that virtually all liver cells are infected during the early stages of infection. This would imply that massive hepatic necrosis should represent a more frequent outcome of an acute hepatitis B.

Animal models

Recent data derived from animal models of HBV infection (such as the chimpanzee and the transgenic mouse models) and from human hepatitis B allow drawing a more complete picture of the cell-mediated immune events occurring during acute and chronic HBV infection. Studies performed in the transgenic mouse model have shown that HBV DNA replicative intermediates can be cleared from the cytoplasm of HBV transgenic hepatocytes as a result of the anti-viral effect of interferon-γ (IFN-γ) and tumour necrosis factor-α (TNF-α) released by infiltrating HBV-specific $CD8^+$[13–16] and $CD4^+$[17] T cells. If this non-cytolytic mechanism of eradication of intracellular virus can also be applied to human HBV infection, it could give an important contribution to viral clearance in hepatitis.

The possibility that these mechanisms are also operative during natural HBV infection is suggested by the analysis of the early events occurring in acutely infected chimpanzees, which develop liver inflammation and mount immune responses against HBV similar to those observed in humans[18]. In this animal model, all intracellular HBV DNA forms peak in the liver approximately 8 weeks after infection and decline rapidly thereafter. The ALT rise and T-cell mRNA in the liver are detectable only at later time points. In particular, CD8 RNA is undetectable when HBV DNA disappears from the liver of the animals[18]. Thus, the decline of HBV DNA from serum and liver seems to precede the appearance of liver damage and massive T-cell infiltration. This suggests that most viral DNA (at least 90% in the chimpanzee model) can be eliminated by non-cytolytic processes that do not require the destruction of liver (Fig. 1). This non-cytolytic mechanism could be triggered by IFN-γ and TNF-α prevalently produced by non-T-cells[19–21], that represent the main population present within the infected liver before evidence of liver damage.

Human infection

In human infection control of HBV replication is also observed before the onset of clinical symptoms when ALT levels are still normal (M. Maini and A. Bertoletti, submitted manuscript). This confirms that HBV is not cytopathic

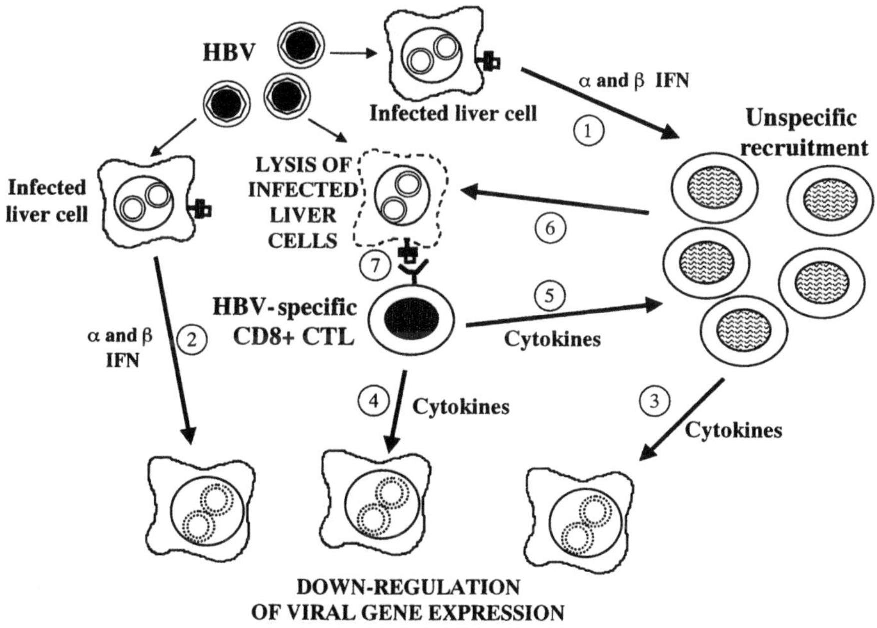

Figure 1 Following HBV infection, interferons released by infected liver parenchymal cells can cause (1) recruitment of virus non-specific mononuclear cells and (2) suppression of HBV gene expression within infected hepatocytes. To this initial suppression of virus replication can also contribute soluble factors released by infiltrating mononuclear cells (3). HBV-specific CTL, after priming in the local lymph nodes and exit from the lymphatic system, reach the blood and, through this route, the infected liver. IFN-γ and TNF-α secreted by HBV-specific CTL can (4) amplify the suppression on viral genes within liver cells and can (5) contribute to the intrahepatic recruitment of HBV non-specific cells. In concert with the effector mechanisms of virus non-specific cells (6), the lytic activity of HBV-specific CTL (7) is believed to be the main responsible for liver cell damage, that eventually contribute to final elimination of residual virus and full control of infection.

and that virus control can be achieved without massive and biochemically detectable destruction of infected liver cells. Interestingly, the peak frequency of circulating HBV-specific CTL coincides with clinical onset of acute hepatitis and ALT elevation[22].

In summary, the concept that emerges from all these studies is that control of viral replication and clearance of most HBV DNA molecules occur before the onset of liver damage and clinical symptoms. These early events are likely caused by suppression of HBV gene expression by soluble cytokines, such as IFN-γ and TNF-α, released by liver-infiltrating lymphomononuclear cells.

At this early stage of infection HBV-specific T-cells can contribute to focus the immune response on the infected organ and to amplify the mechanisms that lead to the recruitment of non-antigen specific mononuclear cells into the inflamed liver. According to this interpretation, liver damage resulting from the immune elimination of infected cells by HBV-specific CTL represents a complementary mechanism operating at later time needed to achieve a full and persistent control of the infection (Fig. 1).

CTL AS MEDIATORS OF VIRUS CONTROL OR PERSISTENT LIVER DAMAGE IN CHRONIC HBV INFECTION

The concept that an effective HBV-specific CD8 response can determine inhibition of virus replication without liver damage is also suggested by studies in chronic healthy HBV carriers. Patients with chronic HBV infection without signs of liver damage have generally been considered to lack an active CTL response against HBV. This view has been challenged by recent studies carried out by tetramer staining and functional analysis of circulating and intrahepatic CTL that show that functionally active HBV-specific CD8 cells are present in the circulation and within the liver of these patients, despite the lack of liver damage[23]. HBV-specific CTL present in the circulation express the phenotype of antigen-primed resting T-cells, can expand efficiently and can exert anti-viral effector function in vitro upon stimulation with viral antigen. Moreover, a high proportion of liver-infiltrating $CD8^+$ T-cells are HBV specific in these patients. Although these data do not allow to totally rule out the possibility that some degree (undetectable by ALT measurement) of liver cell lysis caused by HBV-specific CTL may occur, the sparsely scattered pattern of $CD8^+$ cells within the liver parenchyma suggests that control of virus replication in these patients occurs primarily through the secretion of cytokines by HBV-specific CTL.

In striking contrast to healthy asymptomatic carriers, functionally active HBV-specific CTL are not detectable in the peripheral blood of patients with chronic active hepatitis, who are unable to control the virus and display high degree of liver damage and high levels of HBV replication[23]. In these patients, HBV-specific CTL are detectable only within the liver, where their frequency is low because they are diluted among a large number of virus non-specific T cells, that may play an important role in maintenance of chronic liver cell damage[23].

The behaviour of the CTL response in patients with chronic HBV infection raises the concept that chronic asymptomatic carriers are able to control viral replication by virtue of the antiviral activity of HBV-specific CTL. This control may be primarily exerted, without cell destruction, through the release of cytokines able to efficiently diffuse throughout the liver parenchyma.

Efficient control of virus replication seems to require rapid activation of CD8-mediated effector mechanisms following antigen encounter. This is suggested by the observation that HBV-specific CTL in healthy HBV carriers and patients who successfully recover from acute hepatitis B can efficiently expand and expresses effector function (lytic activity and release of cytokines) upon antigen stimulation in vitro. In contrast, CTL from patients with a chronic active infection, persistent liver damage and active virus replication are generally non-responsive in vitro to exogenous stimulation. Therefore, restoration of the CTL capacity to expand vigorously and to exert efficient effector function represents one of the main objective of antiviral therapies in patients with chronic hepatitis B, to make their CTL functionally similar to those of individuals who are able to control virus replication (healthy carriers and individuals recovered from acute HBV infection). Recent studies show that this objective can be achieved by lamivudine therapy that is able to restore virus-specific helper[24] and CTL (C. Boni et al., submitted manuscript) functions and to render HBV-specific CTL susceptible to exogenous stimulation.

REFERENCES

1. Yewdell JW, Bennink JR. Cell biology of antigen processing and presentation to major histocompatibility complex class I molecule-restricted T lymphocytes. Adv Immunol. 1992;52:1–123.
2. Penna A, Chisari FV, Bertoletti A, Missale G, Fowler P, Giuberti T et al. Cytotoxic T lymphocytes recognize an HLA A2 restricted epitope within the hepatitis B virus nucleocapsid antigen. J Exp Med. 1991;174:1565–70.
3. Bertoletti A, Ferrari C, Penna A, Margolskee R, Schlicht HJ, Fowler P et al. HLA class I restricted cytotoxic T cells in acute viral hepatitis type B. Proc Natl Acad Sci USA. 1991;88:10445–9.
4. Missale G, Redeker A, Person J, Fowler P, Guilhot S, Schlicht HJ et al. HLA-A31 and HLA-Aw68 restricted cytotoxic T cell responses to a single hepatitis B virus nucleocapsid epitope during acute viral hepatitis. J Exp Med. 1993;177:751–62.
5. Nayersina R, Fowler P, Guilhot S, Missale G, Cherny A, Schlicht HJ et al. HLA-A2-restricted cytotoxic T lymphocyte responses to multiple hepatitis B surface antigen epitopes during hepatitis B virus infection. J Immunol. 1993;150:4659–71.
6. Rehermann B, Fowler P, Sidney J, Person J, Redeker A, Brown M et al. The cytotoxic T lymphocyte response to multiple hepatitis B polymerase epitopes during and after acute viral infection. J Exp Med. 1995;181:1047–58.
7. Ferrari C, Penna A, Bertoletti A, Valli A, Degli Antoni A, Giuberti T et al. Cellular immune response to hepatitis B virus (HBV) encoded antigens in acute and chronic HBV infection. J Immunol. 1990;145:3442–9.
8. Jung M-C, Spengler U, Schraut W, Hoffmann R, Zachoval R, Eisenburg J et al. Hepatitis B virus antigen-specific T-cell activation in patients with acute and chronic hepatitis B. J Hepatol. 1991;13:310–17.
9. Ferrari C, Bertoletti A, Penna A, Cavalli A, Valli A, Missale G, Fiaccadori F. Identification of immunodominant T cell epitopes of the hepatitis B virus nucleocapsid antigen. J Clin Invest. 1991;88:214–22.
10. Milich DR, McLachlan A, Thornton GB, Hughes JL. Antibody production to the nucleo capsid and envelope of hepatitis B virus primed by a single synthetic T cell site. Nature. 1987;329:547–9.
11. Rehermann B, Ferrari C, Pasquinelli C, Chisari FV. The hepatitis B virus persists for decades after patients' recovery from acute viral hepatitis despite active maintenance of a cytotoxic T-lymphocyte response. Nature Med. 1996;2:1104–8.

12. Penna A, Artini M, Cavalli A, Levrero M, Bertoletti A, Pilli M et al. Long-lasting memory T cell responses following self-limited acute hepatitis B. J Clin Invest. 1996;98:1185–94.
13. Guidotti LG, Ishikawa T, Hobbs MV, Matzke B, Schreiber R, Chisari FV. Intracellular inactivation of the hepatitis B virus by cytotoxic T lymphocytes. Immunity. 1996;4:25–36.
14. Guidotti LG, Borrow P, Hobbs MV, Matzke B, Gresser I, Oldstone MB, Chisari FV. Viral cross talk: intracellular inactivation of the hepatitis B virus during an unrelated viral infection of the liver. Proc Natl Acad Sci USA. 1996;93:4589–94.
15. Heise T, Guidotti LG, Cavanaugh VJ, Chisari FV. Hepatitis B virus RNA-binding proteins associated with cytokine-induced clearance of viral RNA from the liver of transgenic mice. J Virol. 1999;73:474–81.
16. McClary H, Koch R, Chisari FV, Guidotti LG. Relative sensitivity of hepatitis B virus and other hepatotropic viruses to antiviral effect of cytokines. J Virol. 2000;74:2255–64.
17. Franco A, Guidotti LG, Hobbs MV, Pasquetto V, Chisari FV. Pathogenetic effector function of CD4-positive T helper 1 cells in hepatitis B virus transgenic mice. J Immunol. 1997;159:2001–8.
18. Guidotti LG, Rochford R, Chung J, Shapiro M, Purcell R, Chisari FV. Viral clearance without destruction of infected cells during acute HBV infection. Science. 1999;284:825–9.
19. MacDonald HR, NK1.1+ T cell receptor-a/b + cells: new clues to their origin, specificity and function. J Exp Med. 1995;182:633–8.
20. Ohteki T, MacDonald HR. Major histocompatibility complex class I related molecules control and development of CD4+ and CD4– subsets of natural killer 1.1 + T cell receptor a/b + cells in the liver of mice. J Exp Med. 1994;180:699–704.
21. Doherty DG, Norris S, Madrigal-Estebas L, McEntee G, Traynor O, Hegarty JE, O'Farrel C. The human liver contains multiple populations of NK cells, T cells and CD3+CD56+ natural T cells with distinct cytotoxic activities and Th 1, Th 2 and Th 0 cytokine secretion patterns. J Immunol. 1999;163:2314–21.
22. Maini MK, Boni C, Lee CK, Larrubia JR, Reignat S, Ogg GS et al. Direct ex vivo analysis of hepatitis B virus-specific CD8+ T cells associated with the control of infection. Gastroenterology. 1999;117:1–13.
23. Maini MK, Boni C, Ogg GS, King AS, Reignat S, Lee CK et al. The role of virus-specific CD8(+) cells in liver damage and viral control during persistent hepatitis B virus infection. J Exp Med. 2000;191:1269–80.
24. Boni C, Bertoletti A, Penna A, Cavalli A, Pilli M, Urbani S et al. Lamivudine treatment can restore T cell responsiveness in chronic hepatitis B. J Clin Invest. 1998;102:968–75.

7 Natural history of hepatitis B infection

G. M. DUSHEIKO

Type B hepatitis is a complex disease. Infection with hepatitis B virus (HBV) is characterised by several outcomes ranging from acute infection which can resolve without symptoms, to persistent or even fulminant and fatal disease. The course and outcome of chronic type-B hepatitis is variable. The outcome of both acute and chronic disease is largely related to the host immune response at the onset of infection and during the course of the ensuing chronic infection. Immunogenetic factors may affect the immune response. The major factors to consider in reviewing the natural course and risk factors for disease progression in hepatitis B are factors which affect the likelihood of chronic infection, progression of the disease in children, progression of chronic hepatitis during the course of the disease in later life, progression of cirrhosis to liver failure once cirrhosis has occurred, and progression to hepatocellular carcinoma. Some factors influencing the outcome of infection, and detailing the morbidity and mortality of chronic hepatitis B are known.

OUTCOME AFTER ACUTE HEPATITIS B

Acute hepatitis B in adults usually leads to resolution of the disease due to a complex if as yet poorly understood concerted immune response. The opposite is true in neonates and also in young children in whom acute hepatitis B is not usually accompanied by an symptomatic illness, but leads to persistent viraemia as a result of an impaired immune response.

High rates of chronic infection (> 90%) occur in unvaccinated neonates after maternal infant transmission, and in children. One to 5% of adults, and perhaps less, develops chronic hepatitis B. Following a single source outbreak of hepatitis B among 79 adult women, 3 patients (4%) became chronic carriers of hepatitis B virus[1]. After a single source outbreak following autohaemotherapy, we have observed that 4 of 32 patients infected with the same viral isolate developed chronic hepatitis B. In 3 of these patients infection was acquired when the patient's were receiving corticosteroid therapy for another disease, and the subsequent chronic infection may have been due to their immunosuppressive therapy. The mechanism of development of chronic hepatitis B has not been elucidated. Resolution in part depends upon the development of a hepatitis illness characterised by a discernible increase in the serum aminotransferases. However, viral clearance without cytolysis of infected cells during acute hepatitis B virus infection may be a pivotal first step in resolution of the disease. In acutely infected chimpanzees, hepatitis B DNA has been shown to largely disappear from the liver and blood before maximal CD4+ and CD8+ cell T-cell infiltration of the liver and the onset of hepatitis[2]. These results suggest that non-cytopathic antiviral mechanisms contribute to viral clearance during acute viral hepatitis. Residual hepatitis B DNA declines after a complex antigen-specific CD8 response associated with hepatocyte lysis.

CHRONIC HEPATITIS B

The various categories of hepatitis B can be defined in terms of serological markers (1) HBsAg, HBeAg and anti-HBe, (2) concentration of hepatitis B DNA in serum, (3) hepatic biochemistry (ALT and AST), (4) histological staging and grading, (5) histochemical staining for HBsAg and HBcAg and (6) the state of the hepatitis B genome in hepatocytes (predominantly episomal or integrated). However the latter is not routinely assessed. Two major forms of the disease are recognized, i.e. HBeAg-positive chronic hepatitis and anti-HBe-positive chronic hepatitis.

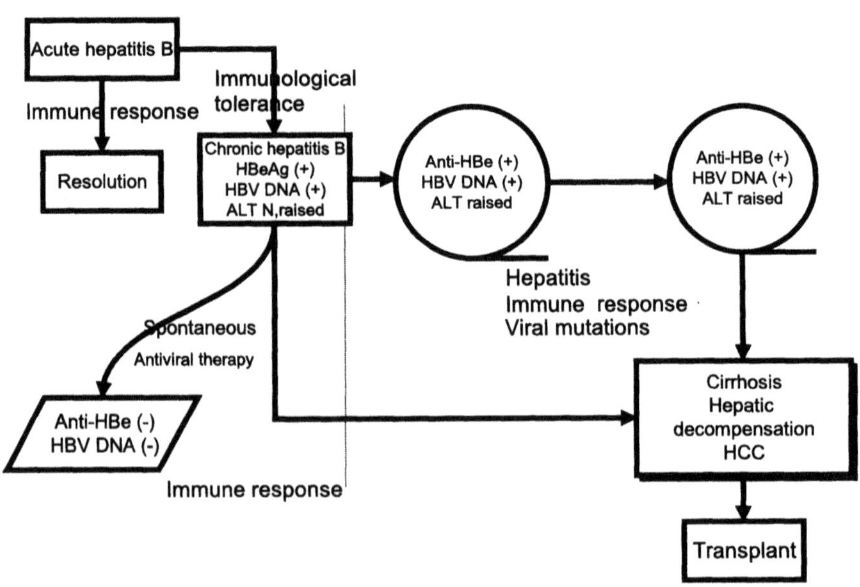

Figure 1. Natural history and immune responses in acute and chronic hepatitis B: implications for antiviral therapy

During the first phase of the illness chronically infected children typically, although not always, have high levels of viraemia and are HBeAg-positive with normal or near normal serum aminotransferases (Figure 1). They constitute an important pool of infection. In a varying percentage of HBeAg-positive patients, spontaneous remission or even resolution of the disease can be observed. Patients with HBeAg in serum may have normal or abnormal serum aminotransferases. They are infected with predominantly "wild type" hepatitis B, expressing HBeAg. During this time there may be an exacerbation of the hepatitis accompanying seroconversion from HBeAg to anti-HBe. Hepatitis B DNA becomes undetectable in serum by hybridisation assays, and patients may have normal serum aminotransferases for many years following spontaneous seroconversion. If these events occur prior to the onset of severe liver injury and fibrosis, the disease can be relatively benign. It is clear, however, that for many patients, this state is not maintained, however, and a proportion of patients may again become HBeAg-positive, or alternatively may have fluctuating titres of HBeAg and anti-HBe, varying levels of viraemia, and intermittently raised serum aminotransferases. Thus for many other patients such a beneficial outcome is not observed and gradual progression of the disease, associated with a remarkably dynamic serological and clinical pattern, may occur over a period of years or decades. These patients may develop periodic episodes of necroinflammatory disease characterised typically by a lobular hepatitis histologically, which appears to be injurious to the liver in the long term.

In several parts of the world, the dominant pattern of chronic disease in adults is characterised by a declining prevalence of HBeAg in serum. This pattern is in part accounted for by a decline in levels of viraemia, and infectivity, explained by integration of hepatitis B genomes within hepatocytes. However, predominant infection with HBeAg-negative variants of hepatitis B, with continuing albeit often lower levels of replication, also explains the mechanism of infection in HBeAg-negative, anti-HBe-positive patients with HBV DNA detectable by hybridization in serum. This is accounted for by a predominance of circulating hepatitis B virus variants which do not express HBeAg; the most common variant is the so-called 'pre-core mutant' with a stop codon at position 1896 leading to a failure of HBeAg expression. This variant is probably selected by an immune response targeted towards variants of HBV expressing HBeAg.

Persistent hepatitis B virus infection of the liver can occur without significant, continuous necroinflammatory disease. These patients have been referred to as 'healthy carriers' but this nomenclature needs review. The diagnosis is based on presence of HBsAg in the serum, with no or only low levels of HBV DNA (although the values are as yet uncertain), persistently normal serum aminotransferase and absence of significant necrosis and inflammation in the liver. Positive HBsAg staining may be found in the liver (ground glass cells may be present) but these patients are negative for HBcAg in the liver by histochemical staining. These patients have predominantly integrated viral genomes within the liver. These patients may have some degree of fibrosis in the liver, if fibrosis accrued during the active phase of the infection, but the disease tends not to progress.

Natural history of chronic hepatitis B in children

The natural history of the disease in children is only partially understood. The outcome of chronic hepatitis B in Caucasian children has been studied after a 20 (mean 13) year follow-up in 185 HBsAg-positive children, 168 of whom were HBeAg-positive. The majority of these children seroconverted to anti-HBe (83.8%) within this period and only a minority (7.5%) remained HBeAg-positive. A small percentage of children (6%) became HBsAg-negative[(3)]. Similarly Ruiz-Moreno[4] followed 103 anti-HBe-positive children with normal serum aminotransferases for a mean period of 6.3 years (range 0.6–12.5 years). Liver biopsies were done in 83 cases. The serum ALT remained normal in 79% of these children throughout follow-up and there appeared to be some improvement in the histology activity index (HAI) and fibrosis scores suggesting a durable, stable outcome after HBeAg seroconversion in children. In contrast Lok *et al.* followed 51 asymptomatic Chinese children for a median period of 4 years. At presentation, 84% were HBeAg-positive and after follow-up the majority of HBeAg-positive children remained HBeAg-positive – only 7% had cleared HBeAg[5]. Serum ALT were normal in 80% initially and remained normal in 60%. These data suggest that there are geographic differences in seroconversion to anti-HBe, which are unexplained. Extra hepatic remissions of polyarteritis and particularly glomerulonephritis have been observed after clearance of HBeAg[6].

Natural history of chronic hepatitis B in adults

The progression of chronic hepatitis in adults is complex and is only partially known. The disease may be variable and can be stable or followed by periodic exacerbations, typified by fluctuations in viral replication, but may be asymptomatic. Variable HBeAg to anti-HBe seroconversion rates have been reported in different parts of the world. Fattovich *et al.* followed 105 patients with chronic hepatitis B. Forty-six had 'chronic persistent hepatitis', 59 had 'chronic active hepatitis'. These patients were followed up for 16 years (mean 5.5 years) with a histological follow-up of 3.7 years (mean). Cirrhosis developed in 21 (20%) with a calculated annual incidence of 5.9%. Several variables were associated with a poor prognosis in this cohort with longer-term follow up. These variables were old age, bridging hepatic necrosis and persistent hepatitis B DNA[7].

Progression to cirrhosis

The most important outcome at this stage of the natural history of hepatitis B is the development of cirrhosis. Liaw *et al.* followed 684 patients, 509 of whom were HBeAg-positive and 175 of whom were anti-HBe-positive[8]. The average follow-up in this mixed cohort of hepatitis B-positive patients was 35.3 months. Approximately 6% of the HBeAg-positive patients developed cirrhosis compared to approximately 4% of the anti-HBe-positive patients. The calculated incidence of cirrhosis was greater in the HBeAg-positive patients (approximately 2.9%). Factors associated with the development of cirrhosis were increasing age, repeated exacerbations associated with bridging hepatic necrosis and exacerbations in which HBeAg seroconversion did not lead to loss of HBeAg and development of anti-HBe.

Hepatitis B sequelae in Alaskans has been studied by McMahon[9,10]. In this study, 1400 HBsAg-positive Alaskans were prospectively followed for sequelae for a total of 7,815 carrier years. Cirrhosis developed in eight cases (5.7%). The incidence of cirrhosis was 107/100,000 men and 95/100,000 women. Hepatocellular carcinoma developed in 20 cases (1.4%) and the incidence of hepatocellular carcinoma was 387/100,000 men and 63/100,000 women. Villeneuve *et al.*[11] followed up 317 asymptomatic HBsAg-positive French Canadian carriers. After a 16-year follow-up, death from cirrhosis had occurred in three. No patient had died from hepatocellular carcinoma and there were nine unrelated deaths. The number of deaths from hepatocellular carcinoma was lower than the rate that would have been expected from Far Eastern patients with hepatocellular carcinoma.

The cumulative probability of exacerbations has been estimated in a large cohort of 388 patients from Hong Kong who were followed for one to five years. The cumulative probability of exacerbation was greater in patients whose serum ALT was greater than 200 (24%) versus patients whose ALT was less then 200 (6.3%). The cumulative probability after four years of follow-up was likewise greater in patients whose serum ALT was greater than 200 (47%) versus 15%[12].

Natural history of chronic hepatitis B after the development of cirrhosis

The next important transition in the natural history of chronic hepatitis B is the natural history of the disease after the development of cirrhosis. Cirrhosis is generally a dynamic and progressive disease but rates of progression vary depending upon the status of the patients. Liaw *et al.* noted exacerbations in 25% of 76 patients with recent onset of cirrhosis who were HBeAg- and/or hepatitis B DNA-positive. However, exacerbations were noted in only 11.9% of patients who were DNA-negative. The annual incidence of decompensation was 2.3%, of variceal bleeding 2.3% and of hepatocellular carcinoma 2.8%. The estimated 5 year survival in this cohort was 80%[13].

Survival has also been studied in Caucasian patients with HBsAg-positive cirrhosis[14]. Three hundred and sixty-six Caucasian patients with hepatitis-B virus infection with proven cirrhosis who had not previously developed clinical decompensation were followed for a mean follow-up of 72 months. Death occurred in 23% of these patients as a result of liver failure in 45 and hepatocellular carcinoma in 23. The estimated five-year survival in this group was 84% and the estimated ten-year survival was 68%. Age, serum albumin, serum platelets, the presence of splenomegaly, bilirubin concentrations, HBeAg-positivity, but not hepatitis-D virus infection, influenced survival in this study.

HEPATOCELLULAR CARCINOMA

Most cases of hepatocellular carcinoma (HCC), but not all, occur after the development of cirrhosis. HCC and decompensation in cirrhosis due to chronic hepatitis B has been studied in 349 Western European patients[15]. The follow-up in this cohort was a mean period of six years. Hepatocellular carcinoma developed in 9% and decompensation occurred in 28%. After a first episode of decompensation, the five-year probability of survival was 35%. Yu *et al.* followed 1506 male asymptomatic HBsAg-positive carriers for a mean of 7.1 years. Hepatocellular carcinoma developed in 16 cases (1%) and cirrhosis in 89 cases (5.9%). Sub-clinical cirrhosis on ultrasound was significantly associated with the later development of hepatocellular carcinoma. The risk factors for cirrhosis in this group were age, HBeAg, elevated serum aminotransferases, smoking, non-A blood types and low educational levels[16]. Several extraneous factors, but importantly aflatoxin ingestion in staple diets in various populations, may profoundly affect the incidence of hepatocellular carcinoma and may be an important oncogenic factor. There is an increased risk of hepatocellular carcinoma in HBsAg-positive men with aflatoxin metabolite M1. Sun *et al.* followed 145 men with chronic hepatitis B who were followed for ten years to determine aflatoxin exposure. Their urine samples were pooled to detect aflatoxin metabolite M1. If an increased AFM1was found, the hepatocellular carcinoma risk was increased 3.3-fold. With concomitant hepatitis C the hepatocellular carcinoma risk was increased 5.8-fold and with a family history of hepatocellular carcinoma the HCC risk was increased 5.6-fold[17].

In a recent study published by DiMarco, 302 HBsAg-positive patients were followed for a median follow-up of 94 months[18]. Eighty-six percent of patients had cirrhosis. One hundred and nine received alpha-interferon. Twenty-eight percent were HBeAg-positive, 26% were HBeAg-negative, 25% were hepatitis D-positive and 14% were co-infected with hepatitis B virus and hepatitis C. Forty-six patients had decompensation and 35 died, with an overall mortality of 5.2 times the expected mortality. Factors associated with survival were young age, the absence of cirrhosis, normal serum aminotransferases and interestingly alpha-interferon treatment. An increasing percentage of patients with dual hepatitis B and hepatitis C may be at risk of severe sequelae of chronic hepatitis[19].

NATURAL HISTORY OF TRANSPLANTATION FOR HEPATITIS B

Fibrosing cholestatic hepatitis is a severe complication of recurrence of hepatitis B in immunosuppressed patients. This has particularly been reported in patients with corticosteroid immunosuppression but is not restricted to this group. The disease is characterized by high levels of HBsAg and may be related to a cytopathic effect or possibly an immune response to the virus. This fortunately has been altered by antiviral therapy or with immunoglobulin prophylaxis. Treatment for post transplant recurrence may also be effective in this group as long as resistance does not develop[20].

Reactivation may occur with immunosuppression and can occur indeed several years after recovery from acute hepatitis B with reduction in CD4 counts and B lymphocyte dysfunction[21].

TREATMENT EFFECTS UPON THE NATURAL HISTORY OF HEPATITIS B

Antiviral treatment of hepatitis B may influence the natural history. A marked influence of pre-treatment ALT has been found to affect seroconversion rates in both alpha-interferon- and lamivudine-treated patients as well as affecting seroconversion rates in untreated patients. For reasons that are not clear, seroconversion rates are accelerated and are higher in treated patients. Survival has been associated with clearance of HBeAg in both treated and untreated patients[22].

VARIANTS OF HEPATITIS B

Several important variants of hepatitis B have been reported. Their influence on the natural history of the disease is uncertain. However, there are important influences upon the serologic changes and the selection of variants in different regions of the world. Nucleotide and amino acid divergences have been reported to be higher in the basic core promoter of HBV in patients with hepatocellular carcinoma, compared with asymptomatic carriers, particularly with respect to the paired 1762 adenine to thymine (1762T) and 1764 guanine to adenine 1764A missense mutations. These have been observed in 66% of patients with hepatocellular carcinoma compared with 11% of asymptomatic carriers[23].

Pre-Core mutant hepatitis B characterized by circulating variants of hepatitis B unable to secrete HBeAg are important. These may be the cause (or result) of more severe disease. Generally this variant is associated with older age of patients and higher histological activity. Seroconversion has been observed in children with both wild type hepatitis-B and mixed viraemia. Seroconversion to anti-HBe has been observed in children with wild type and mixed viraemia (37% vs 33%). In cases with mixed viraemia, seroconversion occurred in four (66%) of six with $HBeAg^{(-)}$ levels lower than 20% of total viraemia but in none of six with higher levels ($p < 0.066$)[24].

Pre-core changes have exclusively been found in patients infected with hepatitis B who have a T at nucleotide 1858 (87% versus 0%)[25]. There are important genotype–subtype associations with genotype F predominant in the Americas and genotype B in East Asia.

Core gene mutations. Changes in the hepatitis B core gene sequence are rarely detected in patients who are still in the immune tolerant phase. Higher rates of change have been found during the immune clearance of chronic hepatitis B[26]. Core promoter changes are significantly more common in patients infected with hepatitis B who have C at nucleotide 1858 (91% versus 27%).

The HBsAg subtype may be significantly associated with HBsAg disappearance and carriers with subtype adr (odds ratio equal 2.87) have an increased probability of clearing HBsAg compared with carriers with subtype adw[27,28].

Polymerase variants. The most important variants currently in hepatitis B are variants in the polymerase selected for by treatment with lamivudine. Although spontaneous seroconversion may still occur following the development of variants, it is premature to believe that such variants will be benign and or less pathogenic than wild type. The influence of these variants on the natural history of both immunosuppressed and non-immunosuppressed patients remains to be clarified but it is important that this outcome is measured at this time. Although the median serum ALT and hepatitis B DNA patients have been reported to be lower than baseline levels in patients with YMDD ariants on lamivudine treatment, it is clear that serum ALT levels and hepatitis B DNA concentrations are higher in patients with these variants.

CO-INFECTION

Occult hepatitis B virus infection has been reported in hepatitis C virus infection[29]. This may be an important pathogenic factor but the mechanism of the pathogenicity of co-infection remains to be determined. Recently 200 patients with chronic hepatitis C liver disease have been followed. In 66 of 200 patients, (33%) hepatitis B virus sequences were found. Forty-six of the 66 were anti-HBc-positive and 20 of the 66 were anti-HBc-negative. Cirrhosis was found in 22 of the 66 (33 %) of patients who had hepatitis B DNA, but was present in 26 of 134 (19 %) without hepatitis B.

Similarly, HIV co-infection has been reported to cause increased viraemia and decreased HBeAg to anti-HBe seroconversion rates[30].

CONCLUSIONS

Thus several key factors have been observed to influence the natural course of chronic hepatitis B. There is a varied risk of progression but the basis for this variation is uncertain. A number of factors involved in the pathogenesis of the disease and hepatic necroinflammatory change, in particular both antigen-specific cytotoxic lymphocyte responses and nonspecific cytokine mediator damage as well as apoptosis are being studied. The events occurring around the time of loss of viral tolerance may shed some light on this apparent beneficial effect (beneficial at least in a proportion of patients) and could lead to better antiviral therapy. The genetic heterogeneity of the immune and inflammatory response needs further study and the influence of HBeAg and HBcAg variants which appear around the time of loss of viral tolerance, or are involved with loss of viral tolerance, require further study.

REFERENCES

1. Heijtink RA, Paulij W, Van Roosmalen M, et al. Characteristics of the early phase of chronicity in acute hepatitis B infection. J Med Virol. 1999;57:331–336.
2. Guidotti LG, Rochford R, Chung J, Shapiro M, Purcell R, Chisari FV. Viral clearance without destruction of infected cells during acute HBV infection. Science. 1999;284:825–829.
3. Bortolotti F, Jara P, Crivellaro C, et al. Outcome of chronic hepatitis B in Caucasian children during a 20-year observation period. J Hepatol. 1998;29:184–190.
4. Ruiz-Moreno M, Otero M, Millán A, et al. Clinical and histological outcome after hepatitis B e antigen to antibody seroconversion in children with chronic hepatitis B. Hepatology. 1999;29(2):572–575.
5. Lok AS, Lai CL. A longitudinal follow-up of asymptomatic hepatitis B surface antigen-positive Chinese children. Hepatology. 1988;8:1130–1133.
6. Gilbert RD, Wiggelinkhuizen J. The clinical course of hepatitis B virus-associated nephropathy. Pediatr Nephrol. 1994;8:11–14.
7. Fattovich G, Brollo L, Giustina G, et al. Natural history and prognostic factors for chronic hepatitis type B. Gut. 1991;32:294–298.
8. Liaw YF, Tai DI, Chu CM, Chen TJ. The development of cirrhosis in patients with chronic type B hepatitis: a prospective study. Hepatology. 1988;8:493–496.
9. McMahon BJ, Alberts SR, Wainwright RB, Bulkow L, Lanier AP. Hepatitis B-related sequelae. Prospective study in 1400 hepatitis B surface antigen-positive Alaska native carriers. Arch Intern Med. 1990;150:1051–1054.

10. McMahon BJ, Lanier AP, Wainwright RB, Kilkenny SJ. Hepatocellular carcinoma in Alaska Eskimos: epidemiology, clinical features, and early detection. Prog Liver Dis. 1990;9:643–655.
11. Villeneuve J-P, Desrochers M, Infante-Rivard C, et al. A long-term follow-up study of asymptomatic hepatitis B surface antigen-positive carriers in Montreal. Gastroenterology. 1994;106:1000–1005.
12. Lok AS, Lai CL. Acute exacerbations in Chinese patients with chronic hepatitis B virus (HBV) infection. Incidence, predisposing factors and etiology. J Hepatol. 1990;10:29–34.
13. Liaw YF, Lin DY, Chen TJ, Chu CM. Natural course after the development of cirrhosis in patients with chronic type B hepatitis: a prospective study. Liver. 1989;9:235–241.
14. Realdi G, Fattovich G, Hadziyannis S, et al. Survival and prognostic factors in 366 patients with compensated cirrhosis type B: A multicenter study. J Hepatol. 1994;21:656–666.
15. Fattovich G, Giustina G, Schalm SW, et al. Occurrence of hepatocellular carcinoma and decompensation in Western European patients with cirrhosis type B. Hepatology. 1995;21:77–82.
16. Yu MW, Hsu FC, Sheen IS, et al. Prospective study of hepatocellular carcinoma and liver cirrhosis in asymptomatic chronic hepatitis B virus carriers. Am J Epidemiol. 1997;145:1039–1047.
17. Sun ZT, Lu PX, Gail MH, et al. Increased risk of hepatocellular carcinoma in male hepatitis B surface antigen carriers with chronic hepatitis who have detectable urinary aflatoxin metabolite M1. Hepatology. 1999;30:379–383.
18. Di Marco V, Lo I, Cammà C, et al. The long-term course of chronic hepatitis B. Hepatology. 1999;30:257–264.
19. Benvegnù L, Fattovich G, Noventa F, et al. Concurrent hepatitis B and C virus infection and risk of hepatocellular carcinoma in cirrhosis: A prospective study. Cancer. 1994;74:2442–2448.
20. Andreone P, Caraceni P, Grazi GL, et al. Lamivudine treatment for acute hepatitis B after liver transplantation. J Hepatol. 1998;29:985–989.
21. Altfeld M, Rockstroh JK, Addo M, et al. Reactivation of hepatitis B in a long-term anti-HBs-positive patient with AIDS following lamivudine withdrawal. J Hepatol. 1998;29:306–309.
22. Niederau C, Heintges T, Lange S, et al. Long-term follow-up of HBeAg-positive patients treated with interferon alpha for chronic hepatitis B. N Engl J Med. 1996;334:1422–1427.
23. Baptista M, Kramvis A, Kew MC. High prevalence of 1762^T 1764^A mutations in the basic core promoter of hepatitis B virus isolated from black Africans with hepatocellular carcinoma compared with asymptomatic carriers. Hepatology. 1999;29(3):946–953.
24. Barbera C, Calvo P, Coscia A, et al. Precore mutant hepatitis B virus and outcome of chronic infection and hepatitis in hepatitis B e antigen-positive children. Pediatr Res. 1994;36:347–350.
25. Chan HL, Hussain M, Lok AS. Different hepatitis B virus genotypes are associated with different mutations in the core promoter and precore regions during hepatitis B e antigen seroconversion. Hepatology. 1999;29:976–984.
26. Bozkaya H, Ayola B, Lok ASF. High rate of mutations in the hepatitis B core gene during the immune clearance phase of chronic hepatitis B virus infection. Hepatology. 1996;24:32–37.
27. Blitz L, Pujol FH, Swenson PD, et al. Antigenic diversity of hepatitis B virus strains of genotype F in Amerindians and other population groups from Venezuela. J Clin Microbiol. 1998;36:648–651.
28. Furusyo N, Hayashi J, Sawayama Y, Kishihara Y, Kashiwagi S. Hepatitis B surface antigen disappearance and hepatitis B surface antigen subtype: A prospective, long-term, follow-up study of Japanese residents of Okinawa, Japan with chronic hepatitis B virus infection. Am J Trop Med Hyg. 1999;60:616–622.
29. Fukuda R, Ishimura N, Niigaki M, Hamamoto S, Satoh S, Tanaka S et al. Serologically silent hepatitis B virus coinfection in patients with hepatitis C virus-associated chronic liver disease: Clinical and virological significance. J Med Virol. 1999;58:201–207.
30. Gilson RJC, Hawkins AE, Beecham MR, et al. Interactions between HIV and hepatitis B virus in homosexual men: Effects on the natural history of infection. AIDS. 1997;11:597–606.

8
Chronic hepatitis B: new therapies

J. M. HOARE, S. J. FORBES and H. C. THOMAS

INTRODUCTION

Advances in molecular biology and immunology have increased our knowledge of chronic hepatitis B and have led to the development of new therapies. Between 50 000 and 100 000 people acquire HBV infection each year in the USA[1] despite the availability of an effective vaccine. The outcome of infection is variable and depends on viral and host factors. It is estimated there are 350 million hepatitis B virus (HBV) carriers world-wide.

CHRONIC HEPATITIS B

The viruses

Two strains of HBV exist: HBe antigen positive and negative viruses[2,3]. Both cause significant liver disease and are candidates for anti-viral therapy. HBe antigen/antibody seroconversion is used as the indicator of clinical response when treating the HBe-positive infection. Response to therapy in HBe-negative patients is monitored with HBV DNA assays and ALT measurements.

Host factors

The outcome of HBV infection may be influenced by host immune responses. Variation of the immune response is dependent on polymorphism of 'immune response genes' within the major histocompatibility complex (MHC). Thursz et al. studied MHC class II genes in Gambia and found that HLA DRB1*1302 was associated with protection against persistent HBV infection in both children and adults[4]. In patients in whom genetic factors underlie viral persistence, stimulation of the host immune response to clear HBV infected cells may not be possible: in such cases viral suppressive therapy may be the way forward.

Treatment

Interferon-α

These have anti-viral and immunostimulatory properties and are currently used as monotherapy for HBV infection. In the future they may be usefully combined with nucleoside analogues to accelerate clearance of HBV infected hepatocytes and to prevent emergence of drug resistant variants.

Interferon-α (IFN) remains first-line treatment for HBeAg-positive HBV carriers but lamivudine is now challenging this position principally because of its equal efficacy combined with fewer side effects. Interferon-α therapy was cost-effective in a meta-analysis study of 552 HBeAg positive patients without cirrhosis[5]. With therapy 45.6% cleared HBeAg and 7.7% cleared HBsAg, compared to 9.1% and 1.7% clearing HBeAg and HBsAg respectively without therapy. Life expectancy increased by 3.1 years with quality adjusted life years increasing by 3.4 years.

Nucleoside analogues

These well-tolerated orally administered viral suppressant agents can be used to suppress HBV infection but drug resistant variants have started to emerge.

Lamivudine, the (–) enantiomer of 3′-thiacytidine, is more potent and less toxic than the (+) enantiomer and acts as a chain terminator of reverse transcriptase and DNA polymerase activity[6]. In a study of 32 chronic HBV patients, lamivudine transiently reduced HBV DNA to undetectable levels following 12 weeks' treatment[7]. In persistently infected patients, studies with lamivudine have found that HBV particles are cleared from the plasma with a half-life of approximately 1 day, implying a 50% daily turnover of the free virus population and total peripheral viral release of 10^{11} particles per day[8]. Twelve months of lamivudine gives sero-conversion rates of about 20%[9,10], consistent with this mathematical prediction and comparable to the results from interferon alpha monotherapy.

Adenine arabinoside 5′ monophosphate administered intramuscularly is a potent DNA polymerase inhibitor. It has a transient antiviral effect unless patients have low HBV replication pre-therapy[11,12]. Treatment is limited by neuropathic side effects, but liver targeting systems are now being developed.

Following 10 days' treatment with famciclovir (FCV), HBV DNA levels decreased by 90% in six of 11 evaluable patients[13]. HBV does not have thymidine kinase activity and it is thought that FCV has an inhibitory effect on HBV polymerase. Longer term therapy is currently being investigated.

One of the cited reasons for IFN treatment failure in HBV is persistence of hepatic supercoiled HBV DNA. Nalidixic acid combined with ganciclovir substantially reduced hepatic levels of viral supercoiled DNA, relaxed circular and single stranded DNA and viral RNA in ducks infected with duck HBV, whereas ganciclovir alone reduced DNA replication but not supercoiled DNA or RNA levels and nalidixic acid alone had no effect[14]. Following liver transplantation ganciclovir has been used to suppress HBV DNA levels[15] but with no established clinical benefit. Other nucleoside analogue studies of prolonged monotherapy or in combination with IFN are being assessed as maintenance therapy following liver transplantation.

Adefovir and lobucavir are new nucleoside analogues which are potent inhibitors of HBV replication[16]. Their role in clinical practice has yet to be established. They may be used as single agents or, more probably, in combination with lamivudine or interferon. Adefovir has activity against lamivudine resistant variants and clinical studies are progressing rapidly.

Fialuridine (FIAU) was discontinued following death in five of 15 patients from multisystem failure[17]. Subsequent studies suggest that FIAU is toxic to mitochondrial DNA[18].

Mathematical modelling and insights into new approaches to treatment

Mathematical modelling[8] has demonstrated that the half-life of the virus in peripheral blood is less than 24 h, but the half life of the virus-infected cell ranges from 10 to 100 days. The protracted half life of the virus-infected cell suggests that even when viral suppressive therapy is 100% effective in inhibition of virion production, cure, which is dependent on the clearance of the last HBV-infected cell, can take between 1 and 10 years, dependent on the infected cell half-life. This will be influenced by the rate of recovery of the endogenous anti-viral immune response[19]. When antiviral therapy is less than 100% effective, protracted periods of treatment with single inhibitors of viral replication often result in the emergence of variants which are resistant to the antiviral drug.

In order to shorten the period of treatment required to produce cure, one needs to add to viral suppressive therapy, agents that have immunostimulatory functions thereby accelerating the rate of lysis of HBV infected cells. Potential approaches include:

- Interferon-α, which has been shown to stimulate both CD4 and CD8 T-cell responses to virus infected antigens, resulting in HBV clearance in a proportion (up to 40%) of cases[20].
- Interleukin 2, which has been tried in small trials as a method of amplifying CD4 helper T-cell responses, but in the main has been of limited value because of the toxicity of this compound.
- Interleukin 12, which has the capacity to amplify TH1/CD8 anti-viral responses. This compound has activity against HBV but is insufficient as monotherapy. In in vitro experiments IL12 requires the presence of IL18 and IL2 to amplify TH1 responses. It remains to be seen whether these approaches can be used successfully with compounds such as interferon alpha or nucleoside analogues such as lamivudine.
- Interleukin 2, 12 and 18 combined with antigen-specific stimulation by co-injection of viral antigens or peptides. Cytokines may also be added to viral DNA vaccines again as a method of amplifying the antiviral immune response accelerating clearance of virus infected cells. DNA vaccines are potent inducers of cellular immunity and may find utility in this role in the therapy of HBV. Current problems include methods of delivery and dosages required to induce appropriate responses.
- The ideal combination may involve viral suppressive therapy combined with immuno stimulatory therapy of the type described. Immunostimulatory approaches may deal with the problem of emergence of drug-resistant variants in that the immune response should be capable of controlling cells supporting replication of these variants as they emerge. This problem may also be

controlled, as has been shown in the case of HIV, by the administration of several viral suppressive drugs simultaneously. Here addition of adefovir to lamivudine may contribute.

- Most of the cytokines which amplify the immune response, including interferon-α, interferon-γ, interleukin-2, interleukin-12 and interleukin-18 are all relatively toxic; this limits their clinical usefulness. Techniques allowing the local production of cytokines within the infected liver would improve this aspect of therapy. Liver specific gene delivery systems could be used for delivery of pro-drug activating enzymes (thymidine kinase for activation of ganciclovir, famciclovir or acyclovir) or cytokines such as interleukin-2, 12 and 18 which amplify the CD4 and CD8 antiviral responses respectively, or interferon α which generates a local antiviral effect.

  A number of methods for gene delivery to liver cells, based on viral and non-viral systems have been investigated. Non-viral delivery systems have tended to have a low efficiency of uptake, e.g. liposomes, or are relatively complex to synthesize, e.g. receptor-mediated uptake. The in vivo transduction efficiencies of retroviruses are at present limited and there are theoretical concerns regarding introducing a second integrating virus into the liver[21]. Adenoviruses have been the hepatotropic vectors most frequently used to date but there is still considerable concern regarding toxicity and inactivation mediated by pre-existing antibodies[22]. An interesting alternative viral vector is the insect baculovirus, *Autographa californica*, which efficiently expresses transgenes in hepatocytes, is unable to replicate in mammalian cells and is not cytopathic; however, its in vivo use is hampered by complement-mediated inactivation[23].
- There are many technical problems to be overcome before liver directed gene therapy against chronic viral hepatitis becomes a practical possibility, and the solution is likely to involve elements from many of the current approaches. An attractive and potentially simpler alternative to provide immunomodulation alongside antiviral therapy is DNA vaccination. In 1994 it was shown that HBV DNA injected into regenerating skeletal muscle was effective at producing a humoral response to HBsAg[24]. Using the duck model of chronic HBV infection, vaccination with DNA coding for envelope proteins has been shown to clear viral particles from the serum[25]. Woodchucks immunized with woodchuck hepatitis core protein developed high antibody titres and were protected against viraemia after challenge with the virus[26]. In viraemic patients preliminary studies indicate that vaccination with HBsAg produces a significant reduction in serum HBV DNA levels in half of recipients[27]. It may be that DNA vaccination into sites remote from the liver overcomes the immune anergy associated with chronic infection by reactivating the TH1-mediated immune response[28].

CHRONIC HEPATITIS D

Superinfection of chronic hepatitis B patients with HDV is seen mainly in intravenous drug users in Northern Europe and in the general population in Mediterranean countries but with decreasing frequency. Since expression of HBs antigen is required to support replication of HDV, therapy of HDV superinfected HBV cases, has been directed to control of HBV with either interferon-α or lamivudine. Results have been disappointing in that relapse rates have been very high after an initial encouraging response[29,30]. Only when HBs antigen is cleared has a durable HDV response been obtained.

Ribozyme approaches are currently being looked at in experimental systems and may eventually be of value in clearing intracellular virus in this and other infections.

CONCLUSIONS

HBV infection remains a major cause of morbidity and mortality, with universal vaccination probably offering the best strategy to eradicate HBV infection both medically and economically. The importance of the HBV surface antigen variants[31] is now becoming evident: 0.8% of vaccinated infants born to HBV-infected mothers develop persistent G145A variant infection[32].

We now have available to us enzyme specific inhibitors of viral replication, recombinant viral proteins, cytokines which selectively amplify TH1 and TH2 responses and potent inducers of cellular antiviral states, and it should be possible to cure an increasing proportion of this large patient population in the coming years. Interferon alpha and lamivudine are now the mainstay of therapy: up to 40% of HBe antigen-positive patients clear HBe antigen and HBV DNA with resolution of their hepatitis: this probably represents a 'sustained response' but emergence of the HBe antigen-negative variant is still a possibility in those that remain HBs antigen positive. Long-term viral suppression with lamivudine or adefovir are alternative experimental approaches but this approach is compromised by the emergence of drug resistant variants. This may be overcome by drug combinations. The most attractive approach combines potent inhibitors of viral replication with immunostimulants.

REFERENCES

1. Moradpour D, Wands JR. Understanding hepatitis B infection. N Engl J Med. 1995;332:1092–3.
2. Carman WF, Jacyna MR, Hadziyannis S, Karaiyannis P, McGarvey MJ, Makris A, Thomas HC. Mutation preventing formation of hepatitis HB e antigen in chronic hepatitis B virus infection. Lancet. 1989;II:588–91.
3. Hadziyannis SJ. Hepatitis B e antigen negative chronic hepatitis B: from clinical recognition to pathogenesis and treatment. Viral Hepatitis Rev. 1995;1:7–36.
4. Thursz MR, Kwiatkowski D, Allsopp CEM, Greenwood BM, Thomas HC, Hill AVS. Association between an MHC class II allele and clearance of hepatitis B virus in the Gambia. N Engl J Med. 1995;332:1065–9.
5. Wong JB, Koff RS, Tine F, Pauker SG. Cost-effectiveness of interferon-alpha 2b treatment for hepatitis B e antigen-positive chronic hepatitis B. Ann Intern Med. 1995;122:664–75.
6. Severini A, Liu XY, Wilson JS, Tyrrell DLJ. Mechanism of inhibition of duck hepatitis B virus polymerase by (–)-beta-L-2′,3′-dideoxy-3′-thiacytidine. Antimicrob Agents Chemother. 1995;39:1430–5.
7. Dienstag JL, Perrillo RP, Schiff ER, Bartholomew M, Vicary C, Rubin M. A preliminary trial of lamivudine for chronic hepatitis B infection. New Engl J Med. 1995;333:1657–61.
8. Nowak MA, Bonhoeffer S, Hill AM, Boehme R, Thomas HC, McDade H. Viral dynamics in hepatitis B infection. Proc Natl Acad Sci USA. 1996;93:4398–402.
9. Nevens F, Main J, Honkoop P, Tyrrell DL, Barber J, Sullivan MT, Fevery J et al. Lamivudine therapy for chronic hepatitis B: a six-month randomized dose-ranging study. Gastroenterology. 1997;113:1258–63.

10. Dienstag JL, Schiff ER, Wright TL, Perrillo RP, Hann HW, Goodman Z et al. Lamivudine as initial treatment for chronic hepatitis B in the United States. N Engl J Med. 1999;341:1256–63.
11. Brook MG, Petrovic L, McDonald JA, Scheuer PJ, Thomas HC. Histological improvement after anti-viral treatment for chronic hepatitis B virus infection. J Hepatol. 1989;8:218–25.
12. Marcellin P, Pouteau M, Loriot MA, Boyer N, Desgos F, Cales P et al. Adenine arabinoside 5′ monophosphate in patients with chronic hepatitis B: comparison of the efficacy in patients with high and low viral replication. Gut. 1995;36:422–6.
13. Main J, Brown JL, Howels C, Galassini R, Crossley M, Karayiannis P et al. A double blind placebo controlled study to assess the effect of famciclovir on viral replication in patients with chronic hepatitis B virus infection. J Viral Hepatitis. 1996;3:211–15.
14. Wang YL, Luscombe C, Bowden S, Shaw T, Locarnini S. Inhibition of duck hepatitis B virus DNA replication by anti-viral chemotherapy with ganciclovir–nalidixic acid. Antimicrob Agents Chemother. 1995;39:556–8.
15. Gish RG, Lau JY, Brooks L, Fang JW, Steady SL, Imperial JC et al. Ganciclovir treatment of hepatitis B infection in liver transplant recipients. Hepatology. 1996;23:1–7.
16. Tsiang M, Rooney JF, Toole JJ, Gibbs CS. Biphasic clearance kinetics of hepatitis B virus from patients during adefovir dipivoxil therapy. Hepatology. 1999;29:1863–9.
17. McKenzie R, Fried MW, Sallie R, Conjeevaram H, Di Biscegli AM, Park Y et al. Hepatic failure and lactic acidosis due to fialuridine (FIAU), an investigational nucleoside analogue for chronic hepatitis B. New Engl J Med. 1995;333:1099–105.
18. Cui L, Yoon S, Schinazi R, Sommadossi JP. Cellular and molecular events leading to mitochondrial toxicity of 1-(2-deoxy-2-fluoro-1-b-d-arabinofuranosyl)-5-idouracil in human liver cells. J Clin Invest. 1995;95:555–63.
19. Ferrari C, Penna A, Bertoletti A, Cavalli A, Missale G, Lamonaca V et al. Antiviral cell-mediated immune responses during hepatitis B and hepatitis C virus infections. Recent Res Cancer Res. 1998;154:330–6.
20. Waters JA, O'Rourke S, Schlict H-J, Thomas HC. Cytotoxic T cell responses in patients with chronic hepatitis B virus infection undergoing HBe antigen/antibody seroconversion. Clin Exp Immunol. 1995;102:314–19.
21. Verma IM, Somia N. Gene therapy – promises, problems and prospects (news). Nature. 1997;389:239–42.
22. Smaglik P. Tighter watch urged on adenoviral vectors. Nature. 1999;402:707.
23. Hofmann C, Strauss M. Baculovirus-mediated gene transfer in the presence of human serum or blood facilitated by inhibition of the complement system. Gene Ther. 1998;5:531–6.
24. Davis HL et al. Direct gene transfer in skeletal muscle: plasmid DNA-based immunisation against the hepatitis B virus surface antigen. Vaccine. 1999;12:1503–9.
25. Triyatni M et al. Protective efficacy of DNA vaccines against duck hepatitis B virus infection. J Virol. 1998;72:84–94.
26. Roos S et al. Protection of woodchucks from infection with woodchuck hepatitis virus by immunization with recombinant core protein. J Gen Virol. 1989;70:2087–95.
27. Pol S et al. Immunotherapy of chronic hepatitis B by anti HBV vaccine. Acta Gastroenterol Belg. 1998;61:228–33.
28. Couillin I et al. Specific vaccine therapy in chronic hepatitis B: induction of T cell proliferative responses specific for envelope antigens. J Infect Dis. 1999;180:15–26.
29. Saracco G, Rizzetto M. A practical guide to the use of interferons in the management of hepatitis virus infections. Drugs. 1997;53:74–85.
30. Lau DT, Doo E, Park Y, Kleiner DE, Schmid P, Kuhns MC, Hoofnagle JH. Lamivudine for chronic delta hepatitis. Hepatology. 1999;30:546–9.
31. Wilson JN, Nokes DJ, Carman WF. The predicted pattern of emergence of vaccine-resistant hepatitis B: a cause for concern? Vaccine. 1999;17:973–8.
32. Zuckerman AJ, Zuckerman JN. Molecular epidemiology of hepatitis B virus mutants. J Med Virol. 1999;58:193–5.

9
Virology and diagnosis of hepatitis C

D. MORADPOUR and H. E. BLUM

Since the identification of the hepatitis C virus (HCV) as the most common cause of post-transfusion and sporadic non-A, non-B hepatitis[1,2] important aspects of the molecular virology, epidemiology and natural course of hepatitis C have been elucidated. In addition, specific and sensitive assays for the diagnosis of HCV infection have been developed. Important aspects of the molecular biology of HCV, the pathogenesis of HCV-induced liver disease as well as many therapeutic and preventive issues of hepatitis C still need to be resolved, however.

It is estimated that 100–200 million people worldwide are infected with HCV. The prevalence of anti-HCV as a marker of past or present HCV infection is about 1% in Western Europe and North America, 3–4% in some Mediterranean and Asian countries and up to 15% in parts of Central Africa and Egypt[3–5]. With the introduction of anti-HCV screening of blood and blood products in 1990 the risk of post-transfusion hepatitis C has decreased from 0.45% to 0.001% per unit of blood transfused[6]. However, spread of the virus through other routes, such as intravenous drug use and rarely sexual transmission, needle stick injuries, mother-to-infant transmission, and iatrogenic routes, including organ transplantation, will continue as long as no protective vaccine is available. For up to 40% of patients with hepatitis C no epidemiological risk factor can be identified (sporadic hepatitis C). In addition, a substantial proportion of the large number of patients with chronic hepatitis C will present with long-term sequelae in the future, resulting among others in an increasing incidence of hepatocellular carcinoma (HCC)[7,8].

In Western countries, HCV infection accounts for approximately 25% of cases of acute sporadic hepatitis[9,10]. After an incubation period of 3–12 weeks HCV infection is usually followed by a clinically inapparent hepatitis. Only about 25% of cases are symptomatic. One of the most important features of hepatitis C is its progression to chronicity in more than 80% of cases. The natural course of chronic hepatitis C is highly variable and may depend on viral (e.g. inoculum size, genotype, and quasispecies complexity) and host factors (e.g. age at the time of infection, gender, major histocompatibility complex (MHC) haplotype, coinfection with hepatitis B virus (HBV) or human immunodeficiency virus

(HIV), and alcohol consumption). Overall, about 20% of patients with chronic hepatitis C will develop liver cirrhosis. Once cirrhosis is established the rate of HCC development is 1–4% per year[11–13].

In the following we will briefly review the current knowledge of the virology and diagnosis of hepatitis C. Also, we will try to provide a perspective on how progress in this field has allowed the identification of novel targets for antiviral intervention.

VIROLOGY OF HEPATITIS C

The structure and replication cycle of HCV are incompletely understood due to the lack of an efficient cell culture system permissive for HCV infection and the low viral titres commonly found in sera and livers of HCV-infected individuals. Nevertheless, considerable progress in the understanding of the virology of hepatitis C has been made using heterologous expression systems[14–16].

Genetic organization and polyprotein processing of HCV

HCV has been classified in the Hepacivirus genus within the Flaviviridae family of viruses which includes the classical flaviviruses, such as yellow fever virus, and the animal pestiviruses (Table 1)[17,18]. All of these viruses are enveloped positive-strand RNA viruses which express their proteins *via* translation of a single long open reading frame (ORF). Only recently has HCV been visualized by electron microscopy as a 50–60 nm particle of spherical shape[19,20].

HCV contains a single-stranded, positive-sense RNA genome of approximately 9600 nucleotides[21–23]. Functional HCV cDNA clones[24–28] and selectable subgenomic replicons[29] have recently been constructed. As in flavi- and pestiviruses, the viral genome is composed of a 5′ non-coding region (5′ NCR), a long ORF encoding a polyprotein precursor of about 3000 amino acids, and a 3′ NCR (Fig. 1). The 5′ NCR is highly conserved among different HCV genotypes and functions as an internal ribosomal entry site (IRES) essential for cap-independent translation of the viral RNA[30,31]. A highly conserved 98 nucleotide RNA element, predicted to form a stable stem-loop structure and likewise found to be required for HCV replication in vivo, has recently been identified at the 3′ terminus of the viral genome[32–34].

Table 1 Classification of flaviviruses

Family	*Genus*	*Species examples*
Flaviviridae	Flavivirus	Yellow fever virus (YFV)
		Tick-borne encephalitis virus (TBEV)
		Japanese encephalitis virus (JEV)
		Dengue virus (DENV-1, -2, -3, -4)
	Pestivirus	Bovine viral diarrhoea virus (BVDV)
		Classical swine fever virus (CSFV)
		Border disease virus (BDV)
	Hepacivirus	Hepatitis C virus (HCV)
	Unassigned	GB viruses (GBV)-A, -B, -C (HGV)

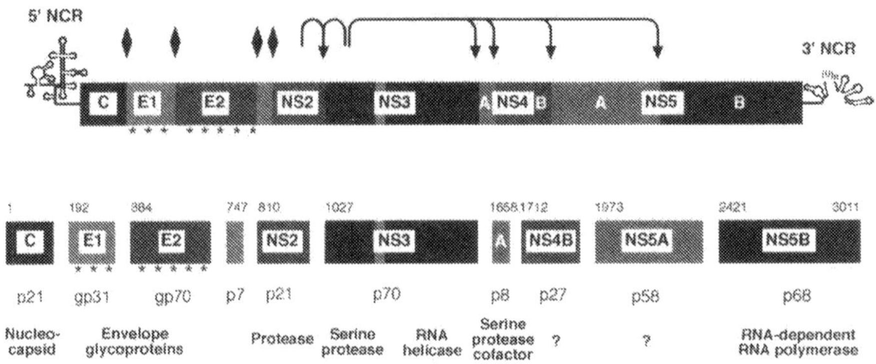

Figure 1 Genetic organization and polyprotein processing of HCV. Asterisks in the E1 and E2 region indicate glycosylation of the envelope proteins. Diamonds denote cleavages of the HCV polyprotein precursor by the ER signal peptidase and arrows indicate cleavages by HCV NS2-3 and NS3 proteases. The position of the first amino acid (Hutchinson strain) is indicated above each protein.

The HCV polyprotein precursor is co- and post-translationally processed by cellular and viral proteases to yield the mature structural and non-structural proteins[35]. The first structural protein encoded by the HCV ORF is the highly basic RNA-binding core protein which presumably forms the viral nucleocapsid[36–38]. This is followed by the envelope proteins E1 and E2 which are glycosylated and form non-covalent heterodimers[39–41]. The structural proteins core, E1, and E2 are released from the polyprotein precursor by the endoplasmic reticulum signal peptidase of the host cell[36,42].

Intriguingly, a number of functional properties have recently been postulated for the core protein. These include among others *trans*-suppression of various promoters[43–45] and of HBV replication[46,47], interaction with tumour necrosis factor-α (TNF-α) receptor family members[48–51], malignant transformation potential[44,45,52–54], induction[50,55] or suppression[56,57] of apoptosis, and immunosuppression[58]. Clearly, the relevance of these in vitro findings for the viral life cycle and the pathogenesis of hepatitis C need to be further investigated.

Recently, the envelope glycoprotein E2 has been reported to interact with CD81 (TAPA-1) as a potential cellular receptor or component of a receptor complex for HCV[59,60]. In addition, E2 has been reported to interact with and repress the catalytic activity of the interferon (IFN)-induced double-stranded RNA-activated protein kinase PKR[61].

The non-structural proteins NS2–NS5 include two viral proteases essential for processing of the polyprotein precursor, an RNA helicase located in the carboxyterminal region of NS3, the NS4A polypeptide, the NS4B and NS5A proteins, and an RNA-dependent RNA polymerase represented by NS5B[62–66]. The non-structural proteins, together with as yet unidentified host cell components, are believed to form a membrane-associated cytoplasmic replication complex[67,68]. Cleavage of the polyprotein precursor at the NS2–NS3 junction is accomplished in cis by an autoprotease encoded by NS2 and the aminoterminal one-third of NS3[69,70]. A distinct serine protease located in the aminoterminal one-third of NS3 is responsible for the downstream cleavages in the non-structural region[71–73]. The crystal structures of the serine protease[74–76] and RNA helicase domains of NS3[77,78] and, more recently, of the entire NS3 protein[79] have been elucidated. In addition, the three-dimensional structure of the RNA-dependent RNA polymerase has been identified[80]. These enzymes have emerged as major targets in the design of novel antiviral agents. The NS4A polypeptide functions as a cofactor for the NS3 serine protease and is incorporated as an integral component into the enzyme core[74,81,82]. The functions of NS4B and NS5A, a serine phosphoprotein[83–85], remain to be established. Similar to E2, NS5A has been reported to interfere with PKR function. A role for NS5A in modulating the IFN-α response was first suggested by studies performed in Japan by Enomoto et al. These investigators found a correlation between mutations within a discrete region of NS5A, termed interferon sensitivity determining region (ISDR), and a favourable response to IFN-α therapy[86,87]. These findings were largely confirmed in Japan, but not in Europe and North America[88]. The reasons for this discrepancy are not understood but may involve both differences in doses and regimens of IFN-α treatment and the low prevalence of 'mutant type' HCV genotype 1b isolates in Western countries[89]. Interestingly, an interaction with and repression of the catalytic activity of PKR by NS5A has been found by biochemical, transfection and yeast functional analyses[90,91]. In addition, disruption of PKR-dependent translational control and apoptotic programs by NS5A has been suggested to confer oncogenic potential to HCV[92]. Finally, a recent study has provided evidence for a src homology 3 (SH3) domain-dependent interaction of NS5A with growth factor receptor-bound protein 2 (Grb2) adaptor protein which could interfere with mitogenic signal transduction pathways[93].

Taken together, the presumed life cycle of HCV includes binding to an as yet unidentified cell surface receptor, internalization into the host cell, cytoplasmic

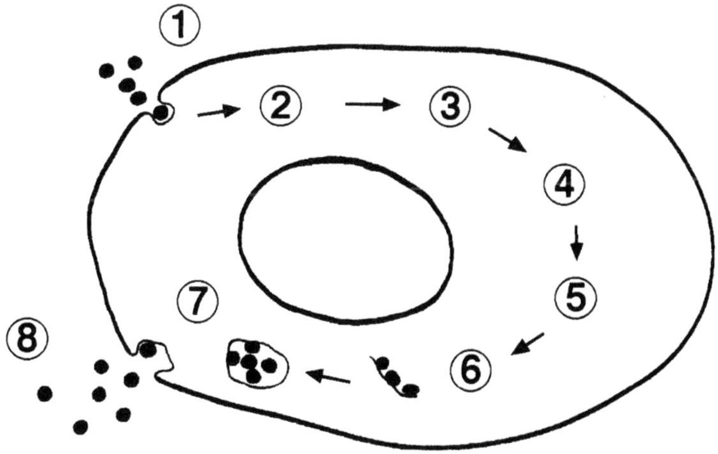

Figure 2 HCV life cycle. (1) Virus binding and internalization, (2) cytoplasmic release and uncoating, (3) IRES-mediated translation, (4) polyprotein processing, (5) RNA replication, (6) packaging and assembly, (7) virion maturation, (8) virion release.

release and uncoating of the viral RNA genome, IRES-mediated translation, polyprotein processing by cellular and viral proteases, RNA replication, packaging and assembly, virion maturation, and release from the host cell (Fig. 2). Particularly the early and late steps of this process are poorly understood due to the lack of efficient cell culture systems. As mentioned above, CD81 (TAPA-1) has recently been identified as potential HCV receptor or component of a receptor complex[59]. In the case of the related tick-borne encephalitis virus the three-dimensional structure of the envelope glycoprotein has been identified and cellular uptake by receptor-mediated endocytosis and endosomal release by pH-dependent fusion have been shown[94,95]. Various members of the Flaviviridae family assemble and mature on intracellular membranes and cytoplasmic vesicles[14,96–99]. Knowledge of these related viruses, for which efficient cell culture systems exist, may facilitate further investigations of the HCV life cycle.

The rapidly increasing knowledge of the HCV life cycle will provide opportunities for the development of innovative therapeutic and preventive strategies. As outlined above, the biochemically well characterized NS3 serine protease, the RNA helicase, and the RNA-dependent RNA polymerase have emerged as major targets in the design of specific inhibitors as antiviral agents. Efforts in this direction have been facilitated by the elucidation of the crystal structures of these essential viral enzymes. In addition to these more classical pharmacological approaches, gene therapeutic strategies aimed at inhibiting HCV gene expression and replication are currently being explored in various experimental systems[100]. These include antisense oligodeoxynucleotides[101–105] and RNA constructs[106], ribozymes[107], a small yeast RNA capable of specifically inhibiting internal ribosome entry site-mediated translation[108], and RNA aptamers[109]. Moreover, based on the concept that a quantitatively and qualitatively insufficient $CD4^+$ and $CD8^+$ T cell response may contribute to viral persistence, immunotherapeutic strategies aimed at enhancing the cellular immune response against HCV are currently being investigated. These include, among others, DNA vaccination[110], peptide or protein vaccines[111], and adoptive immunotherapy.

Genetic variability of HCV

Recent studies have suggested that HCV infection is a highly dynamic process with a viral half-life of only a few hours and average daily virion production and clearance rates of up to more than 10^{12} [112–115]. These findings are similar to the dynamics of HIV infection[116,117] and provide a rationale for the development and implementation of multidrug combination therapies against hepatitis C. In addition, together with the lack of a proof-reading function of the viral RNA-dependent RNA polymerase this high replicative activity provides the basis for the genetic variability of HCV. HCV isolates fall into three major categories, depending on the degree of sequence divergence: genotypes, subtypes, and isolates[118,119]. The term quasispecies refers to the genetic heterogeneity of the population of HCV genomes co-existing in a single infected individual[118,120]. The quasispecies nature of HCV may have important implications for the pathogenesis, natural course and prevention of hepatitis C. Through the acceptance of a nomenclature for HCV genotypes and subtypes, it was possible to systematically collect and compare HCV sequence data[121]. More recently, it was proposed to divide HCV isolates into six phylogenetically distinct groups, termed clades 1–6[18]. Clades 1, 2, 4, and 5 correspond to genotypes 1, 2, 4, and 5 while clade 3 comprises genotypes 3 and 10, and clade 6 comprises genotypes 6, 7, 8, 9, and 11. A database of all available HCV sequences can be found in the internet at http://s2as02.genes.nig.ac.jp/.

Even though mutations have been identified in all regions of the HCV genome, the genes encoding the envelope glycoproteins E1 and E2 appear to be particularly variable. A hypervariable region (HVR) of approximately 28 amino acids in the aminoterminal domain of E2 has been termed HVR1[122,123]. Another HVR within E2 (HVR2) has been observed among certain HCV isolates[122]. Depending on structural and functional constraints, the mutation rate varies significantly in the various regions of the HCV genome, with the NCRs and the core region being the most conserved (< 0.1% changes per site and year) and E1 and E2 being the most variable regions (0.2–0.4% changes per site and year)[124,125].

The relationship between defined genetic HCV variants and their biological or clinical implications has yet to be defined. Several studies have shown that genotype 1 is associated with a poor response to IFN-α therapy[126–128].

Cell culture systems and animal models

Evidence for low-level replication of HCV in cultured cells was obtained in human B and T cell lines[20,129–132], primary human[133,134] and chimpanzee hepatocytes[135], and biliary epithelial cells[136]. In this context, during natural infection in vivo HCV appears to infect not only hepatocytes, but also other cell and tissue types, particularly of the hematopoietic system[137–141]. The frequency and clinical significance of extrahepatic HCV infection in vivo, however, remain to be determined[142]. In terms of demonstrating low-level HCV replication in vitro, specific detection of minus-strand RNA as a HCV replicative intermediate by PCR is problematic. In addition, viral proteins could not be detected consistently in these cell culture systems. A major breakthrough was recently achieved with the construction of selectable subgenomic HCV replicons that efficiently replicate in the human HCC cell line HuH-7[29]. In addition, recombinant cell culture systems are being developed that will allow the investigation of structural and functional properties of HCV proteins, their interactions with cellular proteins and pathways, and the evaluation of novel antiviral strategies against hepatitis C[143–145].

Humans are the only natural host of HCV and chimpanzees are the only established animal model for HCV infection[146–148]. The tree shrew *Tupaia belangeri chinensis* has recently been reported to be susceptible to HCV infection and is currently being investigated as a potentially useful small animal model[149]. A number of transgenic mice expressing either constitutively or inducibly subgenomic HCV sequences have been described[150–155]. In most cases, expression of HCV proteins did not result in any pathological changes in the liver. A sialadenitis histologically resembling Sjögren's syndrome was described in envelope protein transgenic mice[152] and liver steatosis and HCC have been found to develop in certain strains of HCV core transgenic mice[54,155]. Finally, immunodeficient mice may represent an interesting model system to study selected aspects of HCV in vivo[156].

DIAGNOSIS OF HEPATITIS C

Diagnosis of hepatitis C is based on serological assays which detect HCV-specific antibodies (anti-HCV) and on molecular assays which detect HCV RNA. The molecular assays currently available are reverse transcriptase (RT)-PCR and the branched DNA (bDNA) assay. By RT-PCR the viral RNA is reverse transcribed into complementary DNA (cDNA) that is then amplified by PCR. In the bDNA assay the signal resulting from a specific hybridization of capture and detection probes with the viral RNA is amplified.

Serological assays for anti-HCV antibodies were developed based on recombinant structural and non-structural proteins. Using the first generation C-100 anti-HCV test, about 90% of patients with non-A, non-B post-transfusion hepatitis and about 60% of those with sporadic non-A, non-B hepatitis were found to be positive[2]. Subsequently, the sensitivity and specificity of the C-100 anti-HCV test has been improved by the inclusion of additional viral antigens (second and third generation ELISAs) and the development of a supplemental assay (recombinant immunoblot assays, RIBA)[157]. Third-generation anti-HCV tests contain antigens from the HCV core, NS3, NS4, and NS5 genes. No routine serological test for a viral antigen is available as yet. As a potentially major diagnostic advance, an immunoassay based on the use of two high-affinity monoclonal antibodies against core protein to detect and quantitate HCV in serum has been described[158–161]. If validated, this assay system would allow to directly demonstrate viraemia by serology, thereby reducing the need for molecular analyses.

The detection of HCV RNA by RT-PCR amplification clearly has broadened the diagnostic spectrum. With this method HCV is positive as early as 1–2 weeks after infection and 4–6 weeks before anti-HCV seroconversion. The determination of HCV RNA as the only marker of viraemia is, in principle, important for the selection of patients for antiviral therapy and for the assessment of its efficacy[127,128,162]. Optimal PCR assays at present have a sensitivity of less than 100 copies of HCV RNA per milliliter of plasma or serum. RT-PCR amplification, however, is difficult to standardize. Frequent false-positive and/or false-negative results, therefore, represent a major limitation of this technology in clinical practice[163,164]. Standardization and proficiency testing of diagnostic laboratories performing HCV PCR remains an important problem for further study. While the bDNA assay is less sensitive than RT-PCR (200 000 genome equivalents/ml), it is easier to handle, less contamination-prone, and allows the quantitation of viraemia[157,165].

Real-time detection (RTD-) PCR represents a novel highly sensitive and accurate method to quantify HCV viraemia[166]. RTD-PCR takes advantage of the RT and 5′-3′ nuclease activity of *Taq* DNA polymerase to digest a probe labeled with a fluorescent reporter and a quencher dye. This probe is designed to hybridize to a region between the PCR primers and is added directly to the PCR reaction mixture. During PCR, the probe hybridizes to the template and is digested as the Taq DNA polymerase extends the PCR primer. Digestion of the probe releases the fluorescent reporter from the activity of the quencher, and successive PCR cycles result in exponential amplification of the PCR product and fluorescence intensity which can be continuously monitored.

At the tissue level, HCV proteins or RNA can be identified by immunostaining[167], in situ hybridization[168], or in situ RT-PCR[169]. To date, however, these analyses are reserved for selected clinical cases or research purposes[170,171].

Genotypes can be determined by RT-PCR, followed by sequence analysis of regions for which sufficient reference data are available (C, E1, NS5B)[118]. Alternatively, the second round of PCR amplification can be performed with type-specific primers or the amplified segment can be hybridized with type-specific probes (e.g., line probe (LIPA) assay) or analyzed by restriction fragment length polymorphism (RFLP)[118,119]. Serological typing methods are based on the detection of type-specific antibodies to epitopes of HCV that differ between genotypes[118,119]. Based on the results of recent large, randomized, controlled multicenter trials of IFN-α plus ribavirin combination therapy[172–175], discrimination of genotype 1 from genotypes 2 and 3 as well as quantitative determination of viraemia levels has become important for the selection of the optimal treatment regimen[128].

SUMMARY AND PERSPECTIVES

Since the identification of HCV in 1989 important aspects of the virology and diagnosis of hepatitis C have been elucidated. Important steps of the viral life cycle, including IRES-mediated translation and polyprotein processing are now understood in great detail. The function, and in the case of NS3 and NS5B the three-dimensional structure, of most of the viral proteins has been characterized. In addition, functional HCV cDNA clones and selectable subgenomic replicons have been constructed. These advances have allowed the identification of novel antiviral targets such as the viral NS3 serine protease, the RNA helicase, and the RNA-dependent RNA polymerase. In addition, gene therapeutic strategies aimed at inhibiting HCV gene expression and replication as well as immunotherapeutic concepts aimed at enhancing the cellular immune response against HCV are being explored in various experimental systems. These and other novel antiviral strategies may complement the existing therapeutic modalities in the future. Much work remains to be done with respect to HCV virion structure, the early and late steps of the viral life cycle, and the pathogenesis of HCV induced liver disease. Progress in these directions will depend, among others, on the development of efficient cell culture systems and small animal models of hepatitis C. Ultimately, an improved understanding of the viral life cycle should result in innovative therapeutic and preventive modalities for one of the most common causes of chronic hepatitis, liver cirrhosis, and HCC worldwide.

ACKNOWLEDGMENT

The authors acknowledge support by grants Mo 799/1-1 and 799/1-2 from the Deutsche Forschungsgemeinschaft.

REFERENCES

1. Choo Q-L, Kuo G, Weiner AJ, Overby LR, Bradley DW, Houghton M. Isolation of a cDNA clone derived from a blood-borne non-A, non-B viral hepatitis genome. Science. 1989;244:359–62.
2. Kuo G, Choo Q-L, Alter HJ et al. An assay for circulating antibodies to a major etiologic virus of human non-A, non-B hepatitis. Science. 1989;244:362–4.
3. Alter MJ. Epidemiology of hepatitis C. Hepatology. 1997;26(Suppl 1):62S–5S.
4. Heintges T, Wands JR. Hepatitis C virus: epidemiology and transmission. Hepatology. 1997;26:521–6.
5. Alter MJ, Kruszon-Moran D, Nainan OV et al. The prevalence of hepatitis C virus infection in the United States, 1988 through 1994. N Engl J Med. 1999;341:556–62.
6. Schreiber GB, Busch MP, Kleinman SH, Korelitz JJ, Study ftRED. The risk of transfusion-transmitted viral infections. N Engl J Med. 1996;334:1685–90.
7. Deuffic S, Buffat L, Poynard T, Valleron AJ. Modeling the hepatitis C virus epidemic in France. Hepatology. 1999;29:1596–1601.
8. El-Serag HB, Mason AC. Rising incidence of hepatocellular carcinoma in the United States. N Engl J Med. 1999;340:745–50.
9. Alter MJ. Epidemiology of hepatitis C in the West. Semin Liver Dis. 1995;15:5–14.
10. Hoofnagle JH. Hepatitis C: the clinical spectrum of disease. Hepatology. 1997;26(Suppl 1):15S–20S.
11. Kiyosawa K, Sodeyama T, Tanaka E et al. Interrelationship of blood transfusion, non-A, non-B hepatitis and hepatocellular carcinoma: analysis by detection of antibody to hepatitis C virus. Hepatology. 1990;12:671–5.
12. Di Bisceglie AM. Hepatitis C and hepatocellular carcinoma. Hepatology. 1997;26(Suppl 1):34S–8S.
13. Seeff LB. Natural history of hepatitis C. Hepatology. 1997;26(Suppl 1):21S–8S.
14. Rice CM. Flaviviridae: the viruses and their replication. In: Fields BN, Knipe DM, Howley PM, eds. Fields Virology. Third edn. Philadelphia: Lippincott-Raven. 1996: pp. 931–59.
15. Major ME, Feinstone SM. The molecular virology of hepatitis C. Hepatology. 1997;25:1527–38.
16. Reed KE, Rice CM. Molecular characterization of hepatitis C virus. Curr Stud Hematol Blood Transfus. 1998;62:1–37.
17. Wengler G, Bradley DW, Collett MS, Heinz FX, Schlesinger RW, Strauss JH. Family Flaviviridae. In: Murphy FA, Fauquet CM, Bishop DHL et al., eds. Classification and nomenclature of viruses. Sixth report of the International Committee on Taxonomy of Viruses. New York: Springer-Verlag, 1995: pp. 415–27.
18. Robertson B, Myers G, Howard C et al. Classification, nomenclature, and database development for hepatitis C virus (HCV) and related viruses: proposals for standardization. Arch Virol. 1998;143:2493–2503.
19. Kaito M, Watanabe S, Tsukiyama-Kohara K et al. Hepatitis C virus particle detected by immunoelectron microscopy study. J Gen Virol. 1994;75:1755–60.
20. Shimizu YK, Feinstone SM, Kohara M, Purcell RH, Yoshikura H. Hepatitis C virus: detection of intracellular virus particles by electron microscopy. Hepatology. 1996;23:205–9.
21. Kato N, Hijikata M, Ootsuyama Y et al. Molecular cloning of the human hepatitis C virus genome from Japanese patients with non-A, non-B hepatitis. Proc Natl Acad Sci USA. 1990;87:9524–8.
22. Choo Q-L, Richman KH, Han JH et al. Genetic organization and diversity of the hepatitis C virus. Proc Natl Acad Sci USA. 1991;88:2451–5.
23. Takamizawa A, Mori C, Fuke I et al. Structure and organization of the hepatitis C virus genome isolated from human carriers. J Virol 1991;65:1105–13.
24. Kolykhalov AA, Agapov EV, Blight KJ, Mihalik K, Feinstone SM, Rice CM. Transmission of hepatitis C by intrahepatic inoculation with transcribed RNA. Science. 1997;277:570–4.
25. Yanagi M, Purcell RH, Emerson SU, Bukh J. Transcripts from a single full-length cDNA clone of hepatitis C virus are infectious when directly transfected into the liver of a chimpanzee. Proc Natl Acad Sci USA. 1997;94:8738–43.
26. Beard MR, Abell G, Honda M et al. An infectious molecular clone of a Japanese genotype 1b hepatitis C virus. Hepatology. 1999;30:316–24.

27. Hong Z, Beaudet-Miller M, Lanford RE et al. Generation of transmissible hepatitis C virions from a molecular clone in chimpanzees. Virology. 1999;256:36–44.
28. Yanagi M, Purcell RH, Emerson SU, Bukh J. Hepatitis C virus: An infectious molecular clone of a second major genotype (2a) and lack of viability of intertypic 1a and 2a chimeras. Virology. 1999;262:250–63.
29. Lohmann V, Körner F, Koch J-O, Herian U, Theilmann L, Bartenschlager R. Replication of subgenomic hepatitis C virus RNAs in a hepatoma cell line. Science. 1999;285:110–13.
30. Wang C, Siddiqui A. Structure and function of the hepatitis C virus internal ribosome entry site. Curr Top Microbiol Immunol. 1995;203:99–115.
31. Honda M, Brown EA, Lemon SM. Stability of a stem-loop involving the initiator AUG controls the efficiency of internal initiation of translation on hepatitis C virus RNA. RNA. 1996;2:955–68.
32. Tanaka T, Kato N, Cho M-J, Sugiyama K, Shimotohno K. Structure of the 3′ terminus of the hepatitis C virus genome. J Virol. 1996;70:3307–12.
33. Kolykhalov AA, Feinstone SM, Rice CM. Identification of a highly conserved sequence element at the 3′ terminus of hepatitis C virus genome RNA. J Virol. 1996;70:3363–71.
34. Yanagi M, St Claire M, Emerson SU, Purcell RH, Bukh J. In vivo analysis of the 3′ untranslated region of the hepatitis C virus after in vitro mutagenesis of an infectious cDNA clone. Proc Natl Acad Sci USA. 1999;96:2291–5.
35. Grakoui A, Wychowski C, Lin C, Feinstone SM, Rice CM. Expression and identification of hepatitis C virus polyprotein cleavage products. J Virol. 1993;67:1385–95.
36. Santolini E, Migliaccio G, La Monica N. Biosynthesis and biochemical properties of the hepatitis C virus core protein. J Virol. 1994;68:3631–41.
37. Matsumoto M, Hwang SB, Jeng K-S, Zhu N, Lai MMC. Homotypic interaction and multimerization of hepatitis C virus core protein. Virology. 1996;218:43–51.
38. Yasui K, Wakita T, Tsukiyama-Kohara K et al. The native form and maturation process of hepatitis C virus core protein. J Virol. 1998;72:6048–55.
39. Dubuisson J, Hsu HH, Cheung RC, Greenberg HB, Russell DG, Rice CM. Formation and intracellular localization of hepatitis C virus envelope glycoprotein complexes expressed by recombinant vaccinia and Sindbis viruses. J Virol. 1994;68:6147–60.
40. Deleersnyder V, Pillez A, Wychowski C et al. Formation of native hepatitis C virus glycoprotein complexes. J Virol. 1997;71:697–704.
41. Dubuisson J, Rice CM. Hepatitis C virus glycoprotein folding: disulfide bond formation and association with calnexin. J Virol. 1996;70:778–86.
42. Hijikata M, Kato N, Ootsuyama Y, Nakagawa M, Shimotohno K. Gene mapping of the putative structural region of the hepatitis C virus genome by in vitro processing analysis. Proc Natl Acad Sci USA. 1991;88:5547–51.
43. Kim DW, Suzuki R, Harada T, Saito I, Miyamura T. Trans-suppression of gene expression by hepatitis C viral core protein. Jpn J Med Sci Biol. 1994;47:211–20.
44. Ray RB, Steele R, Meyer K, Ray R. Transcriptional repression of p53 promoter by hepatitis C virus core protein. J Biol Chem. 1997;272:10983–6.
45. Ray RB, Steele R, Meyer K, Ray R. Hepatitis C virus core protein represses p21WAF1/Cip1/Sid1 promoter activity. Gene. 1998;208:331–6.
46. Shih C-M, Chen C-M, Chen S-Y, Lee Y-HW. Modulation of the *trans*-suppression activity of hepatitis C virus core protein by phosphorylation. J Virol. 1995;69:1160–71.
47. Shih C-M, Lo SJ, Miyamura T, Chen S-Y, Lee Y-HW. Suppression of hepatitis B virus expression and replication by hepatitis C virus core protein in HuH-7 cells. J Virol. 1993;67:5823–32.
48. Chen C-M, You L-R, Hwang L-H, Lee Y-HW. Direct interaction of hepatitis C virus core protein with the cellular lymphotoxin-β receptor modulates the signal pathway of the lymphotoxin-β receptor. J Virol. 1997;71:9417–26.
49. Matsumoto M, Hsieh T-Y, Zhu N et al. Hepatitis C virus core protein interacts with the cytoplasmic tail of lymphotoxin-β receptor. J Virol. 1997;71:1301–9.
50. Zhu N, Khoshnan A, Schneider R et al. Hepatitis C virus core protein binds to the cytoplasmic domain of tumor necrosis factor (TNF) receptor 1 and enhances TNF-induced apoptosis. J Virol. 1998;72:3691–7.
51. You LR, Chen CM, Lee YHW. Hepatitis C virus core protein enhances NF-kappaB signal pathway triggering by lymphotoxin-beta receptor ligand and tumor necrosis factor alpha. J Virol. 1999;73:1672–81.

52. Ray RB, Lagging LM, Meyer K, Ray R. Hepatitis C virus core protein cooperates with ras and transforms primary rat embryo fibroblasts to tumorigenic phenotype. J Virol. 1996;70:4438–43.
53. Chang J, Yang S-H, Cho Y-G, Hwang SB, Hahn YS, Sung YC. Hepatitis C virus core from two different genotypes has an oncogenic potential but is not sufficient for transforming primary rat embryo fibroblasts in cooperation with the H-*ras* oncogene. J Virol. 1998;72:3060–5.
54. Moriya K, Fujie H, Shintani Y et al. The core protein of hepatitis C virus induces hepatocellular carcinoma in transgenic mice. Nature Med. 1998;4:1065–7.
55. Ruggieri A, Harada T, Matsuura Y, Miyamura T. Sensitization to Fasmediated apoptosis by hepatitis C virus core protein. Virology. 1997;229:68–76.
56. Ray RB, Meyer K, Steele R, Shrivastava A, Aggarwal BB, Ray R. Inhibition of tumor necrosis factor α-mediated apoptosis by hepatitis C virus core protein. J Biol Chem. 1998;273:2256–9.
57. Ray RB, Meyer K, Ray R. Suppression of apoptotic cell death by hepatitis C virus core protein. Virology. 1996;226:176–82.
58. Large MK, Kittlesen DJ, Hahn YS. Suppression of host immune response by the core protein of hepatitis C virus: possible implications for hepatitis C virus persistence. J Immunol. 1999;162:931–8.
59. Pileri P, Uematsu Y, Campagnoli S et al. Binding of hepatitis C virus to CD81. Science. 1998;282:938–41.
60. Flint M, Maidens C, Loomis-Price LD et al. Characterization of hepatitis C virus E2 glycoprotein interaction with a putative cellular receptor, CD81. J Virol. 1999;73:6235–44.
61. Taylor DR, Shi ST, Romano PR, Barber GN, Lai MMC. Inhibition of the interferon-inducible protein kinase PKR by HCV E2 protein. Science. 1999;285:107–10.
62. Behrens S-E, Tomei L, De Francesco R. Identification and properties of the RNA-dependent RNA polymerase of hepatitis C virus. EMBO J. 1996;15:12–22.
63. Lohmann V, Körner F, Herian U, Bartenschlager R. Biochemical properties of hepatitis C virus NS5B RNA-dependent RNA polymerase and identification of amino acid sequence motifs essential for enzymatic activity. J Virol. 1997;71:8416–28.
64. Yamashita T, Kaneko S, Shirota Y et al. RNA-dependent RNA polymerase activity of the soluble recombinant hepatitis C virus NS5B protein truncated at the C-terminal region. J Biol Chem. 1998;273:15479–86.
65. Ferrari E, Wright-Minogue J, Fang JW, Baroudy BM, Lau JY, Hong Z. Characterization of soluble hepatitis C virus RNA-dependent RNA polymerase expressed in *Escherichia coli*. J Virol. 1999;73:1649–54.
66. Oh JW, Ito T, Lai MM. A recombinant hepatitis C virus RNA-dependent RNA polymerase capable of copying the full-length viral RNA. J Virol. 1999;73:7694–702.
67. Lin C, Wu J-W, Hsiao K, Su M-S. The hepatitis C virus NS4A protein: interactions with the NS4B and NS5A proteins. J Virol. 1997;71:6465–71.
68. Koch JO, Bartenschlager R. Modulation of hepatitis C virus NS5A hyperphosphorylation by nonstructural proteins NS3, NS4A, and NS4B. J Virol. 1999;73:7138–46.
69. Grakoui A, McCourt DW, Wychowski C, Feinstone SM, Rice CM. A second hepatitis C virus-encoded proteinase. Proc Natl Acad Sci USA. 1993;90:10583–7.
70. Hijikata M, Mizushima H, Akagi T et al. Two distinct proteinase activities required for the processing of a putative nonstructural precursor protein of hepatitis C virus. J Virol. 1993;67:4665–75.
71. Bartenschlager R, Ahlborn-Laake L, Mous J, Jacobsen H. Nonstructural protein 3 of the hepatitis C virus encodes a serine-type proteinase required for cleavage at the NS3/4 and NS4/5 junctions. J Virol. 1993;67:3835–44.
72. Grakoui A, McCourt DW, Wychowski C, Feinstone SM, Rice CM. Characterization of the hepatitis C virus-encoded serine proteinase: determination of proteinase-dependent polyprotein cleavage sites. J Virol. 1993;67:2832–43.
73. Tomei L, Failla C, Santolini E, De Francesco R, La Monica N. NS3 is a serine protease required for processing of hepatitis C virus polyprotein. J Virol. 1993;67:4017–26.
74. Kim JL, Morgenstern KA, Lin C et al. Crystal structure of the hepatitis C virus NS3 protease domain complexed with a synthetic NS4A cofactor peptide. Cell. 1996;87:343–55.
75. Love RA, Parge HE, Wickersham JA et al. The crystal structure of hepatitis C virus NS3 proteinase reveals a trypsin-like fold and a structural zinc binding site. Cell. 1996;87:331–42.
76. Yan Y, Li Y, Munshi S et al. Complex of NS3 protease and NS4A peptide of BK strain of hepatitis C virus: a 2.2 Å resolution structure in a hexagonal crystal form. Protein Sci. 1998;7:837–47.

77. Yao N, Hesson T, Cable M et al. Structure of the hepatitis C virus RNA helicase domain. Nature Struct Biol. 1997;4:463–7.
78. Kim JL, Morgenstern KA, Griffith JP et al. Hepatitis virus NS3 RNA helicase domain with a bound oligonucleotide: the crystal structure provides insights into the mode of unwinding. Structure. 1998;6:89–100.
79. Yao N, Reichert P, Taremi SS, Prosise WW, Weber PC. Molecular views of viral polyprotein processing revealed by the crystal structure of the hepatitis C virus bifunctional protease-helicase. Structure. 1999;7:1353–63
80. Lesburg CA, Cable MB, Ferrari E, Hong Z, Mannarino AF, Weber PC. Crystal structure of the RNA-dependent RNA polymerase from hepatitis C virus reveals a fully encircled active site. Nature Struct Biol. 1999;6:937–43.
81. Lin C, Rice CM. The hepatitis C virus NS3 proteinase and NS4A cofactor: establishment of a cell-free trans-processing assay. Proc Natl Acad Sci USA. 1995;92:7622–6.
82. Shimizu Y, Yamaji K, Masuho Y et al. Identification of the sequence on NS4A required for enhanced cleavage of the NS5A/5B site by hepatitis C virus NS3 protease. J Virol. 1996;70:127–32.
83. Tanji Y, Kaneko T, Satoh S, Shimotohno K. Phosphorylation of hepatitis C virus-encoded nonstructural protein NS5A. J Virol. 1995;69:3980–6.
84. Reed KE, Xu J, Rice CM. Phosphorylation of the hepatitis C virus NS5A protein in vitro and in vivo: properties of the NS5A-associated kinase. J Virol. 1997;71:7187–97.
85. Reed KE, Gorbalenya AE, Rice CM. The NS5A/NS5 proteins of viruses from three genera of the family flaviviridae are phosphorylated by associated serine/threonine kinases. J Virol. 1998;72:6199–206.
86. Enomoto N, Sakuma I, Asahina Y et al. Comparison of full-length sequences of interferon-sensitive and resistant hepatitis C virus 1b. J Clin Invest. 1995;96:224–30.
87. Enomoto N, Sakuma I, Asahina Y et al. Mutations in the nonstructural protein 5A gene and response to interferon in patients with chronic hepatitis C virus 1b infection. N Engl J Med. 1996;334:77–81.
88. Bréchot C. The direct interplay between HCV NS5A protein and interferon transduction signal: from clinical to basic science. J Hepatol. 1999;30:1152–4.
89. Sarrazin C, Berg T, Lee JH et al. Improved correlation between multiple mutations within the NS5A region and virological response in European patients chronically infected with hepatitis C virus type 1b undergoing combination therapy. J Hepatol. 1999;30:1004–13.
90. Gale M, Jr., Korth MJ, Tang NM et al. Evidence that hepatitis C virus resistance to interferon is mediated through repression of the PKR protein kinase by the nonstructural 5A protein. Virology. 1997;230:217–27.
91. Gale M, Jr., Blakely CM, Kwieciszewski B et al. Control of PKR protein kinase by hepatitis C virus nonstructural 5A protein: molecular mechanisms of kinase regulation. Mol Cell Biol. 1998;18:5208–18.
92. Gale M Jr, Kwieciszewski B, Dossett M, Nakao H, Katze MG. Antiapoptotic and oncogenic potentials of hepatitis C virus are linked to interferon resistance by viral repression of the PKR protein kinase. J Virol. 1999;73:6506–16.
93. Ghosh AK, Steele R, Meyer K, Ray R, Ray RB. Hepatitis C virus NS5A protein modulates cell cycle regulatory genes and promotes cell growth. J Gen Virol. 1999;80:1179–83.
94. Rey FA, Heinz FX, Mandl C, Kunz C, Harrison SC. The envelope glycoprotein from tick-borne encephalitis virus at 2 Å resolution. Nature. 1995;375:291–8.
95. Schalich J, Allison SL, Stiasny K, Mandl CW, Kunz C, Heinz FX. Recombinant subviral particles from tick-borne encephalitis virus are fusogenic and provide a model system for studying flavivirus envelope glycoprotein functions. J Virol. 1996;70:4549–57.
96. Deubel V, Digoutte JP, Mattei X, Pandare D. Morphogenesis of yellow fever virus in *Aedes aegypti* cultured cells. Am J Trop Med Hyg. 1981;30:1071–7.
97. Chambers TJ, Hahn CS, Galler R, Rice CM. Flavivirus genome organization, expression, and replication. Annu Rev Microbiol. 1990;44:649–88.
98. Westaway EG, Mackenzie JM, Kenney MT, Jones MK, Khromykh AA. Ultrastructure of Kunjin virus-infected cells: colocalization of NS1 and NS3 with double-stranded RNA, and of NS2B with NS3, in virus-induced membrane structures. J Virol. 1997;71:6650–61.
99. Mackenzie JM, Jones MK, Westaway EG. Markers for trans-Golgi membranes and the intermediate compartment localize to induced membranes with distinct replication functions in flavivirus-infected cells. J Virol. 1999;73:9555–67.

100. von Weizsäcker F, Wieland S, Köck J et al. Gene therapy for chronic viral hepatitis: ribozymes, antisense oligonucleotides, and dominant negative mutants. Hepatology. 1997;26:251–5.
101. Wakita T, Wands JR. Specific inhibition of hepatitis C virus expression by antisense oligodeoxynucleotides. J Biol Chem. 1994;269:14205–10.
102. Alt M, Renz R, Hofschneider PH, Paumgartner G, Caselmann WH. Specific inhibition of hepatitis C viral gene expression by antisense phosphorothioate oligodeoxynucleotides. Hepatology. 1995;22:707–17.
103. Hanecak R, Brown-Driver V, Fox MC et al. Antisense oligonucleotide inhibition of hepatitis C virus gene expression in transformed hepatocytes. J Virol. 1996;70:5203–12.
104. Lima WF, Brown-Driver V, Fox M, Hanecak R, Bruice TW. Combinatorial screening and rational optimization for hybridization to folded hepatitis C virus RNA of oligonucleotides with biological antisense activity. J Biol Chem. 1997;272:626–38.
105. Zhang H, Hanecak R, Brown-Driver V et al. Antisense oligonucleotide inhibition of hepatitis C virus (HCV) gene expression in livers of mice infected with an HCV-vaccinia virus recombinant. Antimicrob Agents Chemother. 1999;43:347–53.
106. Wakita T, Moradpour D, Tokushige K, Wands JR. Antiviral effects of antisense RNA on hepatitis C virus RNA translation and expression. J Med Virol. 1999;57:217–22.
107. Lieber A, He C-Y, Polyak SJ, Gretch DR, Barr D, Kay MA. Elimination of hepatitis C virus RNA in infected human hepatocytes by adenovirus-mediated expression of ribozymes. J Virol. 1996;70:8782–91.
108. Das S, Ott M, Yamane A et al. A small yeast RNA blocks hepatitis C virus internal ribosome entry site (HCV IRES)-mediated translation and inhibits replication of a chimeric poliovirus under translational control of the HCV IRES element. J Virol. 1998;72:5638–47.
109. Kumar PKR, Machida K, Urvil PT et al. Isolation of RNA aptamers specific to the NS3 protein of hepatitis C virus from a pool of completely random RNA. Virology. 1997;237:270–82.
110. Inchauspé G. DNA vaccine strategies for hepatitis C. J Hepatol. 1999;30:339–46.
111. Maertens G, Ducatteeuw A, Priem S et al. Therapeutic vaccination of chronically infected chimpanzees with the HCV E1 protein. Hepatology. 1998;28:398A.
112. Fukumoto T, Berg T, Ku Y et al. Viral dynamics of hepatitis C early after orthotopic liver transplantation: evidence for rapid turnover of serum virions. Hepatology. 1996;24:1351–4.
113. Zeuzem S, Schmidt JM, Lee J-H, Rüster B, Roth WK. Effect of interferon alfa on the dynamics of hepatitis C virus turnover in vivo. Hepatology. 1996;23:366–71.
114. Lam NP, Neumann AU, Gretch DR, Wiley TE, Perelson AS, Layden TJ. Dose-dependent acute clearance of hepatitis C genotype 1 virus with interferon alfa. Hepatology. 1997;26:226–31.
115. Neumann AU, Lam NP, Dahari H et al. Hepatitis C viral dynamics in vivo and the antiviral efficacy of interferon-alpha therapy. Science. 1998;282:103–7.
116. Wei X, Ghosh SK, Taylor ME et al. Viral dynamics in human immunodeficiency virus type 1 infection. Nature. 1995;373:117–22.
117. Ho DD, Neumann AU, Perelson AS, Chen W, Leonard JM, Markowitz M. Rapid turnover of plasma virions and CD4 lymphocytes in HIV-1 infection. Nature. 1995;373:123–6.
118. Bukh J, Miller RH, Purcell RH. Genetic heterogeneity of hepatitis C virus: quasispecies and genotypes. Semin Liver Dis. 1995;15:41–63.
119. Simmonds P. Variability of hepatitis C virus. Hepatology. 1995;21:570–83.
120. Martell M, Esteban JI, Quer J et al. Hepatitis C virus (HCV) circulates as a population of different but closely related genomes: quasispecies nature of HCV genome distribution. J Virol. 1992;66:3225–9.
121. Simmonds P, Alberti A, Alter HJ et al. A proposed system for the nomenclature of hepatitis C viral genotypes. Hepatology. 1994;19:1321–4.
122. Hijikata M, Kato N, Ootsuyama Y, Nakagawa M, Ohkoshi S, Shimotohno K. Hypervariable regions in the putative glycoprotein of hepatitis C virus. Biochem Biophys Res Commun. 1991;175:220–8.
123. Weiner AJ, Brauer MJ, Rosenblatt J et al. Variable and hypervariable domains are found in the regions of HCV corresponding to the flavivirus envelope and NS1 proteins and the pestivirus envelope glycoproteins. Virology. 1991;180:842–8.
124. Ogata N, Alter HJ, Miller RH, Purcell RH. Nucleotide sequence and mutation rate of the H strain of hepatitis C virus. Proc Natl Acad Sci USA. 1991;88:3392–6.
125. Okamoto H, Kojima M, Okada S-I et al. Genetic drift of hepatitis C virus during an 8.2-year infection in a chimpanzee: variability and stability. Virology. 1992;190:894–9.

126. Yoshioka K, Kakumu S, Wakita T et al. Detection of hepatitis C virus by polymerase chain reaction and response to interferon-α therapy: relationship to genotypes of hepatitis C virus. Hepatology. 1992;16:293–9.
127. National Institutes of Health consensus development conference panel statement: management of hepatitis C. Hepatology. 1997;26(Suppl 1):2S–10S.
128. Consensus Statement. European Association for the Study of the Liver. J Hepatol. 1999;30:956–61.
129. Shimizu YK, Iwamoto A, Hijikata M, Purcell RH, Yoshikura H. Evidence for in vitro replication of hepatitis C virus genome in a human T-cell line. Proc Natl Acad Sci USA. 1992;89:5477–81.
130. Shimizu YK, Purcell RH, Yoshikura H. Correlation between the infectivity of hepatitis C virus in vivo and its infectivity in vitro. Proc Natl Acad Sci USA. 1993;90:6037–41.
131. Mizutani T, Kato N, Saito S, Ikeda M, Sugiyama K, Shimotohno K. Characterization of hepatitis C virus replication in cloned cells obtained from a human T-cell leukemia virus type 1-infected cell line, MT-2. J Virol. 1996;70:7219–23.
132. Nakajima N, Hijikata M, Yoshikura H, Shimizu YK. Characterization of longterm cultures of hepatitis C virus. J Virol. 1996;70:3325–9.
133. Ito T, Mukaigawa J, Zuo J, Hirabayashi Y, Mitamura K, Yasui K. Cultivation of hepatitis C virus in primary hepatocyte culture from patients with chronic hepatitis C results in release of high titre infectious virus. J Gen Virol. 1996;77:1043–54.
134. Iacovacci S, Manzin A, Barca S et al. Molecular characterization and dynamics of hepatitis C virus replication in human fetal hepatocytes infected in vitro. Hepatology. 1997;26:1328–37.
135. Lanford RE, Sureau C, Jacob JR, White R, Fuerst TR. Demonstration of in vitro infection of chimpanzee hepatocytes with hepatitis C virus using strand-specific RT/PCR. Virology. 1994;202:606–14.
136. Loriot MA, Bronowicki JP, Lagorce D et al. Permissiveness of human biliary epithelial cells to infection by hepatitis C virus. Hepatology. 1999;29:1587–95.
137. Lerat H, Berby F, Trabaud M-A et al. Specific detection of hepatitis C virus minus strand RNA in hematopoietic cells. J Clin Invest. 1996;97:845–51.
138. Bronowicki JP, Loriot MA, Thiers V, Grignon Y, Zignego AL, Bréchot C. Hepatitis C virus persistence in human hematopoietic cells injected into SCID mice. Hepatology. 1998;28:211–18.
139. Laskus T, Radkowski M, Wang LF, Vargas H, Rakela J. Search for hepatitis C virus extrahepatic replication sites in patients with acquired immunodeficiency syndrome: specific detection of negative-strand viral RNA in various tissues. Hepatology. 1998;28:1398–401.
140. Lerat H, Rumin S, Habersetzer F et al. In vivo tropism of hepatitis C virus genomic sequences in hematopoietic cells: influence of viral load, viral genotype, and cell phenotype. Blood. 1998;91:3841–9.
141. Sansonno D, Lotesoriere C, Cornacchiulo V et al. Hepatitis C virus infection involves CD34(+) hematopoietic progenitor cells in hepatitis C virus chronic carriers. Blood. 1998;92:3328–37.
142. Lanford RE, Chavez D, Chisari FV, Sureau C. Lack of detection of negative-strand hepatitis C virus RNA in peripheral blood mononuclear cells and other extrahepatic tissues by the highly strand-specific rTth reverse transcriptase PCR. J Virol. 1995;69:8079–83.
143. Moradpour D, Kary P, Rice CM, Blum HE. Continuous human cell lines inducibly expressing hepatitis C virus structural and nonstructural proteins. Hepatology. 1998;28:192–201.
144. Duvet S, Pillez A, Cocquerel L et al. Hepatitis C virus glycoprotein complex localization in the endoplasmic reticulum involves a determinant for retention and not retrieval. J Biol Chem. 1998;273:32088–95.
145. Heim MH, Moradpour D, Blum HE. Expression of hepatitis C virus proteins inhibits signal transduction through the Jak-STAT pathway. J Virol. 1999;8469–75.
146. Walker CM. Comparative features of hepatitis C virus infection in humans and chimpanzees. Springer Semin Immunopathol. 1997;19:85–98.
147. Prince AM, Brotman B. Biological and immunological aspects of hepatitis C virus infection in chimpanzees. Curr Stud Hematol Blood Transfus. 1998;62:250–65.
148. Major ME, Mihalik K, Fernandez J et al. Long-term follow-up of chimpanzees inoculated with the first infectious clone for hepatitis C virus. J Virol. 1999;73:3317–25.
149. Xie ZC, Riezu-Boj JI, Lasarte JJ et al. Transmission of hepatitis C virus infection to tree shrews. Virology. 1998;244:513–20.

150. Koike K, Moriya K, Ishibashi K et al. Expression of hepatitis C virus envelope proteins in transgenic mice. J Gen Virol. 1995;76:3031–8.
151. Wakita T, Taya C, Yonekawa H et al. Liver injury with apoptotic cell death in HCV transgenic mice with Cre/loxP switching system. Hepatology. 1996;24:366A.
152. Koike K, Moriya K, Ishibashi K et al. Sialadenitis histologically resembling Sjögren's syndrome in mice transgenic for hepatitis C virus envelope genes. Proc Natl Acad Sci USA. 1997;94:233–6.
153. Kawamura T, Furusaka A, Koziel MJ et al. Transgenic expression of hepatitis C virus structural proteins in the mouse. Hepatology. 1997;25:1014–21.
154. Pasquinelli C, Shoenberger JM, Chung J et al. Hepatitis C virus core and E2 protein expression in transgenic mice. Hepatology. 1997;25:719–27.
155. Moriya K, Yotsuyanagi H, Shintani Y et al. Hepatitis C virus core protein induces hepatic steatosis in transgenic mice. J Gen Virol. 1997;78:1527–31.
156. Galun E, Burakova T, Ketzinel M et al. Hepatitis C virus viremia in SCID → BXR mouse chimera. J Infect Dis. 1995;172:25–30.
157. de Medina M, Schiff ER. Hepatitis C: diagnostic assays. Semin Liver Dis. 1995;15:33–40.
158. Tanaka T, Lau JYN, Mizokami M et al. Simple fluorescent enzyme immunoassay for detection and quantification of hepatitis C viremia. J Hepatol. 1995;23:742–5.
159. Orito E, Mizokami M, Tanaka T et al. Quantification of serum hepatitis C virus core protein level in patients chronically infected with different hepatitis C virus genotypes. Gut. 1996;39:876–80.
160. Tanaka E, Kiyosawa K, Matsumoto A et al. Serum levels of hepatitis C virus core protein in patients with chronic hepatitis C treated with interferon alfa. Hepatology. 1996;23:1330–3.
161. Shiratori Y, Kato N, Yokosuka O et al. Quantitative assays for hepatitis C virus in serum as predictors of the long-term response to interferon. J Hepatol. 1997;27:437–44.
162. Gretch DR. Diagnostic tests for hepatitis C. Hepatology 1997;26(Suppl 1):43S–7S.
163. Zaaijer HL, Cuypers HT, Reesink HW, Winkel IN, Gerken G, Lelie PN. Reliability of polymerase chain reaction for detection of hepatitis C virus. Lancet. 1993;341:722–4.
164. Damen M, Cuypers HT, Zaaijer HL et al. International collaborative study on the second EUROHEP HCV-RNA reference panel. J Virol Methods. 1996;58:175–85.
165. Hayashi J, Yoshimura E, Kishihara Y et al. Hepatitis C virus RNA levels determined by branched DNA probe assay correlated with levels assessed using competitive PCR. Am J Gastroenterol. 1996;91:314–18.
166. Takeuchi T, Katsume A, Tanaka T et al. Real-time detection system for quantification of hepatitis C virus genome. Gastroenterology. 1999;116:636–42.
167. Krawczynski K, Beach MJ, Bradley DW et al. Hepatitis C virus antigen in hepatocytes: immunomorphologic detection and identification. Gastroenterology. 1992;103:622–9.
168. Nouri Aria KT, Sallie R, Sangar D et al. Detection of genomic and intermediate replicative strands of hepatitis C virus in liver tissue by in situ hybridization. J Clin Invest. 1993;91:2226–34.
169. Nuovo GJ, Lidonnici K, MacConnell P, Lane B. Intracellular localization of polymerase chain reaction (PCR)-amplified hepatitis C cDNA. Am J Surg Pathol. 1993;17:683–90.
170. Guido M, Thung SN. The value of identifying hepatitis C virus in liver pathology specimens. Hepatology. 1996;23:376–9.
171. Lau JY, Krawczynski K, Negro F, Gonzalez-Peralta RP. In situ detection of hepatitis C virus – a critical appraisal. J Hepatol. 1996;24:43–51.
172. Davis GL, Esteban-Mur R, Rustgi V et al. Interferon alfa-2b alone or in combination with ribavirin for the treatment of relapse of chronic hepatitis C. International Hepatitis Interventional Therapy Group. N Engl J Med. 1998;339:1493–9.
173. McHutchison JG, Gordon SC, Schiff ER et al. Interferon alfa-2b alone or in combination with ribavirin as initial treatment for chronic hepatitis C. Hepatitis Interventional Therapy Group. N Engl J Med. 1998;339:1485–92.
174. Poynard T, Marcellin P, Lee SS et al. Randomised trial of interferon alpha2b plus ribavirin for 48 weeks or for 24 weeks versus interferon alpha2b plus placebo for 48 weeks for treatment of chronic infection with hepatitis C virus. International Hepatitis Interventional Therapy Group. Lancet. 1998;352:1426–32.
175. Reichard O, Norkrans G, Fryden A, Braconier JH, Sonnerborg A, Weiland O. Randomised, double-blind, placebo-controlled trial of interferon alpha-2b with and without ribavirin for chronic hepatitis C. The Swedish Study Group. Lancet. 1998;351:83–7.

10
Hepatitis C – immunopathogenesis

U. SPENGLER, F. L. DUMOULIN, R. WOITAS, L. LEIFELD, A. SCHNEIDERS, B. LANGHANS, S. SCHWEITZER, U. DÜESBERG, M. LECHMANN and T. SAUERBRUCH

DEFINING A ROLE FOR THE IMMUNE SYSTEM IN HEPATITIS C VIRUS INFECTION

The mechanisms for tissue injury in hepatitis C virus (HCV) infection are not well understood. However, there is circumstantial evidence that the immune response is critically involved. First, the observations from various expression systems (cell culture or transgenic mice) indicate that HCV is not cytopathic. Second, liver cell damage is always associated with the presence of an intrahepatic inflammatory infiltrate, and hepatocellular damage coincides with the onset of an immune response during acute infection but not viral replication[1]. Furthermore, viral replication can occur in the absence of a detectable inflammatory reaction[2,3]. With the exception of HIV infection immunosuppression is associated with transient amelioration of the inflammatory activity and hepatocellular damage, whereas viraemia increases[3]. An exacerbation of hepatitis C is frequently noted, when immunosuppressive therapy is terminated[4–6]. Finally, there are numerous reports that link the outcome of hepatitis C infection to various immunogenetic factors, in particular HLA class II alleles[7–19]. Despite this ample evidence for activation of the immune system HCV can persist and establish chronic hepatitis in the majority of infected patients. It is a key feature of HCV related immunity that the presence of a HCV-specific immune response, which would be protective in other infectious diseases, does not prevent reinfection in the chimpanzee model nor man.

Fundamentally the immune system can control an infection via two effector pathways (Fig. 1): (1) the humoral response which involves antibodies neutralizing circulating pathogens, and (2) the cellular immune response, which can eliminate intracellular pathogens mainly via MHC class I restricted $CD8^+$ cytolytic T cells (CTLs). Both effector arms of immunity are regulated by the activity of $CD4^+$ T helper cells.

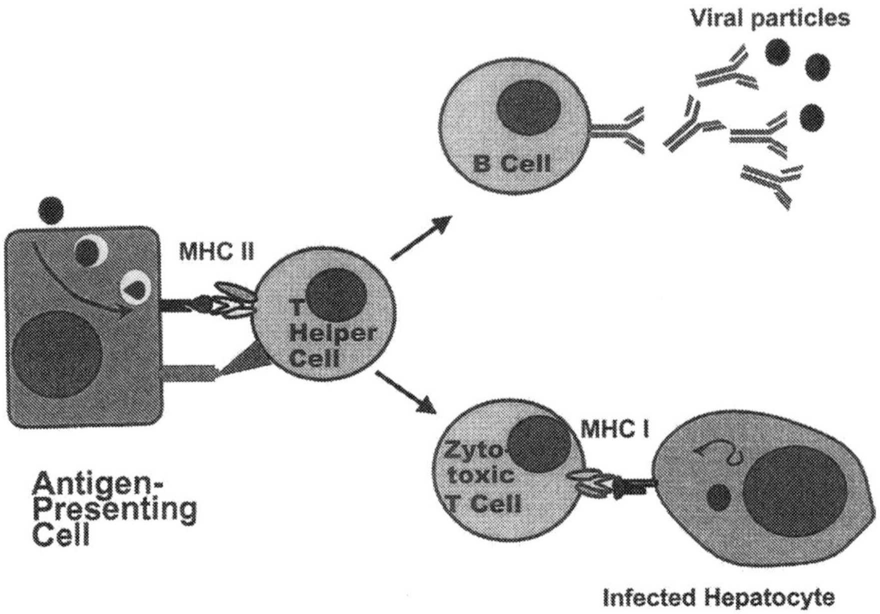

Figure 1 Principal mechanisms of the antiviral immune response in hepatitis C virus infection

HUMORAL IMMUNITY IN HEPATITIS C INFECTION

Antibodies can be readily detected by enzyme-linked immunoassays or Western blot in hepatitis C infection, and their presence forms the basis for serological diagnosis and epidemiological studies. However, HCV antibodies do not provide protection as both experiments in the chimpanzee as well as observations in man indicate that reinfection can take place with different isolates[20–22].

It is further discussed controversially whether antibodies, in particular those directed against the putative envelope protein E2, have a role in the elimination of HCV infection[23]. On the other hand, it is quite clear that HCV antibodies are involved in the immunopathogenesis of HCV disease, as they can form immune complexes with HCV antigens. This process can lead to type II mixed cryoglobulinemia, glomerulonephritis, vasculitis and arthritis[24].

Finally anti-E2 antibodies may also contribute to intrahepatic pathology. Viral proteins such as core and E2 can bind to the cell membranes of various cell types, which then become coated by the corresponding antibodies. Preliminary experiments from our laboratory indicate that cells coated by E2, which need not necessarily be infected, can be killed by antibody-dependent cellular cytotoxicity (Fig. 2). As the required type of E2 antibody is found both in patients with acute resolving hepatitis C or previous self-limited HCV infection and in patients with chronic infection (A. Schneiders, personal communication), E2-specific antibody dependent cellular cytotoxicity is probably not pivotal for elimination of HCV infection but may also cause damage to cells coated by viral proteins which are not infected.

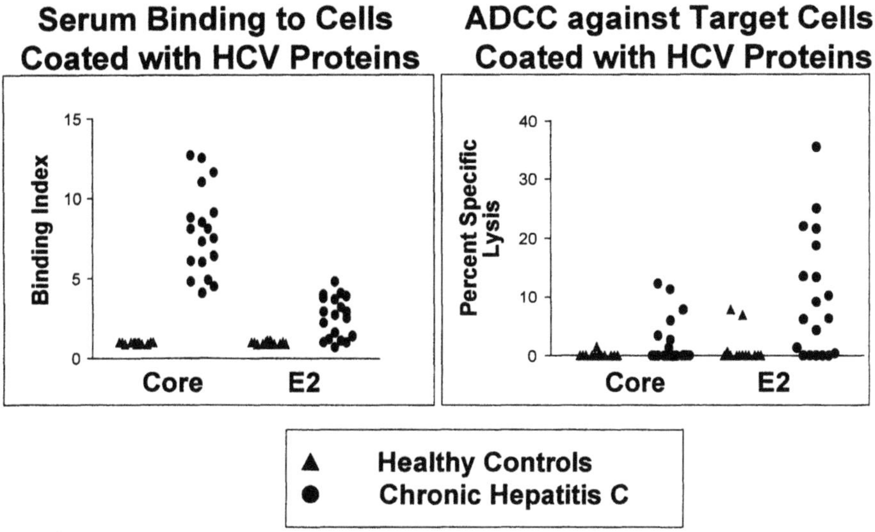

Figure 2 Binding and antibody dependent cellular cytotoxicity to HCV core and E2 protein-coated target cells

THE ANTIVIRAL HCV RESPONSE OF CD8+ CYTOLYTIC T LYMPHOCYTES

HLA class I-restricted $CD8^+$ cytolytic T lymphocytes (CTL) are the major defence mechanism in most viral infections. They recognize small linear peptides 8–11 amino acids in length that are intracellularly processed from the original viral protein and presented on the cell surface in association with self HLA class I molecules. CTL mediate lysis of virus-infected host cells. However, even if viral clearance is not achieved, as occurs frequently in HCV infection, CTL can cause extended tissue injury[25] because they not only lyse virus-infected cells but also innocent bystander hepatocytes due to the release of proapoptotic mediators such as Fas ligand or tumour necrosis factor (TNF)[26].

The spectrum of CTL isolated from infected patients indicates that the response is directed against conserved and variable epitopes both in peripheral blood and in the liver[27–36]. Moreover, the CTL response is usually multispecific and many epitopes can be presented in association with different HLA alleles[37]. A recent study using soluble HLA–peptide constructs as novel sensitive probes to detect and quantitate HCV-specific CTL has indicated at least 10-fold enrichment of NS3-specific CTL in the liver[38]. Similar compartmentalization may occur with $CD8^+$ lymphocytes, which have specificity for other viral proteins (Fig. 3). Finally, several groups have reported an inverse relationship between the strength of the CTL response and the viral loads[39–41] suggesting that in principle it is possible for CTL to control HCV infection[42]. However, HCV is not cleared in most patients, indicating that the immune response is not sufficient to eradicate the virus but, on the other hand, leads to an increased intrahepatic production of proinflammatory cytokines, tissue destruction and the development of cirrhosis[43,44].

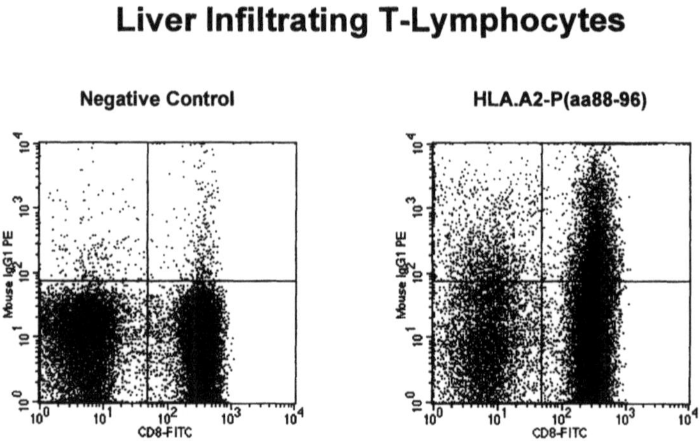

Figure 3 Flowcytometric identification of intrahepatic CD8+ T cells with T cell receptors that recognize the antigenic HCV peptide aa 88-96 in association with HLA-A2

THE ANTIVIRAL HCV RESPONSE OF CD4+ T HELPER LYMPHOCYTES

CD4+ T helper lymphocytes function primarily as immunoregulatory cells which secrete lymphokines that activate B lymphocytes for antibody production or induce the proliferation and maturation of specific cytotoxic T lymphocytes. T helper cells can be classified into at least two distinct populations according to their cytokine production[45]. TH1 cells secrete interleukin (IL)-2, interferon-γ and lymphotoxin (TNF-β), whereas TH2 cells produce IL-4, -5, -6, and -13. Although IL-10 was originally described as a TH2-like cytokine, it is now clear that IL-10 can also be secreted by TH1 cells and macrophages[46]. Type 1 cytokines enhance cellular immune responses, while type 2 cytokines contribute to T-cell help for antibody production[47,48]. An important role of the balance between type 1 and type 2 cytokine secretion for the pathogenesis of human infectious diseases is proposed by findings in leprosy, in which type 1 cytokine formation is associated with the tuberculoid form and predominant type 2 cytokine production with lepromatous lesions[49]. In HIV infection and leishmaniasis, a shift towards type 2 cytokine profiles has been observed, which was proposed to be a pivotal step for pathogenesis and disease progression[50,51].

CD4+ T lymphocytes are triggered by short antigenic peptides which are processed from exogenous antigens by so-called antigen presenting cells (dendritic cells, macrophages, B lymphocytes) and presented in the antigen-binding groove of MHC class II molecules on the cell surface. The function of CD4+ T lymphocytes is usually assessed by [^{3}H]thymidine uptake in response to recombinant proteins. According to our findings, the HCV proteins core, NS3 and NS4 were most reactive in this type of assay[52].

Several groups have observed that proliferative responses of CD4+ T lymphocytes are considerably stronger in patients with self-limited infection than in those with chronic hepatitis C[52–57]. Once a vigorous antigen-specific T cell proliferative response has been established in HCV infection, it usually persists and can be detected even decades after an HCV infection has been cleared. Further observations suggest an important role of Th1-like responses of the $CD4^+$ T helper cells in the recovery from HCV-infection, and there is accumulating evidence that sufficient type 1 cytokine responses are not achieved in the patients with chronic hepatitis C: serum levels of TH2 cytokines were found to be increased in chronic hepatitis C and decreased during IFN-α treatment[58]. Preferential induction of IFN-γ and IL-2 producing lymphocytes in non-viraemic patients as well as higher numbers of type 2 cytokine producing cells in patients with chronic hepatitis C have been reported[59–64]. Recent data from our laboratory suggest that patients with persistent viraemia and chronic liver disease have less PBMC showing type 1 cytokine (IL-2, IFN-γ) responses to the HCV core protein in the sensitive ELISpot assay than patients with self-limited HCV infection[65] (Fig. 4). Although a clear-cut shift from TH1 towards TH2 cytokines was not noted with this assay, in terms of positive responses, more patients with chronic hepatitis showed a peptide-specific IL-10 response than patients with self-limited hepatitis C. Thus, patients with chronic hepatitis C are characterized by an overall weak HCV-specific T-cell response with production of fewer type 1 cytokines than patients who controlled their HCV infection. Therefore, it is an attractive hypothesis that despite abundant recruitment of specific CTL in chronic hepatitis C their effector function is insufficient because the help from the $CD4^+$ T helper lymphocytes is too weak.

T helper cell responses are determined to a large extent during priming and activation of the T-cells by the antigen presenting cells. For the generation of an effective immune response antigen presenting cells must express co-stimulatory molecules and secrete stimulatory cytokines in addition to presentation of antigenic peptides[66]. Triggering of T lymphocytes in the absence of sufficient co-stimulatory activity may result in anergy and apoptosis instead of activation.

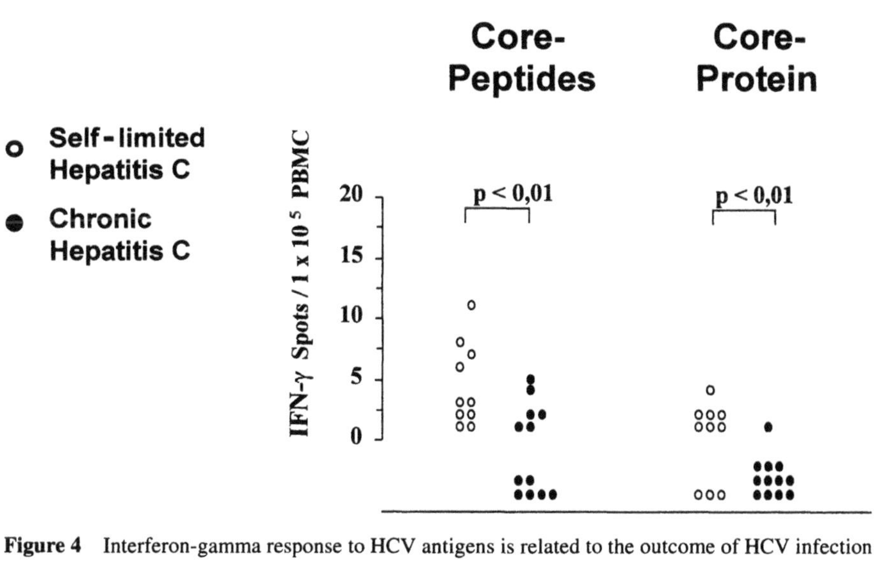

Figure 4 Interferon-gamma response to HCV antigens is related to the outcome of HCV infection

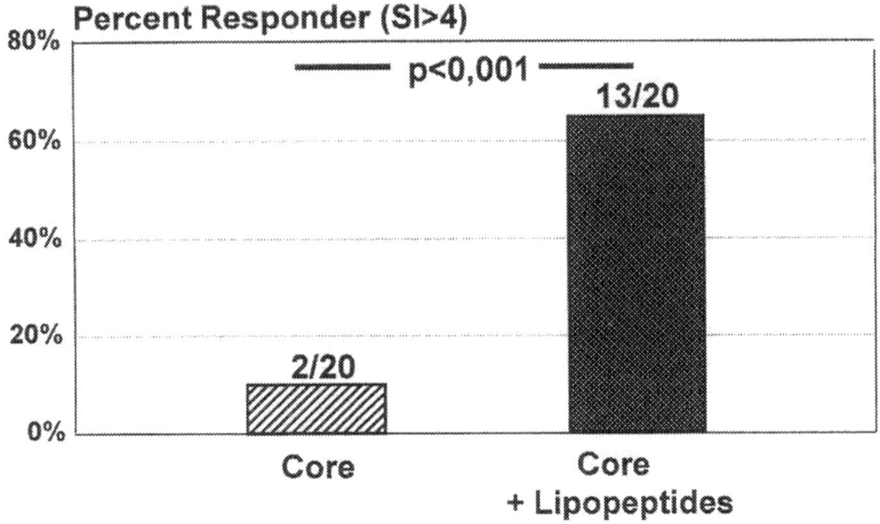

Figure 5 Superior antigenicity of HCV antigens coupled to a lipid moiety as a potential principle to improve HCV-specific immunity in chronic HCV infection

HCV infection may interfere with T helper cell activation at the level of the antigen presenting cells. In this context it is interesting that we found a peptide fragment derived from the core protein that can apparently inhibit processing of HCV core[67]. Furthermore, impaired allostimulatory capacity of peripheral blood dendritic cells has been reported in hepatitis C[68], and reduced production of monokines was observed both in the peripheral blood and the livers of patients with chronic hepatitis C[69,70]. T-cell proliferative responses can be markedly strengthened, when the HCV antigens are delivered as lipopeptides, which can activate antigen presenting cells via Toll-like receptors in addition to providing the antigenic peptide[71,72] (Fig. 5). To date it is not clear whether this lipopeptide effect can be used clinically to overcome HCV infection.

POTENTIAL MECHANISMS FOR VIRAL PERSISTENCE

Numerous nucleotide sequences have been obtained from HCV isolates all over the world, which indicate that HCV mutates rapidly. Different viral sequences (quasispecies) have been isolated from the same patient in serial samples. This fact has prompted the idea that HCV might evade immune surveillance via selection of immune escape mutations. However, this hypothesis is quite unlikely considering the fact that the immune response to HCV infection is not restricted to limited epitopes but is polyclonal and multispecific. Furthermore, a recent paper failed to demonstrate the accumulation of immune escape mutations at epitope sites of the HCV core and envelope proteins[73].

The enormous replication rate of HCV, which exceeds even that of HIV infection, has been taken as an explanation why HCV may spread more rapidly than can be controlled by the antiviral immune response[74,75]. However, kinetic considerations cannot explain the transient and prolonged suppression of pre-existing HCV-specific T-cell proliferative responses which we observed in one patient with previous self-limited HCV infection. This patient was studied during reinfection with a different HCV isolate[76]. The follow-up of this patient suggests that HCV may encode one or more gene products that can inhibit the antiviral immune response, e.g. interactions between viral proteins and the host cell have been demonstrated for the HCV core[77–80], E2[81], NS3[82] and NS5[83,84] proteins, and causing cell death and resistance against viral infection. HCV has also been demonstrated to infect immunocompetent cells; and direct immunosuppression[85] or interference with important signalling pathways of the immune system[86,87] have been reported for the HCV core protein. Moreover, stimulation of T lymphocytes with HCV core antigens results in the preferential induction of CD30, a member of the death receptor superfamily, in patients with chronic hepatitis C but not in patients with self-limited HCV infection[60], and it is the $CD30^+$ T lymphocyte subset which exhibits markers of apoptotic commitment such as increased annexin V binding after HCV-specific stimulation (R. Woitas, unpublished observation).

Thus, although not identified in detail yet, HCV may have evolved effective strategies to specifically counteract the host's immune response by either antigen presentation, by influencing the secretion of cytokines, or by neutralizing their antiviral effects, or by direct induction of selective immunosuppression similar to what has been reported for other viruses in their quest for survival[88–91]. Clarifying the precise role of these mechanisms in future studies will contribute considerably to our understanding of the immunopathogenesis in HCV infection.

REFERENCES

1. Farci P, Alter HJ, Shimoda A, Govindarajan S, Cheung LC, Melpolder JC et al. Hepatitis C virus-associated fulminant hepatic failure. N Engl J Med. 1996;335:631–4.
2. Brillanti S, Foli M, Gaiani S, Masci C, Miglioli M, Barbara L. Persistent hepatitis C viraemia without liver disease. Lancet. 1993;341:464–5.
3. Alberti A, Morsica G, Chemello L, Cavaletto D, Noventa F, Pontisso P, Ruol A. Hepatitis C viremia and liver disease in symptom-free individuals with anti-HCV. Lancet. 1992;340:697–8.
4. Collier J, Heathcote J. Hepatitis C viral infection in the immunosuppressed patient. Hepatology. 1998;27:2–6.
5. Gruber A, Lundberg LG, Bjorkholm M. Reactivation of chronic hepatitis C after withdrawal of immunosuppressive therapy. J Intern Med. 1993;234:223–5.
6. Fan FS, Tzeng CH, Hsiao KI, Hu ST, Liu WT, Chen PM. Withdrawal of immunosuppressive therapy in allogeneic bone marrow transplantation reactivates chronic viral hepatitis C. Bone Marrow Transplant. 1991;8:417–20.
7. Manns MP, Krüger M. Immunogenetics of chronic liver diseases. Gastroenterology. 1994;106:1676–97.
8. Czaja AJ, Carpenter H, Santrach PJ, Moore SB. DR human antigens and disease severity in chronic hepatitis C. J Hepatol. 1996;24:666–73.
9. Zavaglia C, Bortolon C, Ferrioli G, Rho A, Mondazzi L, Botelli R et al. HLA typing in chronic type B, D and C hepatitis. J Hepatol. 1996;24:658–65.
10. Tibbs C, Donaldson P, Underhill J, Thomson L, Manabe K, Williams R. Evidence that the HLA DQA1*03 allele confers protection from chronic HCV-infection in northern European Caucasoids. Hepatology. 1996;24:1342–5.
11. Thrusz MR, Mantafounis D, Yallop RM, Hewitt PE, Thomas HC. MHC class II and self limiting hepatitis C virus infection. Hepatology. 1996;24:382A [Abstract].

12. Kuzushita N, Hayashi N, Moribe T, Katayama K, Kanto T, Nakatani S et al. Influence of HLA haplotypes on the clinical courses of individuals infected with hepatitis C virus. Hepatology. 1998;27:240–4.
13. Alric L, Fort M, Izopet J, Vinel JP, Charlet JP, Selves J et al. Genes of the major histocompatibility complex class II influence the outcome of hepatitis C virus infection. Gastroenterology. 1997;113:1675–81.
14. Zavaglia C, Martinetti M, Silini E, Bottelli R, Daielli C, Asti M et al. Association between HLA class II alleles and protection from or susceptibility to chronic hepatitis C. J Hepatol. 1998;28:1–7.
15. Aikawa T, Kojima M, Onishi H, Tamura R, Fukuda S, Suzuki T et al. HLA DRB1 and DQB1 alleles and haplotypes influencing the progression of hepatitis C. J Med Virol. 1996;49:274–8.
16. Yasunami R, Miyamoto T, Kanda T. HLA-DRB1 is related to the pathological changes of the liver in chronic hepatitis C. Hepatol Res. 1997;7:3–12.
17. Congia M, Clemente MG, Dessi C, Cucca F, Mazzoleni AP, Frau F et al. HLA class II genes in chronic hepatitis C virus – infection and associated immunological disorders. Hepatology. 1996;24:1338–41.
18. Höhler T, Gerken G, Notghi A, Knolle P, Lubjuhn R, Taheri H et al. MHC class II genes influence the susceptibility to chronic active hepatitis C. J Hepatol. 1997;27:259–64.
19. Lechmann M, Schneider EM, Giers G, Kaiser R, Dumoulin FL, Sauerbruch T, Spengler U. Increased frequency of the HLA-DR15 (B1*15011) allele in German patients with self-limited hepatitis C virus infection. Eur J Clin Invest. 1999;29:337–43.
20. Farci P, Alter HJ, Govindarajan S, Wong DC, Engle R, Lesniewski RR et al. Lack of protective immunity against reinfection with hepatitis C virus. Science. 1992;258:135–40.
21. Lai ME, Mazzoleni AP, Argiolu F, De Virgilis S, Balestrieri A, Purcell RH et al. Hepatitis C virus in multiple episodes of acute hepatitis in polytransfused thalassaemic children. Lancet. 1994;343:388–90.
22. Cooper S, Erickson AL, Adams EJ, Kansopon J, Weiner AJ, Chien DY et al. Immunity. 1999;10:439–49.
23. Rosa D, Campagnoli S, Moretto C, Guenzi E, Cousens L, Chin M et al. A quantitative test to estimate neutralizing antibodies to the hepatitis C virus: cytofluorometric assessment of envelope glycoprotein-2 binding to target cells. Proc Natl Acad Sci USA. 1996;93:1759–63.
24. Dumoulin FL, Spengler U, Sauerbruch T. Hepatitis C virus-associated mixed cryoglobulinemia. Eur J Gastroenterol Hepatol. 1997;9:1063–5.
25. Doherty PC, Zinkernagel RM. T cell-mediated immunopathology in viral infections. Transplant Rev. 1974;19:89–120.
26. Ando K, Hiroishi K, Kaneko T, Moriyama T, Muto Y, Kaygaki N et al. Perforin, Fas/Fas ligand, and TNF pathways as specific and bystander killing mechanisms in hepatitis C virus-specific human CTL. J Immunol. 1997;158:5283–91.
27. Koziel MJ, Dudley D, Wong JT, Dienstag J, Houghton M, Ralston R, Walker ED. Intrahepatic cytotoxic T lymphocytes specific for hepatitis C virus in persons with chronic hepatitis. J Immunol. 1992;149:3339–44.
28. Koziel MJ, Dudley D, Afdahl N, Choo QL, Houghton M, Ralston R, Walker BD. Hepatitis C virus (HCV)-specific cytotoxic T lymphocyte recognize epitopes in the core and envelope proteins of HCV. J Virol. 1993;67:7522–32.
29. Cerny A, McHutchinson G, Pasquinelli C, Brown ME, Brothers MA, Grabscheid B et al. Cytotoxic T lymphocyte response to hepatitis C virus-derived peptides containing the HLA A2.1 binding motif. J Clin Invest. 1995;95:521–30.
30. Battegay M, Fikes J, Di Bisceglie AM, Wentworth PA, Sette A, Celis E et al. Patients with chronic hepatitis C have circulating cytotoxic T cells which recognize hepatitis C virus-encoded peptides binding to HLA A2.1 molecules. J Virol. 1995;69:2462–70.
31. Kita H, Hiroishi K, Moriyama T, Okamoto H, Kaneko T, Ohnishi S et al. A minimal and optimal cytotoxic T cell epitope within hepatitis C virus nucleoprotein. J Gen Virol. 1995;76:3189–93.
32. Wentworth PA, Sette A, Celis E, Sidney J, Southwood S, Crimi C et al. Identification of A2-restricted hepatitis C virus-specific cytotoxic T lymphocyte epitopes from conserved regions of the viral genome. Int Immunol. 1996;8:651–9.
33. Kaneko T, Nakamura I, Kita H, Hiroishi K, Moriyama T, Imawari M. Three new cytotoxic T cell epitopes identified within the hepatitis C virus nucleoprotein. J Gen Virol. 1996;77:1305–9.

34. Chang KM, Rehermann B, McHutchinson JG, Pasquinelli C, Southwood S, Sette A, Chisari FV. Immunological significance of cytotoxic T lymphocyte epitope variants in patients chronically infected by the hepatitis C virus. J Clin Invest. 1997;100:2376–85.
35. Koziel MJ, Walker BD. Characteristics of the intrahepatic cytotoxic T lymphocyte response in chronic hepatitis C virus infection. Springer Semin Immunopathol. 1997;19:69–83.
36. Wong DK, Dudley DD, Afdahl NH, Dienstag J, Rice CM, Wang L et al. Liver-derived CTL in hepatitis C virus infection: breadth and specificity of responses in a cohort of persons with chronic infection. J Immunol. 1998;160:1479–88.
37. Schweitzer S, Langhans B, Kraus W, Jung G, Inchauspé G, Vidalin O et al. Limited repertoire of HCV core CTL epitopes in man. Cytokine, 2000 (in press).
38. He XS, Rehermann B, Lopez-Labrador FX, Boisvert J, Cheung R, Mumm J et al. Quantitative analysis of hepatitis C virus-specific CD8(+) T cells in peripheral blood and liver using peptide-MHC tetramers. Proc Natl Acad Sci USA. 1999;96:5692–7.
39. Rehermann B, Chang KM, McHutchinson J, Kokka R, Houghton M, Rice CM, Chisari FV. Differential cytotoxic T-lymphocyte responsiveness to the hepatitis B and C viruses in chronically infected patients. J Virol. 1996;70:7092–102.
40. Hiroishi K, Kita H, Kojima M, Okamoto H, Moriyama T, Kaneko T et al. Cytotoxic T lymphocyte response and viral load in hepatitis C virus infection. Hepatology. 1997;25:705–72.
41. Nelson DR, Marousis CG, Davis GL, Rice CM, Wong J, Houghton M, Lau JY. The role of hepatitis C virus specific cytotoxic T lymphocytes in chronic hepatitis C. J Immunol. 1997;158:1473–81.
42. Koziel MJ, Wong DKH, Dudley D, Houghton M, Walker BD. Hepatitis C virus-specific cytolytic T lymphocyte and T helper cell responses in seronegative persons. J Infect Dis. 1997;176:859–66.
43. Dumoulin FL, Bach A, Leifeld L, El Bakri M, Fischer HP, Sauerbruch T, Spengler U. Semiquantitative analysis of intrahepatic cytokine mRNAs in chronic hepatitis C. J Infect Dis. 1997;175:681–5.
44. Napoli J, Bishop GA, McGuinness PH, Painter DM, McCauchghan GW. Progressive liver injury in chronic hepatitis C infection correlates with increased intrahepatic expression of Th1-associated cytokines. Hepatology. 1996;4:759–65.
45. Mosmann TR, Cherwinski H, Bond MW, Giedlin MA, Coffman RL. Two types of murine helper T cell clone I. Definition according to profiles of lymphokine activities and secreted proteins. J Immunol. 1986;136:2348–57.
46. Sornasse T, Larenas PV, Davis KA, deVries JE, Yssel HJ. Differentiation and stability of T helper 1 and 2 cells derived from naive human neonatal CD4+ T cells, analyzed at the single-cell level. J Exp Med. 1996;184:473–83.
47. Mosmann TR, Coffman RL. TH1 and TH2 cells: Different patterns of lymphokine secretion lead to different functional properties. Annu Rev Immunol. 1989;7:145–73.
48. Bottomly K. A functional dichotomy in CD4+ T lymphocytes. Immunol Today. 1988;9:268–74.
49. Yamamura M, Uyemura K, Deans RJ, Weinberg K, Rea TH, Bloom BR, Modlin RL. Defining protective responses to pathogens: cytokine profiles in leprosy lesion. Science. 1991;254:277–80.
50. Clerici M, Shearer GM. A TH1→TH2 switch is a critical step in the etiology of HIV infection. Immunol Today. 1993;14:107–11.
51. Sher A, Coffman RL. Regulation of immunity to parasites by T cells and T cell-derived cytokines. Annu Rev Immunol. 1993;10:384–409.
52. Lechmann M, Ihlenfeldt HG, Braunschweiger I, Giers G, Jung G, Matz B et al. T and B cell responses to different hepatitis C virus antigens in patients with chronic hepatitis and healthy anti-HCV positive blood donors without viremia. Hepatology. 1996;24:790–5.
53. Botarelli P, Brunetto MR, Minutello MA, Calvo P, Unutmaz D, Weiner AJ et al. T-lymphocyte response to hepatitis C virus in different clinical courses of infection. Gastroenterology. 1993;104:580–7.
54. Ferrari C, Valli A, Galati L, Penna A, Scaccaglia P, Giuberti T et al. T cell response to structural and nonstructural hepatitis C virus antigen in persistent and self-limited hepatitis C virus infections. Hepatology. 1994;19:286–95.
55. Hoffmann RM, Diepolder HM, Zachoval R, Zwiebel FM, Jung MC, Scholz S et al. Mapping of immunodominant CD4+ T lymphocyte epitopes of hepatitis C virus antigens and their relevance during the course of chronic infection. Hepatology. 1995;21:632–8.

56. Missale G, Bertoni R, Lamonaca V, Valli A, Massari M, Mori C et al. Different clinical behaviours of acute hepatitis C virus infection are associated with different vigor of the antiviral cell-mediated immune response. J Clin Invest. 1996;98:706–14.
57. Diepolder HM, Gerlach JT, Zachoval R, Hoffmann RM, Jung MC, Wierenga EA et al. Immunodominant CD4+ T-cell epitope within nonstructural protein 3 in acute hepatitis C virus infection. J Virol. 1997;71:6011–19.
58. Cacciarelli TV, Martinez OM, Gish RG, Villanueva JC, Krams SM. Immunoregulatory cytokines in chronic hepatitis C virus infection: pre- and posttreatment with interferon alfa. Hepatology. 1996;24:6–9.
59. Tsai S-L, Liaw Y-F, Chen M-H, Huang C-Y, Kuo GC. Detection of type 2-like T-helper cells in hepatitis C virus infection: implication for hepatitis C chronicity. Hepatology. 1997;25:449–58.
60. Woitas R, Lechmann M, Jung G, Kaiser R, Sauerbruch T, Spengler U. CD30 induction and cytokine profiles in HCV core-specific peripheral blood T lymphocytes. J Immunol. 1997;159:1012–18.
61. Reiser M, Marousis CG, Nelson DR, Lauer G, Gonzalez-Peralta RP, Davis GL, Lau JYN. Serum interleukin 4 and interleukin 10 levels in patients with chronic hepatitis C virus infection. J Hepatol. 1997;26:471–8.
62. Malaguarnera M, Di Fazio I, Laurino A, Pistone G, Restuccia S, Trovato BA. Decrease of interferon gamma serum levels in patients with chronic hepatitis C. Biomed Pharmacother. 1997;51:391–6.
63. Osna N, Silonova G, Vigert N, Hagina E, Kuse V, Giedratis V et al. Chronic hepatitis C: T-helper 1/T-helper 2 imbalance could cause virus persistence in peripheral blood. Scand J Clin Lab Invest. 1997;57:703–10.
64. Fan XG, Liu WE, Li CZ, Wang ZC, Luo LX, Tan DM et al. Circulating Th1 and Th2 cytokines in patients with hepatitis C virus infection. Mediators Inflamm. 1998;7:295–7.
65. Lechmann M, Woitas RP, Langhans B, Kaiser R, Ihlenfeldt HG, Jung G et al. Decreased frequency of HCV core-specific peripheral blood mononuclear cells with type 1 cytokine secretion in chronic hepatitis C. J Hepatol. 1999;31:871–8.
66. Schwartz RH. Costimulation of T lymphocytes: the role of CD28, CTLA-4, and B7/BB1 in interleukin 2 production and immunotherapy. Cell. 1992;71:1065–8.
67. Langhans B, Lechmann M, Bär S, El Bakri M, Woitas R, Leifeld L et al. A hepatitis C virus (HCV) core protein derived peptide inhibits core specific cellular immune responses. J Hepatol. 1996;25:75A [Abstract].
68. Kanto T, Hayashi N, Takehara T, Tatsumi T, Kuzushita N, Ito A et al. Impaired allostimulatory capacity of peripheral blood dendritic cells recovered from hepatitis C virus-infected individuals. J Immunol. 1999;162:5584–91.
69. Pasi KJ, Evans JA, Wadwa M, Thorpe R, Hill FGH. Association of changes in monocyte antigen presentation and cytokine production in haemophiliac boys with treatment and blood-borne infections. Br J Haematol. 1995;91:191–6.
70. Dumoulin FL, Leifeld L, Honecker U, Sauerbruch T, Spengler U. Intrahepatic expression of interleukin-1 beta and tumor necrosis factor alpha in chronic hepatitis C. J Infect Dis. 1999;180:1704–8.
71. Langhans B, Braunschweiger B, Schweitzer S, Jung G, Inchauspé G, Sauerbruch T, Spengler U. Hepatitis C virus (HCV) core-derived T helper lipopeptides improve HCV specific lymphocyte proliferation. 2000. Submitted.
72. Aliprantis AO, Yang RB, Mark MR, Sugget S, Devaux B, Radolf JD et al. Cell activation and apoptosis by bacterial lipoproteins through Toll-like receptor-2. Science. 1999;285:736–9.
73. Christie JML, Chapel H, Chapman RW, Rosenberg WMC. Immune selection and genetic sequence variation in core and envelope regions of hepatitis C virus. Hepatology. 1999;30:1037–44.
74. Lam NP, Neumann AU, Gretch DR, Wiley TE, Perelson AS, Layden TJ. Dose-dependent acute clearance of hepatitis genotype 1 virus with interferon-alfa. Hepatology. 1997;26:226–31.
75. Neumann AU, Lam NP, Dahari H, Gretch TR, Wiley TE, Layden TJ, Perelsen AS. Hepatitis C viral dynamics in vivo and the antiviral efficacy of interferon-alpha therapy. Science. 1998;282:103–7.
76. Düesberg U, Kaiser R, Brackmann HH, Matz B, Sauerbruch T, Spengler U. Viral clearance associated with transient loss of peripheral blood T cell reactivity in a patient with HCV reinfection – a case report. 2000. Submitted.

77. Ruggieri A, Harada T, Matsuura Y, Miyamura T. Sensitization to Fas-mediated apoptosis by hepatitis C virus core protein. Virology. 1997;229:68–76.
78. Zhu N, Khoshnan A, Schneider R, Matsumo M, Dennert G, Ware C, Lai MM. Hepatitis C virus core protein binds to the cytoplasmic domain of tumor necrosis factor (TNF) receptor 1 and enhances TNF-induced apoptosis. J Virol. 1998;72:3691–7.
79. Meyer RBK, Steele R, Shrivastava A, Aggarwal BB, Ray R. Inhibition of tumor necrosis factor (TNF-alpha)-mediated apoptosis by hepatitis C virus core protein. J Biol Chem. 1998;273:2256–9.
80. Marusawa H, Hijikata M, Chiba T, Shimotohno K. Hepatitis C virus core protein inhibits Fas- and tumor necrosis factor alpha-mediated apoptosis via NF-kappaB activation. J Virol. 1999;73:4713–20.
81. Tayor DR, Shi ST, Romano PR, Barber GN, Lai MMC. Inhibition of the interferon-inducible protein kinase PKR by HCV E2 protein. Science. 1999;285:107–10.
82. Borowski P, Heiland M, Feucht H, Laufs R. Characterisation of the non-structural protein 3 of the hepatitis C virus as modulator of protein phosphorylation mediated by PKA and PKC: evidence for action on the level of substrate and enzyme. Arch Virol. 1999;144:687–701.
83. Polyak SJ, Paschal DM, McArdle S, Gale MJ, Moradpour D, Gretch DR. Characterization of the effects of hepatitis C virus nonstructural 5A protein expression in human cell lines and on interferon-sensitive virus replication. Hepatology. 1999;29:1262–71.
84. Gale M, Blakely CM, Kwieciszewski B, Tan SL, Dossett M, Tang NM et al. Control of PKR protein kinase by hepatitis C virus nonstructural 5A protein: molecular mechanism of kinase regulation. Mol Cell Biol. 1998;18:5208–18.
85. Large MK, Kittleson DJ, Hahn YS. Suppression of the host immune response by the core protein of hepatitis C virus: possible implications for hepatitis C virus persistence. J Immunol. 1999;162:931–8.
86. Matsumo M, Hsieh N, Zhu T, Van Arsdale T, Hwang SB, Jeng KS et al. Hepatitis C virus core protein interacts with the cytoplasmic tail of lymphotoxin-B receptor. J Virol. 1997;71:1301–7.
87. Chen CM, You LR, Hwang LH, Lee YH. Direct interaction of hepatitis C virus core protein with the cellular lymphotoxin-β receptor modulates the signal pathway of the lymphotoxin-β receptor. J Virol. 1997;71:9417–22.
88. Gooding LR. Virus proteins that counteract the host immune defenses. Cell. 1992;71:5–7.
89. Barry M, McFadden G. Virus encoded cytokines and cytokine receptors. Parasitology. 1997;115:S89–100.
90. Davis-Poyntner NJ, Farell HE. Masters of deception: a review of herpes virus immune evasion strategies. Immunol Cell Biol. 1996;74:513–22.
91. Hengel H, Koszinowski UH. Interference with antigen processing by viruses. Curr Opin Immunol. 1997;9:470–6.

11
Natural history of hepatitis C virus infection – risk factors for disease progression

S. K. SARIN and D. KAPOOR

Infection with hepatitis C virus (HCV) causes acute and chronic hepatitis with attending sequelae of cirrhosis and primary hepatocellular carcinoma (HCC). Approximately 4 million people in the US and probably more than 100 million people worldwide are infected with this virus[1]. According to the estimates from the Centres for Disease Control and Prevention (CDC), of the 1.8% Americans infected with this agent, about 10 000 succumb to the consequences of this infection every year[2]. While the natural history of hepatitis C has been extensively studied, it still remains unclear how the disease will progress in a given individual. Patients who clear the virus after an acute infection constitute a small percentage of those who get infected with hepatitis C. Those who go on to the chronic course rarely manifest features of chronic hepatitis and often may insidiously progress to cirrhosis and ultimately HCC. It is however not known whether the sequelae of chronic hepatitis C are inevitable in every person infected with this agent and whether there is a linear or a predictable course to any of these events[3]. To make matters more complex, a subset of patients remain apparently 'stable' even in the stages of chronic hepatitis and cirrhosis – they are asymptomatic, have persistently normal aminotransferases, and in the former category, even a mildly abnormal liver histology[4] (Fig. 1). Thus, it has been exceedingly difficult to accurately define outcomes in patients infected with HCV.

From an epidemiologist's standpoint, the requirements of an ideal natural history study of HCV infection have not been possible because of several limitations:

- The precise time of onset of infection is often unknown and inference regarding duration of infection is drawn from an event such as blood transfusion, surgery, intravenous drug abuse (IVDA), etc.
- The acute infection is symptomatic in less than 20% of cases; patients are, therefore, missed at this stage, thus preventing a complete assessment of this cohort.

- Those who harbor the infection chronically are also quite often asymptomatic, making it difficult to determine the full spectrum of chronic illness.
- Parallel studies on a 'control group' of subjects not infected with HCV have been woefully few in numbers. This is because the acute onset of illness can often not be defined. This is far more important as the disease course is greatly modified by 'non-agent factors' such as age, sex of host, alcohol abuse or IVDA.
- Lack of data from controlled studies on the clinical outcome of the infection treated *vis-à-vis* untreated patients. In the former group too, the fate of the disease may largely be governed by success or failure of therapy. At the present time, it might be unethical to conduct natural history studies on patients denied treatment, as new and more effective therapies get added to the armamentarium against this agent.

To circumvent some of these problems, investigators have tried to come up with mathematical models or statistical projections to define the magnitude of the problem in a given patient or a community. Deuffic et al. tried to devise a model based on 'back calculation' to predict the outcome of chronic HCV infection in France[5]. They project that the HCC related mortality (predominantly due to

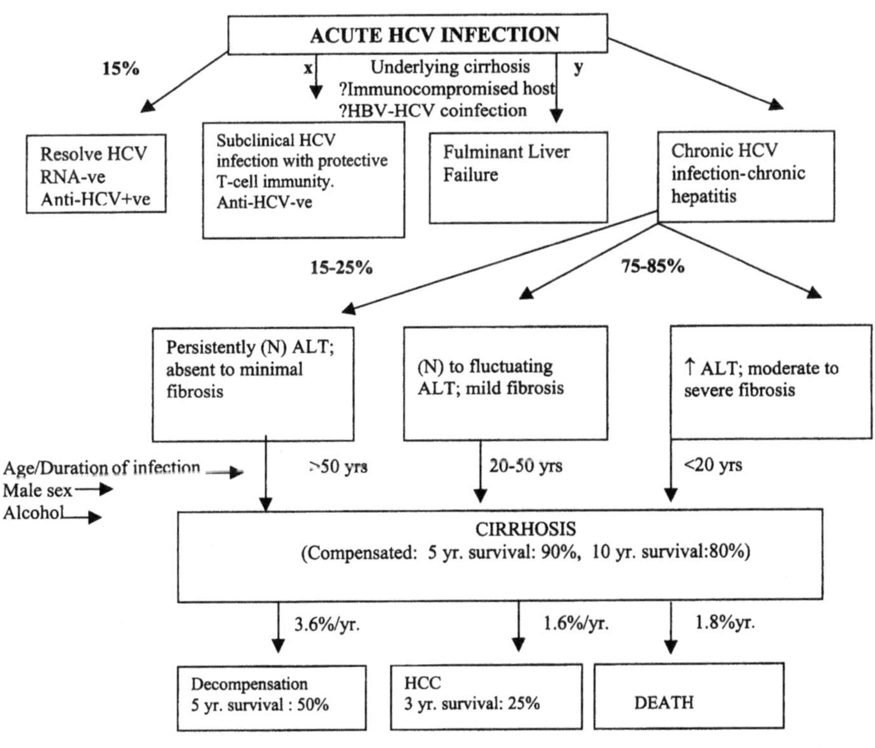

Figure 1 Natural history of HCV infection. 'x' and 'y' represent poorly defined outcomes. Arrows represent synergistic factors.

HCV) will continue to rise through 2020 in the absence of successful therapy, leading to a 150% increase in the yearly incidence among men and 200% among women. In spite of the apparent 'fit' of their calculations with known epidemiological data on the course of chronic infection, there are certain flaws in their projections, the most important being that they have considered only age and sex as the main variables determining the progression from stage of chronic hepatitis to cirrhosis. This underscores the fact that no matter how careful the attempt, the study of a disease whose course is governed by so many variables is not going to be easy.

As is evident from Figure 1, the possible outcomes after infection with HCV can be conveniently categorized into:

(I) Subclinical HCV infection with protective immunity;
(II) Outcomes after acute hepatitis C (AHC);
(III) Outcomes after chronic hepatitis C (CHC);
(IV) Outcomes after liver cirrhosis (LC).

The reason for classifying these events as above is to draw meaningful conclusions from different studies which have taken patients at any of these stages as the cohort and then tried to define their course. In most of these categories, one can draw upon studies which have prospectively, retrospectively or retrospectively–prospectively followed the patients over a period of time. These study prototypes deserve special mention as these are the studies with the largest sample size and in which a cohort of subjects or patients who had experienced a well defined clinical event in the past are traced from specific registries and then tracked many years or decades later to ascertain how they are faring.

SUBCLINICAL HCV INFECTION WITH PROTECTIVE T-CELL IMMUNITY

A group of individuals who are repeatedly exposed to HCV infection, possibly in small doses, may have self-limited clinically covert infections. These subjects are seronegative (i.e. do not produce any anti-HCV antibodies in spite of normal immune status) and yet their T-cells (especially CD 8 cells) are able to mount a vigorous cytotoxic T lymphocyte (CTL) response against multiple HCV epitopes in vitro[6]. These individuals are generally the family contacts of patients with apparent or inapparent chronic HCV infection. The awareness regarding this group is increasing and study of these subjects may help elucidate mechanisms of viral clearance better in the future. The long-term outcome of these subjects is currently unknown.

OUTCOMES AFTER ACUTE HEPATITIS C (AHC)

Most studies which have dealt with the problem of AHC have drawn upon patients from three main groups: transfusion recipients, intravenous drug abusers and sporadic cases. The data show that most of these patients have subclinical infection[7]. The incubation period may vary according to the mode of trans-

Table 1 Progression of acute NANBH to chronicity based on mode of transmission

Mode of transmission	*Acute HCV*	*Chronic HCV (%)*[a]
Blood Transfusion	21	14 (67)
IVDA	20	18 (60)
Occupational exposure	5	3 (60)
Sexual/household contact	6	5 (83)
Low socio-economic status	28	17 (61)
None	7	3 (43)
Total	97	60 (62)

[a] Data modified from Ref. 8
Chronic HCV based on ALT > ULN at least 9 months after acute infection

mission and is higher for post-transfusion (5–12 weeks) than for nosocomial non-A, non-B hepatitis (NANBH) (~ 4 weeks) and NANBH in recipients of coagulation factors (~ 1 week)[7]. The hepatitic illness in those who become symptomatic is milder than that seen with the other causes of acute hepatitis, with peak serum bilirubin and ALT levels generally remaining lower than 12 mg/dl and 600 IU/L. The progression to chronic course may also depend on the initial mode of transmission, being lower for sporadic NANBH (~30–40%) than post-transfusion NANBH (60–70%)[8] (Table 1).

The pattern of ALT abnormalities after AHC may show one of the following features:

- Recurrent elevations interspersed with normal or near normal values (which may occur over weeks or months).
- Monophasic rapid increase to peak ALT followed by rapid decline to normal, only to increase after months or years.
- Moderate increase in ALT which plateaus off at that or slightly lower level.

None of these patterns can determine whether or not a patient would progress to the stage of chronicity[8,9].

The course of acute (post-transfusion) hepatitis C, with respect to viral clearance was studied by Tremolada in a group of 117 patients. These workers showed that HCV RNA is cleared from the serum in 15% of cases while 85% of the cases remain viraemic – 12% with normalized ALT and 73% with raised/fluctuating ALT[10].

The course of acute hepatitis C with respect to histological progression and well defined clinical outcomes has shown that the frequency of cirrhosis is 8–24%, while that of HCC is 0.7–1.3%[10–12], and of liver related deaths 1.6–6.0% after a mean follow-up of 7.6–14 years. The results from one such well defined prospective study are diagrammatically shown in Fig. 2.

Four landmark retrospective–prospective (non-concurrent prospective) studies have contributed greatly to our understanding of HCV infection[13–16]. These studies have been vital, as they have followed up individuals for a long period after they developed AHC. The results of these studies have been

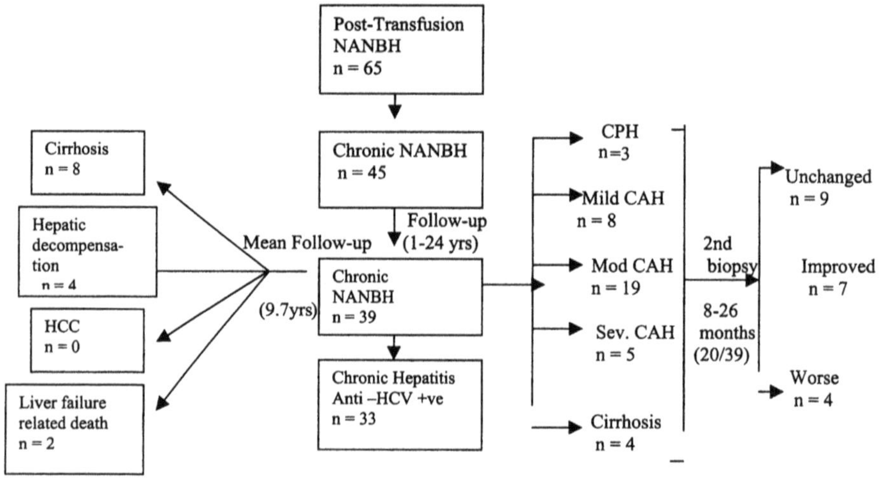

Figure 2 Outcome after acute post transfusion hepatitis (data from Ref. 11).

highlighted in Table 2. Taken together, the data from these studies would suggest that benign outcome is quite common after HCV infection and of the 15–20% of persons who develop serious sequelae, cirrhosis is the critical arbiter of a poor outcome. To counter the impression of a seemingly benign outcome of HCV infection derived from these studies, some authorities believe that the patient population in these studies were young, female patients with low or absent alcohol consumption and who might have received small inocula of the virus at the outset.

OUTCOMES AFTER CHRONIC HEPATITIS C (CHC)

The clinical course of chronic hepatitis C is generally long and indolent and a fair number of patients remain 'stable' even when CHC has progressed to liver cirrhosis. Roughly 50% of these patients are asymptomatic. A large proportion of these patients are now coming to the fore during routine testing of blood donors or have vague complaints including right upper quadrant pain/discomfort or malaise/fatiguability or on incidental detection of elevated transaminases.

Before discussing the results of large prospective and retrospective studies of outcome of CHC, it is worth addressing the issue of patients who are asymptomatic or have persistently normal ALT. Alberti et al.[17] found nine out of 16 patients with normal ALT and no symptoms to have chronic hepatitis on biopsy. All these patients were HCV RNA positive. Gholson et al.[18] studied 50 patients with persistently normal ALT. Although only a few were symptomatic, abnormal histological features were seen in 46 (92%). While 60% of this study population had a grade and/or stage of liver disease ≤ 2, seven were cirrhotic (14%), which underscores the point of stable but significant liver disease mentioned above. At the other end of the spectrum are studies which moot the concept of 'HCV carrier state'. Naito et al.[19] studied 22 HCV RNA positive

Table 2 Long-term outcome of chronic HCV infection: data from retrospective–prospective studies

Author; No. Patients	*Source of infection*	*Follow-up (years)*	*Symptoms*	*Passed ALT*	*CPH*	*CAH*	*Cirrhosis*	*HCC*	*Death due to liver disease*
Seef et al.[13] n = 568	Blood/Igs	18	–	–	–	–	–	–	19 (3.3%)[a]
Muller et al.[14b] n = 152	Anti-D Igs	15	–	–	83 (55%)	0	0	0	0
Walsh et al.[15] n = 376	Anti-D Igs	17	304 (81%)	47%	HAI < 4 in 43% No/2 fibrosis in 49%		7 (2%)[c]	–	–
Rodger et al.[16d] n = 35	Community acquired	20	–	16 (44%)	–	–	2 (6%)	0	–

[a] Compared to 15 deaths in 984 control ($p = 0.033$). Of the 19 deaths in the NANBH group, 2 deaths were due to liver cancer, 11 due to cirrhosis and the rest due to miscellaneous causes. Extended follow up of 23 years showed similar trends
[b] 65% completely recovered; 4 had normal ALT but were HCV RNA positive
[c] Two of the 7 cirrhotics had excessive alcohol consumption
[d] Case control study with most patients having history of IVDA; 60% of those with raised ALT abused alcohol

Table 3 Features of chronic HCV infection in patients with normal ALT[19]

Parameter	*Normal histology*	*Mild CPH*	*Moderate CPH*
Age	42.3 ± 18.5	45.8 ± 10.7	50.9 ± 9.3
ALT (IU/L)	15.3 ± 10.4	21.5 ± 5.4	21.1 ± 3.9
HCV RNA (log^{10} copies/ml)	4.3 ± .2	6.4 ± .8*	7.1 ± 5*

* $p < 0.05$ w.r.t. patients with normal liver biopsy
None of the patients had CAH or LC

subjects who had persistently normal ALT for ≥ 12 months. These workers found a low probability of significant histological lesions, despite the fact that 20 of the 22 patients had genotype Ib (Table 3). However, with advancing age, there was a tendency to more severe histological lesions. Morisco et al.[20] studied 27 anti-HCV-positive subjects for a mean of 2–6 years. The follow-up (biochemical) showed that the ALT levels remained steady in these subjects. Of the 15 HCV RNA positive subjects in this cohort, the mean ALT was <0.6 times the upper limit of normal (ULN) while in the 12 RNA-negative subjects, it was <0.4 × ULN. The steady ALT levels cut across various viral loads and genotypes. The main flaws in this study were, however, that all the study subjects had no history of blood transfusion, IVDA or alcohol consumption, i.e., the study population was a well selected one. In addition, histological disease was assessed in a small number of subjects only. A more important message from this study is that the HCV RNA-positive subjects continued to remain so at the end of follow-up. Similar results were shown by Yokusuka et al.[21], in a much larger study population (n = 320), followed up for more than 3 years. In their study of untreated patients, only 2% of the cases became RNA negative at the end of follow-up, and even in those who normalized ALT (3.5%), the RNA levels remained positive.

New terminology for chronic HCV carrier

The data shown above clearly indicate that the patients who are viraemic with normal ALT do continue to have ongoing liver injury, albeit mild. Since HCV infection is a dynamic process, ALT levels may fluctuate. The term 'carrier' is misleading as it connotes a benign state in which there is no harm being done to the subject carrying the virus. Based on an International Consensus Conference, the term HCV carrier was found unsatisfactory and was replaced by chronic HCV infection[22]. Such subjects could be further divided into four categories (Table 4).

Group I: Anti HCV +ve, HCV RNA –ve, ALT normal;
Group II: Anti HCV +ve, HCV RNA +ve, ALT normal;
Group III: Anti HCV +ve, HCV RNA +ve, ALT raised;
Group IV: Anti HCV –ve, HCV RNA +ve, ALT normal.

Some patients in group I may not have chronic hepatitis C virus infection. It would need a liver biopsy to determine whether HCV RNA is present in the liver

Table 4 Approach to subjects with chronic HCV infection

	Anti-HCV (+) HCV RNA (–) Normal ALT (Group I)	*Anti-HCV (+) HCV RNA (+) Normal ALT (Group II)*	*Anti-HCV (+) HCV RNA (+) Elevated ALT (Group III)*	*Anti-HCV (–) HCV RNA (+) (Group IV)*
Approach				
Repeat anti-HCV	Yes	No	No	No
RIBA	No	No	No	No
Liver biopsy	No	Yes[a]	Yes	Yes
Follow-up				
Clinical	12–24 months	6–12 months	Consider as chronic hepatitis C	As for Group III Subjects
ALT	12–24 months	6–12 months		3–6 months
HCV RNA	12 months	12–24 months		Yes[b]
Alpha fetoprotein	No	Yes, baseline		Yes
Ultrasonography	No	Yes, baseline		Yes
Upper GI endoscopy	No	Yes, baseline		Yes
Liver biopsy	No	No consensus		Yes[b]
Management	No treatment	Depends on biopsy (under protocol)	Treat with interferon + ribavirin	Yes[c]

[a] To be performed only if clinical, biochemical, radiological evidence of liver disease is present or under a research protocol prior to therapy
[b] If therapy has to be instituted
[c] Needs to be individualized. It is unsatisfactory in the post-transplant scenario

tissue or not. Otherwise, a positive anti-HCV in subjects belonging to this group may simply reflect evidence of past HCV infection only. A minimum of two negative HCV RNA results, performed 6 months apart, would be necessary to constitute the HCV RNA-ve group I. By 'normal ALT', it is implied in all the groups that the ALT values (determined by using a standardized analyzer) remains persistently normal for a period of at least 6 months. At least three ALT values should be available during this period. Patients belonging to group IV are generally immunosuppressed, and cannot mount an adequate and strong antibody response. Hence, they are anti-HCV negative but HCV RNA positive. A high index of suspicion is needed to detect them in the specialized group. This terminology is being recently adopted by the Asian Pacific Association for Study of the Liver (APASL).

Three large, retrospective studies have addressed the issue of the natural course of CHC; two defining clinical outcomes[23,24] (Table 5) and one addressing the histological and biochemical course[25]. In the first two studies, transfusion was the exclusive source of infection while only about ~35% of the study population in the last had received blood transfusion. Of the 100 patients followed for a mean of 5 years by Takahatashi et al.[25], sustained normalization of ALT was seen in only four cases. Forty-two of these cases progressed to LC from the initial

Table 5 Progression of chronic hepatitis C data from retrospective studies

		Time (mean ± s.d.) (years)		
Study	*Source of infection*	*Chronic hepatitis*	*Cirrhosis*	*HCC*
Kiyosawa et al.[23] (n = 89)	Transfusion	10.0 ± 11.3	21.2 ± 9.6	29.0 ± 13.2
Tong et al.[24] (n = 131)	Transfusion	13.7 ± 10.9	20.6 ± 10.1	28.3 ± 11.5
Takahashi et al.[25] (n = 333)	transfusion 116 (35%) unknown in 217 (65%)	12 ± 12 – CPH[a] 18 ± 12 – CAH2A[b] 23 ± 9 – CAH2B[b]	24 ± 8	See text

[a] Chronic hepatitis amongst those with h/o transfusion
[b] CAH2A corresponds to moderate CAH and CAH2 B to severe CAH

histological diagnosis after a mean interval of 8 ± 6 years. Nineteen of the 100 patients developed HCC, after a mean period of 3 years from the diagnosis of LC.

The largest well defined prospective study on the course of CHC was reported from Germany[26]. The study was conducted at two referral hospitals and enrolled 838 anti-HCV-positive and HCV RNA-positive patients between 1987 and 1997. It was also able to address the issue of response to therapy which was instituted in about a half of these patients. About 32% of the study population had received transfusion, 16% were IVDAs and in 41% the source of infection was unknown. The salient features studied were age at entry, duration of infection and presence or absence of cirrhosis. These parameters were used to compare all cause and specific cause mortality in the study cohort and the general population matched for age and sex. The salient results from this study are highlighted in Tables 6

Table 6 Age and duration of HCV infection in function of liver histology and HCC in CHC patients[26]

Parameter	*Number of patients*	*Mean duration of infection (years)*	*Mean age at entry (years)*
Stage*			
Neither firbrosis nor cirrhosis	362	9.0	46.3
Fibrosis	88	13.1	53.7
Cirrhosis	130	16.2	57.8
Inflammatory Activity			
No hepatitis/minimal hepatitis	68	13.4#	47.3#
Chronic hepatitis	518	11.8	50.7
Total no. of patients with initial biopsy	586	11.3	50.3
HCC*			
HCC during follow-up	17	21.8	62.2
No HCC during follow-up	821	10.1	49.1
Total no. of patients	838	10.3	49.4

* $p < 0.001$ by ANOVA
\# $p < 0.05$ for age at entry and $p > 0.05$ for duration of infection when patients with histological evidence of CH compared with those without

Table 7 Determinants of mortality in patients with chronic HCV infection[26]

Standardized mortality ratio	*Age*	*Age*	*Duration (years)*		*Cirrhosis*	
	<50	*≥50*	*<15*	*≥15y*	*Present*	*Absent*
0.7	Any	age	+			+
2.5*	Any	age	+		+	
1.2	Any	age		+		+
4.8*	Any	age		+	+	
3.1*	+		Any duration			+
26.2*	+		Any duration		+	
1.9	+		+			+
22.5*	+		+			+
15.5*	+			+	Any histology	
9.1*	+			+		+
30.6*	+			+	+	
0.6		+	Any duration			+
2.8*		+	Any duration		+	
0.5		+	+		+	
1.3		+	+		+	
2.0*		+		+	Any histology	
0.8		+		+		+
3.9*		+		+	+	

* Statistically significant
Note that in those ≥50 years of age but duration of disease <15 years, SMR is not high even if liver histology shows cirrhosis IVDA was an independent factor for high mortality

and 7. After a mean follow-up of 50.2 ± 26.9 months, 62 patients died (31 from liver disease and 31 from other causes). Using multivariate regression analysis, survival was decreased by cirrhosis, long duration of disease, history of IVDA and excessive alcohol consumption, while interferon therapy improved survival. ALT, bilirubin, sex and genotype had no effect on survival. With respect to HCC, the risk was increased by cirrhosis, long duration of disease and high bilirubin but interferon therapy, genotype and other factors had no impact.

Taking into account the results of all the studies, it can be inferred that duration of infection is a critical factor in determining the outcome and that the histological progression of disease occurs with time, albeit in a non-normal distribution pattern. Since HCV infection is a dynamic disease, the term carrier is misleading and should be replaced by chronic HCV infection[22].

OUTCOMES AFTER LIVER CIRRHOSIS (LC)

Two large retrospective studies have addressed the problem of compensated type C cirrhosis: EUROHEP study[27] and the Single Centre French study[28]. Both the studies had strict inclusion criteria for patient entry as LC and excluded patients with seromarkers for HBV or excessive alcohol intake (≥ 80 g/day). The main clinical outcomes were decompensation, HCC and survival. The results are shown in Tables 8 and 9. The foregoing account underscores the fact that HCV

Table 8 Outcome after liver cirrhosis in patients with chronic HCV infection

Study (n)	*Follow-up*	*Liver decompensation*	*HCC*	*Survival*	*Death during follow-up*
EUROHEP[27] (n = 384)	5 years	18%	7%	91%	51 (13%)*
FRENCH STUDY[27] (n = 103)	4 years	20%	11.5%	84%	16(6%)#

36 patients* and 15 patients#, respectively, died due to liver disease related causes

Table 9 Factors governing outcome of liver cirrhosis[26,27]

Univariate analysis	*Multivariate analysis*
Referral pattern*	Age > 54 years
Source of infection	S. bilirubin > 17 mmol/l
Alcohol intake (>80 g/day)	Platelet count <130 × 10^9/l
AST > 1.5 × ULN	Hepatic stigmata
AST/ALT > 1	
S. albumin <3.5 g/dl	
Prothrombin time prolongation >30%	
IFN therapy	

* Patients presenting with transaminasaemia or those followed from stage of CHC fared better than those who had LC at the outset
# IVDAs and those with history of transfusion had better survival than those whose source of infection was unknown
$ 15% and 5% of patients in the 2 studies showed sustained virological responses to IFN. In the French study, treatment with IFN was a significant factor even on multivariate analysis

related liver disease can have serious morbidity and mortality and that the effects may occur many years after the onset of infection.

FACTORS AFFECTING PROGRESSION OF CHRONIC HEPATITIS C

As already mentioned, the rate of progression of disease following HCV infection is highly variable, in part due to various agent and host factors. Some of the important factors are discussed below (Table 10).

Age and gender

Numerous studies have shown that older age and male sex are predictive of a greater chance to progression to cirrhosis in chronic hepatitis C. The older age may indirectly be a reflection of a longer duration of infection with HCV. Mattson et al.[29] noted that out of 92 patients with CHC, 64% of patients above 30 years of age had CAH while only 33% of those younger than 30 years had

Table 10 Variables affecting the outcome of chronic hepatitis C virus infection

Host	*Viral*	*Co-factors*	*Miscellaneous*
Age*	Viral load	Alcohol*	Initial histology*
Race	Genotype	HBV*	Antiviral therapy*
Gender*	Quasispecies	HIV*	
Immune response		Comorbid conditions	
HFE gene		(haemodialysis haemophilia, thalassaemia etc.)	

* Well established variables

this lesion. Wejstal et al.[9] reported in their series of 127 patients that the mean age of patients with CPH was 29.7 years while that of patients with CAH or LC was 46.8 years. The mean time to LC after blood transfusion in the EUROHEP study[27] was 5.7 years in those >50 years of age and 15.8 years in those ≤ 50 years. However, the survival in the two age groups was not statistically different. The benign outcome of HCV infection in young female patients from the large retrospective–prospective immunoglobulin studies has already been alluded to[14,15].

In a well designed analysis of progression of liver fibrosis in CHC patients, Poynard et al.[30] showed that only three independent factors were associated with an increased rate of fibrosis: age >40 years, male sex and daily alcohol consumption >50 g. According to them, the rate of fibrosis progression per year was 0.091 in those ≤ 20 years and 0.333 in those >50 years, thus implying progression to cirrhosis in 44 years and 12 years in the two groups respectively. The fibrosis progression in female patients was 0.111/year and in males, 0.154/year, with the two groups of patients expected to reach the stage of LC in 36 years and 26 years respectively (Fig. 3).

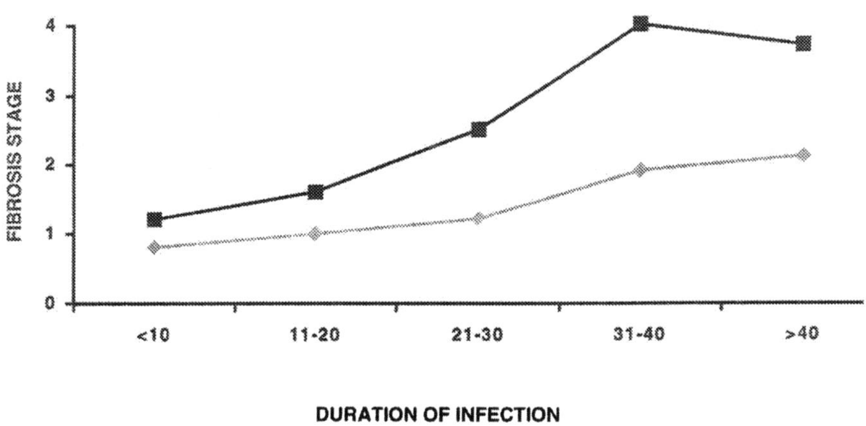

Figure 3 Association between fibrosis stage and duration of HCV infection. Note the steep increase in slope of the graph after 20 years of infection (data from Ref. 30).

Table 11 Estimated clinical outcome in subjects infected with HCV at age 30 and 50 years[5]

	Age at infection (years)	*Percentiles in men*			*Percentiles in women*		
		10	*50*	*90*	*10*	*50*	*90*
Time to cirrhosis (years)	30	22	32	42	27	44	55
	50	3	13	22	11	25	36
Time to HCC (years)	30	26	39	50	31	47	58
	50	8	19	30	15	29	40
Time to death from HCC (years)	30	28	41	53	33	49	60
	50	10	21	33	17	31	41

The two parameters, sex and age, were used to calculate the probability of progression to LC from CHC in the back-calculation model by Deuffic et al.[5]. They showed that at any age the annual probability of progression to cirrhosis is 10 times greater for men than women. For men aged 61–70 years this probability is 300 times greater than that for men aged 21–40 years (Table 11).

Immune response

It has long been known that the CTL response is quite vigorous in patients with CHC, in sharp contrast to patients with chronic hepatitis B. In spite of this, viral clearance occurs in only a small percentage of patients acutely infected with HCV. Missale et al.[31] studied 21 subjects with acute hepatitis C and followed them sequentially for 44 weeks. Twelve patients normalized their ALT and 10 of these also became HCV RNA negative. The T-cell proliferative response to core, E2, NS3, NS4 and NS5 recombinant antigens and synthetic peptides was more vigorous and frequently detectable in this subset of patients rather than in nine patients who failed to normalize ALT or clear the virus. Thus, these early responses are extremely crucial in viral clearance. The host immune response comes to the fore even at the stage of CHC, when patients are retreated with antiviral agents such as interferon (IFN). Lohr et al.[32] showed that T cells from 16 of the 24 HLA-A2-positive, but none of the six HLA-A2-negative patients with CHC lysed targets primed with antigenic peptides. The CTL frequency in patients who had sustained response to IFN was higher than that in non-responders. Thus, the host immune response is a key determinant of outcome after HCV infection.

Viral factors

As has already been mentioned, the viral titres in a given patient with chronic HCV infection may remain steady over prolonged periods. Some authors have shown no correlation between the viral load and severity of liver disease[33] while others have observed a correlation between the height of viral titre and the stage of liver disease[34].

The influence of viral genotype on the outcome of chronic HCV infection is rather controversial: in most studies where genotype 1b was shown to be associated with more severe liver disease there were confounding factors like longer duration of infection, higher viral loads or studies being conducted at referral hospitals. Indeed, it has been shown that genotype 2 might be more prevalent in the community and this genotype is associated with an indolent course of the disease[35]. Poynard et al. found no association between fibrosis progression and HCV genotype[30]. Niederau et al.[26] also showed that the age, duration of infection, ALT levels and cirrhosis to be comparable in patients with genotype 1 and 2. Genotypes 3 and 4 were associated with younger age of patients and shorter disease duration.

The association between genotype 1b and HCC is also equivocal, with some studies reporting a marginally increased relative risk[36], while others showed no such relationship[26,37]. The importance of HCV genotyping has gained recent interest, since results of large trials have shown that response to antiviral therapy is better in non-1 genotypes[38]. The patients with other genotypes have a higher chance of attaining a sustained response and may be treated for even shorter periods (6 months).

The relationship between the degree of diversity of hepatitis C virus quasispecies and progression of liver disease is complex. Honda et al.[39] showed nucleotide diversity in the core and envelope region of the virus to steadily increase from stage of CPH through CAH to LC. This intra-patient variation in nucleotides correlated with the serum levels of ALT. However, such a correlation may not be really straightforward, as the circulating viral population may be different from the hepatic one and it is the latter which governs the extent of liver injury. Recently, Nagayama et al. have also reported certain sequences of the HCV-1b genome which may be related to progression of chronic hepatitis C[40].

Alcohol

In patients with alcoholic liver disease, the prevalence of HCV positivity varies from 15% to 35%, the serological test being more likely to be positive in those with severe histologic liver disease. Takase et al.[41] showed that the anti-HCV positivity was ~5% in patients with alcoholic fibrosis, 31% with cirrhosis and 79% in those with HCC. HCV RNA is detected in about 95% of these anti-HCV-positive patients. In alcoholics, the possible routes of infection are the high risk behaviors like IVDA, sexual promiscuity or rarely, blood transfusion.

Cromic et al.[42] showed that after 4 months of alcohol-free diet, serum HCV RNA levels fell from 2.1×10^6 copies/ml to 0.8×10^6 copies/ml in 15 patients who consumed <10 g/day of ethanol. The fall was more dramatic ($2.6–0.42 \times 10^6$/ml) in those imbibing 70 g/day of alcohol. Similar results were shown by Pessione et al.[43] in a much larger study of 233 patients with CHC. In this study, the RNA levels were three times higher in those consuming >210 g/day of alcohol than in those not taking it.

Transaminase levels (especially ALT) are higher in alcoholics infected with HCV than in those seronegative for HCV. Also, the former group has a histologically more active disease (with respect to inflammation and fibrosis) and lymphoid aggregates on liver biopsy in an alcoholic patient with liver disease may point to concurrent HCV infection. Wiley et al.[44] showed that fibrosis progression in patients with HCV infection alone was lower (0.3 ± 0.007/year) than those also consuming >40 g/day of alcohol (0.5 ± 0.13 year). In this series, the

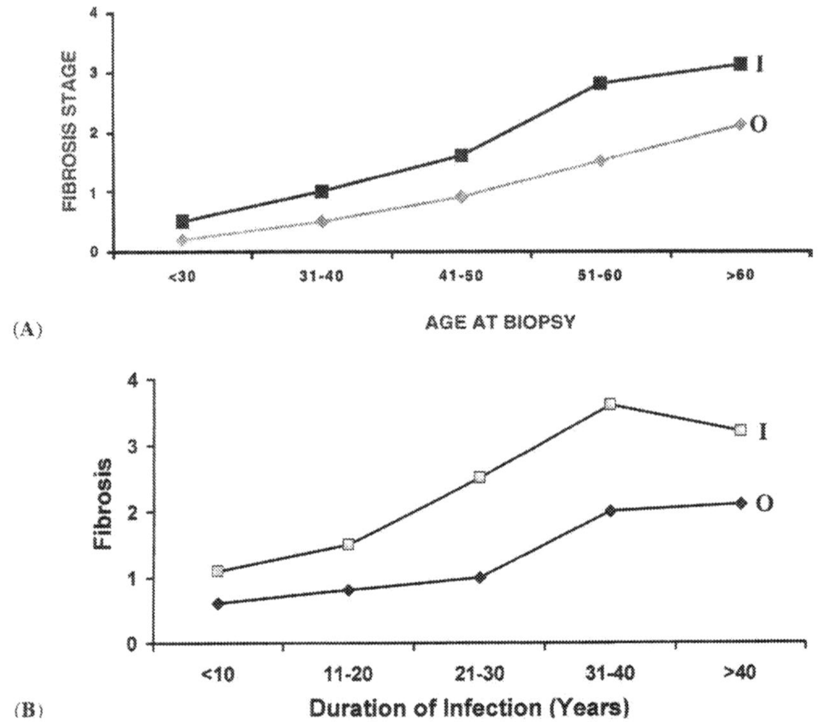

Figure 4 Association between fibrosis stage and (A) Age at biopsy and (B) Duration of HCV infection in the presence (I) and absence (O) of alcohol. Note that alcohol consumption > 50 g/day shifts the curve to the left (data from Ref. 30).

estimated incidence of cirrhosis in the 2 groups after 1, 2, 3 and 4 decades of follow up was 6% and 18%, 12% and 58%, 31% and 64% and 40% and 83%, respectively. Similar results were shown by Poynard et al.[30] (Fig. 4). There is controversy regarding additive risk to development of HCC in HCV infected patients imbibing alcohol, but the bulk of current evidence does point to the synergistic effect.

Another impact of alcohol on outcome of CHC is the poor response to IFN, seen in patients consuming large amounts of alcohol. This might in part be due to the higher RNA levels seen in these patients (see above). Indeed Okazaki et al.[45] showed a lower sustained response to IFN therapy in those taking >60 g/day of alcohol.

HIV co-infection

Both HCV and HIV share the same routes of transmission and are common in those prone to high risk activities such as IVDA. Indeed, in the Euro SIDA cohort, of the 3048 HIV-positive patients, 33% were also anti-HCV positive and this proportion rose to 75% in those with history of IVDA[46].

HIV can accelerate the course of HCV infection, and in the series by Soto et al.[47] cirrhosis developed in 25% of HIV-positive IVDAs, in contrast to 6.5% of patients who were HIV negative. Serum HCV RNA levels are higher in these patients and tend to rise further as the CD4 counts fall. Over the last few years, with the use and success of highly active anti-retroviral therapies (HAART), the longevity of HIV-infected patients has increased, and in this new scenario HCV has emerged as a major cause of liver disease-related morbidity and mortality in these patients. In addition, significant hepatotoxicity due to HAART may occur in patients co-infected with HCV, in part due to restoration of immune competence by these drugs and resultant hepatocytolysis in response to HCV infection in these patients[48].

The response to IFN in patients with HIV/HCV co-infection is similar to that seen in HIV-negative subjects with respect to end-of-treatment (ETR) response as well as sustained response (SR). However, the response rates tend to decrease with falling $CD4^+$ counts[49]. Currently, trials are on to assess the response rate to combination therapy (IFN + ribavirin) in these patients, but caution needs to be exercised in those receiving zidovudine (a nucleoside analogue which may cause bone marrow suppression) as it may accelerate the haemolytic anaemia caused by ribavirin.

HBV co-infection

Due to common routes of transmission, dual infection with HBV and HCV are frequent. Zarski et al.[50] compared 23 patients (HBsAg positive and anti-HCV positive) with 69 age- and sex-matched HBsAg-negative, anti-HCV-positive patients, HCV RNA levels were lower in members of the former group who were HBV DNA positive, thus implying inhibition of HCV replication by HBV in this group. The liver disease in the former group was histologically more severe with respect to cirrhosis, fibrosis, piecemeal necrosis and Knodell score.

The impact of dual infection on HCC is more controversial. Shiratori et al.[51] found dual infection in only 2% of 368 HCC patients *vis-à-vis* 1% of 119 patients with cirrhosis and 1% of 549 patients with CHC. In sharp contrast is the data of Kew et al.[52] from South Africa, who showed a relative risk for HCC of 23 in HBsAg-positive patients, 5 in anti HCV-positive patients but 82.5 in those with dual infection. Thus, in some geographical areas, the two viruses may have a synergistic role in disease progression.

Haemodialysis and renal transplantation

There is a wide range of reported prevalence of HCV infection in patients on maintenance hemodialysis (MHD). The seroprevalence of anti-HCV positivity in patients on MHD is declining but is still quite significant. As per the statement of European Dialysis and Transplant Association (EDTA), the prevalence declined from 21% in 1992 to 17.7% in 1993. In a recent study from Germany involving 2780 patients from 43 centres, HCV viraemia was seen in 3.7% of patients, representing a five times higher risk than in the general population[53]. About 18% of viraemic patients had normal ALT and/or anti-HCV negativity. This underscores the importance of a high index of suspicion and the need to use HCV RNA in addition to ALT and anti-HCV for testing these patients.

The risk factors for HCV infection among dialysis patients are:

(i) Number of blood transfusions. Since the use of erythropoeitin and stringent screening of donor blood, this factor is becoming less important.
(ii) Duration of dialysis. Even in those who have not received transfusion or have no history of IVDA or parenteral exposure, the prevalence of HCV infection with time has been shown to increase. Hardy et al.[54] found this rate of increase as 10%/year of MHD.
(iii) Mode of dialysis. Patients on peritoneal dialysis are at a lower risk for HCV infection than those on MHD. In a group of 129 anti HCV negative patients on chronic dialysis, the seroconversion rate was 0.15%/patient year in those on MHD and 0.03/patient year in those on peritoneal dialysis[55]. This may be because of lower transfusion requirement in the latter group, absence of vascular access site and extracorporeal blood circuit in PD, and possibly most importantly, because peritoneal dialysis is a home procedure preventing the nosocomial transmission of HCV.
(iv) Nosocomial transmission. This constitutes a major cause of HCV transmission in these patients. This may be because of a higher prevalence of HCV infection in dialysis staff which is, in turn, transmitted to non-infected patients. The staff may become infected by needle-stick injury from infected patients, breakdown in standard infection control practices and by physical proximity to infected patients. The role of dialysis machines, dialysis membrane and haemodialysis ultrafiltrate in infection is controversial. As regards reprocessing the dialysers, the risk of HCV transmission is not increased if dialysers from anti-HCV positive patients are processed in rooms different from those used for processing dialysers from uninfected patients.

It has been suggested that anti HCV+ve patients who undergo renal transplantation have an accelerated course. This may in fact be because of the immune depressed status of these patients and the use of immunosuppressive agents (like anti-lymphocyte and anti-thymocyte globulin, OKT3) in these patients, which causes increase in viral replication. The New England Organ Bank study[56] showed that anti-HCV positivity at the time of referral for transplantation was associated with increased mortality which was seen in patients who received a renal allograft or were continuing on dialysis. A more recent French study[57] with 29% of its 834 study subjects testing anti-HCV positive showed that the 5-year survival in those infected was not different from those not infected (85% vs. 87%), but at 10 years this difference became significant (65% vs. 80%). The infected group also had a lower graft survival. At 5 years the survival of those anti-HCV-positive subjects who had cirrhosis was similar to those who had lesser degrees of fibrosis, but at 10 years this difference became significant (33% vs. 69%). In those who had cirrhosis at the time of renal transplantation, the 10 year survival was a meager 26%. These authors thus support the view that all anti-HCV-positive subjects who are candidates for renal transplant should undergo a liver biopsy and presence of cirrhosis on histology should be a contraindication to transplantation.

Multiply transfused patients

The common categories of these patients are haemophiliacs, thalassaemics and those with hypogammaglobulinaemia. An elegant study from UK showed that mortality from liver disease in haemophiliac males was 16.7 times higher than that in the general population, and that from liver cancer was 5.6 times higher[58]. The risk of liver disease (including HCC)-related mortality increased with increasing age of first exposure to the blood products as well as concomitant infection with HIV. The same features apply to polytransfused thalassaemics, in whom the prevalence of HCV infection is quite high. Of the 75 thalassaemic children studied by us, anti-HCV positivity was seen in 68% cases[59]. Serum ferritin as well as ALT levels were higher in those infected than those who were uninfected. Indeed, iron may theoretically potentiate liver injury in this group of patients. Another interesting characteristic of the clinical course in this setting is the possibility of multiple episodes of acute attacks of hepatitis, possibly due to different genotypes[60].

In patients with congenital or acquired hypogammaglobulinaemia, use of contaminated intravenous immunoglobulin is responsible for high seroprevalence of HCV[61]. These patients often have biochemical and histological evidence of liver disease early in the clinical course. In the study by Bjoro et al.[62] nearly one-third of patients had histological evidence of cirrhosis which had developed 1–8 years following first exposure to contaminated immunoglobulins. These patients also face a management problem, as they show a poor sustained response to IFN therapy[63].

Initial histology and outcome of hepatitis C infection

A lot of recent work has highlighted the importance of liver histology early in the course of CHC as a prognostic factor for progression to more severe grades of chronic hepatitis or cirrhosis.

In the study by Di Bisceglie et al.[11] a second liver biopsy was performed in 20 of the 39 patients with chronic NANB hepatitis, about 8–26 months after the first biopsy (Fig. 2). The histology remained unchanged in nine, worsened in four (in three cirrhosis developed during this period) and improved in seven cases. Sanchez-Tapias et al.[64] found that in their study cohort of 306 patients, 7% of patients with CPH, 33% with moderate CAH and 47% of those with severe CAH developed cirrhosis after a mean of 8 years. Hopf et al.[65], in their study of 86 patients with post-transfusion or sporadic chronic hepatitis C infection followed for a mean of 8 years, found that none of the patients with initial histological evidence of CAH moved to the stage of CPH or normal histology, but 53 of those with initial severe CAH progressed to cirrhosis. Similarly, Takahashi et al.[24] reported progression from stages of CPH, moderate CAH (CAH 2A) and severe CAH (CAH 2B) to LC after a mean period of 11, 9 and 7 years respectively.

In an elegant study by Yano et al.[66] 70 patients with chronic HCV infection underwent an average of 3.9 biopsies over a mean follow-up period of 8.8 years. The grade of initial biopsy was scored against a maximum score of 8 (0–4 points for portal/periportal inflammation and 0–4 for lobular inflammation) and the stage (signifying fibrosis) against a maximum score of 4 points. Overall,

35 patients (i.e 50% of cases) progressed to LC. All patients with initial grade score ≥ 5 progressed to LC over 10 years; 96% of those with initial inflammatory score between 3.5 and 4.9 developed LC after 17 years and 30% of those with a score ≤ 3.4 developed LC after a mean of 13 years. Similarly, all patients with initial stage of septal fibrosis with incomplete nodularity (score 3–3.4) progressed to LC over 10 years.

The foregoing account lends credence to the observation that chronic HCV infection follows a rapidly progressive course in a subset of chronic hepatitis C, especially if the initial histological lesion is already significant.

IFN therapy and the outcome of chronic HCV infection

From the discussion thus far, it is amply clear that both necroinflammatory changes and fibrosis on liver histology determine the progression to cirrhosis in patients with CHC. So, it would be logical to assume that antiviral therapy which ameliorates these events should have a salutary effect on disease outcome. This beneficial effect of IFN is also noted in patients with dual infection due to hepatitis B and C[67].

The effect of IFN therapy can be broadly classified into:

(1) Effect on fibrosis: A number of studies have addressed this issue. Suou et al.[68] showed a decrease in levels of N-terminal propeptide of type III procollagen (P-III-NP) in 178 patients treated with IFN-alpha. This effect was seen in patients who had a sustained or a non-sustained response to therapy and lasted for at least 1 year. No change in the levels of P-III-NP were seen in the 45 untreated patients. The decrease was also seen to be independent of the biochemical response.

   Manabe et al.[69] showed decrease in total liver collagen content by a colorimetric method in those treated even with 1 MU of IFN. In those treated with placebo, the collagen content increased. Similar results were shown by Hiramatsu et al.[70], who showed a beneficial effect on necro-inflammatory activity too (in addition to fibrosis), the patients losing HCV-RNA standing to gain the most from therapy.

(2) Effect on cirrhosis: The results of two major studies[27,28] have already been mentioned elsewhere in this review. In the study by Fattoviich et al.[27] benefit from IFN therapy on survival was significant only on univariate analysis. Serfaty et al.[28] showed beneficial effect of IFN therapy on survival, hepatic decompensation and development of HCC on both univariate and multivariate analysis.

(3) Effect on HCC: Two large multicentric studies have addressed this issue: The International Interferon Alfa Hepatocellular Carcinoma Study[71] and the Inhibition of Hepatocarcinogenesis by Interferon Therapy (IHIT) study[72]. In the first of these studies, 943 patients with biopsy proven cirrhosis were either treated with interferon (n = 380; 42%) or followed without treatment (n = 533; 58%). Each patient was followed for a period of at least 3 years. Although the study enrolled patients with both HBV and HCV related LC, only results on the subset of patients with HCV infection will be discussed. The authors found that significant risk factors for the development of HCC were age, male sex and features of portal hypertension. When all patients

who were anti HCV positive were analysed with respect to development of HCC, that 48 of the 259 (18.5%) untreated and 21 of the 232 (9.1%) treated patients developed HCC (RR;3.14; 95% CI: 1.09–3.64). In the subset of patients who were anti-HCV positive and anti-HBc-negative, the results were even more surprising: 29 of the 129 untreated (20%) and 6 of the 116 treated (5%) developing HCC (RR 6.28; 95% CI 1.65–23.8). The authors found that iron stores, alcohol intake, fibrosis stage and inflammatory grade had no effect on the outcome. Overall, only 15% of the study subjects showed a sustained virological response.

In the much larger IHIT study[72] involving 2890 patients, 2400 patients received treatment with IFN and 490 were followed without treatment for a mean follow-up period of 4.3 years. The response to therapy was measured as biochemical and virological response and correlated with the fibrosis score at the initial histology. The risk of development of HCC was significantly reduced even in patients in whom there was no sustained virological response and only a biochemical response was achieved. The results of this study are shown in Tables 12 and 13. These studies drive home the point that IFN therapy even at the stage of compensated LC can significantly mould the outcome of chronic HCV infection, the factors leading to favourable outcome being anti-inflammatory and anti-fibrosis potential of IFN. There may be some other as yet unidentified mechanisms

Table 12 Results of inhibition of hepatocarcinogenesis by interferon therapy (IHIT) study[72]

	Patients with sustained virological response (n = 789)	*Patients with nonsustained virological response (n = 1568)*
Normal ALT	724 (91.7%)	260 (16.6%)
ALT <2 × ULN	59 (7.5%)	592 (37.8%)
ALT >2 × ULN	6 (0.8%)	716 (30.6%)
No. of HCC	10	76
Risk Ratio for HCC* (overall)	0.197 (p < 0.001)	0.631 (p = 0.016)

* Risk ratio for HCC: 145 events – 86 in the treated group and 59 in untreated group (see text)

Table 13 Risk factors for development of HCC: multivariate analysis[72]

Parameter	*Risk ratio*	*p*
Sex (male vs. female)	1.551	0.012
Age (by every 1 year)	1.063	<0.001
Stage of fibrosis (compared with stage F0/F1)		
F2	4.43	0.002
F3	13.10	<0.001
F4	24.01	<0.001
Treatment with IFN	0.52	<0.001

too. Why the same effects do not translate into benefit with respect to HCC development in patients with HBV related cirrhosis, is a still debatable issue[71].

This review has systematically tried to highlight the known facts regarding the natural history and course of HCV infection. It is appropriate to change the term HCV carrier to chronic HCV infection to highlight the ongoing hepatocellular injury. However, in spite of extensive research going into the mechanisms of disease caused by this agent discovered only a decade ago, the lacunae in our knowledge of the same are many. The complexities of host, agent and comorbid factors prevent any simple conclusions to be drawn and much effort needed in future to unravel the enigma of HCV.

REFERENCES

1. Lam NP. Hepatitis C. Natural history, diagnosis and management. Am J Health Syst Pharm. 1999;56:961–73.
2. Alter MJ. Epidemiology of hepatitis C. Hepatology. 1997;26(suppl 1):62S–5S.
3. NIH conference: Pathogenesis, natural history, treatment and prevention of hepatitis C. Ann Intern Med. 2000;132:296–305.
4. Seeff LB. Natural history of hepatitis C. Am J Med. 1999;107:10–15.
5. Deuffic S, Buffat L, Poynard T, Valleron AJ. Modeling the C virus epidemic in France. Hepatology. 1999;29:1596–601.
6. Scognamiglio P, Accapezzato D, Casciaro MA et al. Presence of effector CD8+ T cells in hepatitis C virus exposed healthy seronegative donors. J Immunol. 1999;162:6681–9.
7. Esteban JI, Cordoba J, Sauleda S. The clinical picture of acute and chronic hepatitis C. Curr Stud Hematol Blood Transf. 1998;62:102–18.
8. Alter MJ, Margolis HS, Krawczynski K et al. The natural history of community acquired hepatitis C in the United States. N Engl J Med. 1992;327:1899–905.
9. Wejstal R, Hermodsson S, Norkrans G. Long term follow up of chronic hepatitis non-A, non-B with special reference to hepatitis C. Liver. 1991;11:143–8.
10. Tremoloda F, Casarin C, Alberti A et al. Long term follow up of NANB (type C) post transfusion hepatitis. J Hepatol. 1992;16:273–81.
11. Di Bisceglie AM, Goodman ZD, Ishak KG, Hoofnagle JH, Melpolder JJ, Alter HJ. Long term clinical and histopathological follow up of chronic post transfusion hepatitis. Hepatology. 1991;14:969–74.
12. Koretz FL, Abbey H, Coleman E, Gitnick G. Non-A, non-B post transfusion hepatitis: looking back in the second decade. Ann Intern Med. 1993;119:110–15.
13. Seeff LB, Bales ZB, Wright EC et al. Long term mortality after transfusion associated non-A, non-B hepatitis. N Engl J Med. 1993;327:1906–11.
14. Muller R. The natural history of hepatitis C: clinical experiences. J Hepatol. 1996;24:52–4.
15. Walsh EK. Clinical outcomes after hepatitis C infection from contaminated anti-D immune globulin. N Engl J Med. 1999;40:1228–33.
16. Rodger AJ, Thomson JA, Thompson S et al. Assessment of long term outcomes of hepatitis C virus infection in a cohort of patients with acute hepatitis in 1971–1975: results of a pilot study J Gastroenterol Hepatol. 1999;14:269–73.
17. Alberti A, Morisca G, Chemello L et al. Hepatitis C viremia and liver disease in symptom free individuals with anti-HCV. Lancet. 1997;340:697–8.
18. Gholson CF, Morgan K, Catinis G et al. Chronic hepatitis C with normal aminotransferase levels: A clinical histologic study. Am J Gastroenterol. 1997;92:1788–92.
19. Naito M, Hayashi N, Hagiwara H et al. Serum hepatitis C virus RNA quantity and histological features of hepatitis C virus carriers with persistently normal ALT levels. Hepatology. 1994;19:81–5.
20. Morisco F, Blanco GDV, Tuccillo C, Galli C, Cirino S, Caporaso N. Long term observation of HCV positive patients with normal ALT values. Persistence of a clinically healthy state. Res Virol. 1998;149:277–82.

21. Yokusuka O, Kojima H, Imazeki F et al. Spontaneous negativation of serum hepatitis C virus RNA is a rare event in type C chronic liver disease: analysis of HCV RNA in 320 patients who were followed for more than 3 years. J Hepatol. 1999;31:394–9.
22. Indian association for study of the Liver (INASL), changing terminology of hepatitis B and C carrier: Consensus statement. Ind J Gastroenterol. 1999;18(suppl 1):515–20.
23. Kiyosawa K, Sodeyama T, Tanaka E et al. Interrelationship of blood transfusion, non-A, non-B hepatitis: a 13 year follow up study of hepatitis C virus markers. Liver. 1993;13:274–8.
24. Tong MJ, El-Farra NS, Reikes AR, Co RL. Clinical outcomes after transfusion associated hepatitis C. N Engl J Med. 1995;332:1463–6.
25. Takahashi M, Yamada G, Miyamoto R, Doi T, Endo H, Tsuji T. Natural course of chronic hepatitis C. Am J Gastroenterol. 1993;88:240–3.
26. Niederau C, Lange S, Heintges T et al. Prognosis of chronic hepatitis C: results of a large, prospective cohort study. Hepatology. 1998;28:1687–95.
27. Fattovich G, Giustina G, Degos F et al. Morbidity and mortality in compensated cirrhosis type C: A retrospective follow up study of 384 patients. Gastroenterology. 1997;112:463–72.
28. Serfaty L, Aumaitre H, Chazouilleres O et al. Determinants of outcome of compensated hepatitis C virus related cirrhosis. Hepatology. 1998;27:1435–40.
29. Mattson L, Weiland D, Glaumann H. Chronic non-A, non-B hepatitis developed after transfusion, illicit self injections or sporadically. Outcome during long term follow-up. A comparison. Liver. 1989;9:120–7.
30. Poynard T, Bedossa P, Opolon P. Natural history of liver fibrosis progression in patients with chronic hepatitis C. Lancet. 1997;349:825–32.
31. Missale G, Bertoni R, Lamonaca V et al. Different clinical behaviours of acute hepatitis C virus infection are associated with different vigor of the anti viral cell mediated immune response. J Clin Invest. 1996;98:706–14.
32. Lohr HF, Schmitz D, Arenz M et al. The viral clearance in interferon treated chronic hepatitis C is associated with increased cytotoxic T-cell frequencies. J Hepatol. 1999;31:407–15.
33. Lan JYN, Davis GL, Kniffen J et al. Significance of serum hepatitis C virus RNA levels in chronic hepatitis C. Lancet. 1993;341:1501–4.
34. Gretch D, Corey L, Wilson J et al. Assessment of hepatitis C virus RNA levels by quantitative competitive RNA polymerase chain reaction: high titre viremia correlates with advanced stage of disease. J Infect Dis. 1994;169:1219–25.
35. Puoti C, Magrini A, Stati T et al. Clinical, histological and virological features of hepatitis C virus carriers with persistently normal or abnormal alanine transaminase levels. Hepatology. 1997;26:1393–8.
36. Silini E, Bottelli R, Asti M et al. Hepatitis C virus genotypes and risk of hepatocellular carcinoma in cirrhosis: a case controlled study. Gastroenterology. 1996;111:199–205.
37. Naoumov NV, Chokshi S, Metivier E, Maertens G, Johnson PJ, Williams R. Hepatitis C virus infection in the development of hepatocellular carcinoma in cirrhosis. J Hepatol. 1997;27:331–6.
38. Poynard T, Marcellin P, Lee SS et al. Randomised trial of interferon alfa 2 b plus ribavarin for 48 weeks or for 24 weeks versus interferon alfa 2 b plus placebo for 48 weeks for treatment of chronic infection with hepatitis C virus. International Hepatitis International Therapy Group (IHIT). Lancet. 1998;352:1426–32.
39. Honda M, Kaneko S, Sakai A, Unoura M, Murakami S, Kobayashi K. Degree of diversity of hepatitis C virus quasispecies and progression of liver disease. Hepatology. 1994;20:1144–51.
40. Nagayama K, Kurosakki M, Enomoto N, Miyasaka Y, Masumo F, Sato C. Characteristics of hepatitis C viral genome associated with disease progression. Hepatology. 2000;31:745–50.
41. Takase S, Takada N, Sawada M, Tsutsumi M, Takada A. Relationship between alcoholic liver disease and HCV infection. Alcohol Alcohol. 1993;28:77–84.
42. Cromic SL, Jenkins PJ, Bowden DS, Dudely FJ. Chronic hepatitis C: effect of alcohol on hepatitic activity and viral titre. J Hepatol. 1996;25:821–6.
43. Pessione F, Degos F, Marcellin P et al. Effect of alcohol consumption on serum hepatitis C virus RNA and histological lesions in chronic hepatitis C. Hepatology. 1998;27:1717–22.
44. Wiley TE, McCarthy M, Breidi L, McCarthy M, Layaden TJ. Impact of alcohol on the histological and clinical progression of hepatitis C infection. Hepatology. 1998;27:1730–5.
45. Okazaki T, Yoshihara H, Suzuki K et al. Efficacy of interferon therapy in patients with chronic hepatitis C. Scand J Gastroenterol. 1994;29:1039–43.

46. Stubbe L, Soriano V, Antunes F et al. Hepatitis C in the EuroSIDA cohort of European HIV infected patients: prevalence and prognostic value. 12th World AIDS conference Geneva, July 1998.
47. Soto B, Sanchez-Quijano A, Rodrigo L, Leal M, Lissen E. HIV infection modifies the natural history of chronic parenterally acquired hepatitis C with an unusually rapid progression to cirrhosis. A multicentre study on 547 patients. J Hepatol. 1997;26:1–5.
48. Soriano V, Rodriguez-Rosado R, Garcia-Samaniego J. Management of chronic C hepatitis C in HIV infected patients. AIDS. 1999;13:539–46.
49. Soriano V, Garcia-Samaniego J, Bravo R et al. Interferon alfa for the treatment of chronic hepatitis C in patients infected with human immunodeficiency virus. Clin Infect Dis. 1996;23:585–91.
50. Zarski JP, Bohn B, Bastie A et al. Characteristics of patients with dual infection by hepatitis B and C viruses. J Hepatol. 1998;28:27–33.
51. Shiratori Y, Shiina S, Zhang PY et al. Does dual infection by hepatitis B and C viruses play an important role in the pathogenesis of hepatocellular carcinoma in Japan? Cancer. 1997;80:2060–7.
52. Kew MC, Yu MC, Kedda MA, Coppin A, Sarkin A, Hodkinson J. The relative roles of hepatitis B and C viruses in the etiology of hepatocellular carcinoma in southern African blacks. Gastroenterology. 1997;112:184–7.
53. Hinrichsen H, Schrader H, Steagen G, Leimenstoll G, Folsch UR, Schmidt WE. Prevalence of hepatitis C in hemodialysis patients: viremia without detectable levels of HCV-antibodies. Hepatology. 1998;28:A1631.
54. Hardy NM, Sandroni S, Danielson S, Wilson WJ. Antibody to hepatitis C virus increases with time on dialysis. Clin Nephrol. 1992;38:44–8.
55. Cendoroglo Neto M, Manzano SI, Canziani ME et al. Environmental transmission of hepatitis B and hepatitis C viruses within hemodialysis unit. Artif Organs. 1995;19:251–5.
56. Pereira BJG, Natov SN, Bouthort BA et al. Effect of hepatitis C infection and renal transplantation on survival in end stage renal disease. Kidney Int. 1998;53:1374–81.
57. Mathurian P, Mouquet C, Poynard T et al. Impact of hepatitis B and C virus on kidney transplantation outcome. Hepatology. 1999;29:259–63.
58. Darby SC, Ewart DW, Giangrande PL et al. Mortality from liver cancer and liver disease in hemophiliac men and boys in UK given blood contaminated with hepatitis C. Lancet. 1997;350:1425–31.
59. Thakur V, Guptan RC, Motwani J, Chopra K, Sarin SK. High frequency of hepatitis B and C virus dual infection in thalassemic children in India. JAPI. 1998;46:856–9.
60. Lai ME, Mazzoleni AP, Argiolu F et al. Hepatitis C virus in multiple episodes of acute hepatitis in polytransfused thalassemic children. Lancet. 1994;343:388–90.
61. Rossi G, Tucci A, Cariani E et al. Outbreak of hepatitis C virus infection in patients with hematologic disorders treated with intravenous immunoglobulins: different prognosis according to immune status. Blood. 1997;90:1309–14.
62. Bjoro K, Froland SS, Yun Z, Samdal HH, Haaland T. Hepatitis C infection in patients with primary hypogammaglobulinemia after treatment with contaminated immune globulin. N Engl J Med. 1994;331:1607–11.
63. Christie J, Healey C, Watson J et al. Clinical outcome of hypogammaglobulinemic patients following outbreak of acute hepatitis C: 2 year follow up. Clin Exp Immunol. 1997;110:4–8.
64. Sanchez-Tapias JM, Barrera J, Costa J et al. Hepatitis C virus infection in patients with non-alcoholic chronic liver disease. Ann Intern Med. 1990;112:921–4.
65. Hopf U, Moller B, Kuther D et al. Long term follow up of post transfusion and sporadic chronic hepatitis non-A, non-B and frequency of circulating anti-bodies to hepatitis C virus (HCV). J Hepatol. 1990;10:69–76.
66. Yano M, Kumada H, Kage M et al. The long term pathological evolution of chronic hepatitis C. Hepatology. 1996;23:1334–40.
67. Guptan RC, Trakun V, Raina V, Sarin SK. Alpha interferon therapy in chronic hepatitis due to active dual infection with hepatitis B and C viruses. J Gasteroenterol Hepotol. 1999;14:796–801.
68. Suou T, Hosho K, Kishimoto Y, Horie Y, Kawasakai H. Long term decrease in serum N-terminal propeptide of type III procollagen in patients with chronic hepatitis C treated with interferon alfa. Hepatology. 1995;22:426–31.

69. Manabe N, Chevallier M, Chossegros Ph et al. Interferon alfa 2b therapy reduces liver fibrosis in chronic non-A, non-B hepatitis. A quantitative histological evaluation. Hepatology. 1993;18:1344–9.
70. Hiramatsu N, Hayashi N, Kasahara A et al. Improvement of liver fibrosis in chronic hepatitis C patients treated with natural interferon alfa. J Hepatol. 1995;22:135–42.
71. Branetto MR, Oliveri F, Kochler M, Zahm F, Bonino F. Effect of interferon-alfa on progression of cirrhosis to hepatocellular carcinoma: a retrospective cohort study. Lancet. 1998;351:1535–9.
72. Yoshida H, Shiratori Y, Moriyama M et al. Interferon therapy reduces the risk for hepatocellular carcinoma: National surveillance program of cirrhotic and noncirrhotic patients with chronic hepatitis C in Japan. Ann Intern Med. 1999;131:174–81.

12
Hepatitis C: therapeutic challenges

C. TREPO, P. MIAILHES and F. ZOULIM

INTRODUCTION

Since the first study by Hoofnagle in 1986, interferon-α (IFN) has been thoroughly evaluated and has been actually confirmed as the pivotal treatment for hepatitis C[1]. However, its efficacy remains unsatisfactory[1,2]. While many patients treated with IFN do normalize their ALT and improve their liver histology, fewer clear the virus[2].

Ribavirin is the second drug which proved to be able to improve liver function tests but its kinetic of action proved to be much slower than the swift impact of IFN on ALT levels and it did not significantly reduce viraemia. Ribavirin failed, therefore, to satisfy the criteria for registration although it was apparent that liver histology was improved in the 50% of patients who normalized their ALT. Indeed HCV RNA levels had become at this time a key reference point in evaluating the efficacy of drugs against HCV.

Although the natural history of hepatitis C and its long-term sequelae start to be documented, its physiopathology remains poorly understood. It is clear that HCV, like HBV, is not cytopathic by itself and that the liver lesions are immunologically mediated. More than 20% of HCV-infected individuals do not show disease progression despite high levels of circulating virus. HCV RNA by itself is, therefore, not a good enough marker for measuring drug activity in this disease. When the first therapeutic studies with IFN in hepatitis C were conducted and registration granted, HCV RNA monitoring was not yet available[1]. End points used for clinical trials were therefore liver function tests and especially AST/ALT and liver histology.

More recently ribavirin has emerged as potentially the second most effective therapy. It is an oral broad spectrum antiviral agent that has activity against many RNA and DNA viruses in vivo and in vitro[2–4]. In studies with chronic hepatitis C, ribavirin therapy was associated with reduction in serum aminotransferases but induced little change in HCV RNA levels in the serum[5–7] and the duration of the treatment was limited to 6–9 months.

As with other chronic conditions one should distinguish in hepatitis between two strategies: eradicating the virus on the one hand or suppressing the liver disease activity on the other. The second goal could be a more reasonable choice under certain conditions when eradicating the virus is not feasible.

THE CLASSICAL APPROACH: AIMING AT INHIBITING HCV REPLICATION

HCV replication dynamics

New assays have changed our views and understanding of infection dynamics. The ability to predict treatment outcome prior to, or early in the course of, therapy has important therapeutic implications for the patient, as well as economic implications for the healthcare system.

A major impact of HCV RNA technology has been, as for HIV, the understanding of HCV replication kinetics[8]. To better understand the dynamics of hepatitis C virus and the antiviral effect of IFN-α 2b, viral decline in 23 patients during therapy was analysed using a mathematical model. The analysis indicates that the major initial effect of IFN-α is to block virion production or release, with blocking efficacies of 81, 95, and 96% for daily doses of 5, 10 and 15 million international units, respectively. The estimated virion half-life (t1/2) was, on average, 2.7 hours, with pre-treatment production and clearance of 10^{12} virions per day. The estimated infected cell death rate exhibited large interpatient variation (corresponding t1/2 = 1.7 to 70 days), was inversely correlated with baseline viral load, and was positively correlated with alanine aminotransferase levels. Fast cell death rates were predictive of virus being undetectable at 3 months.

Genetic diversity is key to pathogenesis and six major genotypes and over 70 subtypes have been described. The presence of a genotype other than type 1 (or specifically type 1b in some cases) has been associated with a greater response to IFN compared with other genotypes. Genotype is also important in predicting response to combination IFN/ribavirin therapy[9,10]. Among patients with chronic hepatitis C, 48 weeks of treatment with combination therapy produced a mean response rate of 28% (n = 166) among those with genotype 1 and 66% (n = 61) among patients with other genotypes. Similar differences between genotype 1 and other genotypes were found for combination therapy among patients who had relapsed following previous IFN therapy[10]. Viral load prior to treatment has been clearly shown to be predictive of response to IFN alpha treatment, with increased viral load associated with decreased rates of response. These findings show that infection with hepatitis C virus is highly dynamic and that early monitoring of viral load can help guide therapy. Studies have also shown that declines in HCV levels in the first 2–4 weeks after initiation of IFN appear predictive of therapeutic efficacy.

Efficacy of interferon + ribavirin

IFN-α was until recently the only licensed treatment for patients with chronic hepatitis C. Forty percent of patients have an initial response to this therapy, but most subsequently relapse. Fortunately ribavirin appears to act synergistically with it, as confirmed first in relapse patients in whom sustained virological response was observed in 49% of the combination therapy group, but in only 5% in the IFN group after 6 months of therapy[10].

The same approach was tested in interferon naive patients with 6 or 12 months' therapy[9]. The rate of sustained virological response was higher among patients who received combination therapy for either 24 weeks (31%), or 48 weeks (38%) than among patients who received IFN alone (6% or 13%)[11]. Among genotype 1 patients, the best response occurred at 48 weeks. In patients non-responsive to IFN, a second course of treatment by IFN alone has no beneficial effect whereas combination therapy may give a 25% response. In conclusion, it is clear that combination therapy should be given in all situations. Viral eradication should not be the only objective of the treatment, since histological improvement may be obtained despite persisting viral replication.

As noted previously, treatment with IFN is associated with only modest efficacy. Predictive factors will also identify subsets of the patient population who are likely to benefit from standard interferon treatments. The development of regimens that produce more sustained pressure on HCV may offer new avenues into the treatment of the disease. The *pegylation* of interferons may represent one approach. Antiviral activity is greater with pegylated IFN than with standard IFN and this activity is maintained for at least a week[12].

The challenge of the IFN non-responder

The enhanced efficacy of the IFN–ribavirin combination was first observed in a study including non-responders[13]. In a meta-analysis of individual patient data of six randomized controlled trials comprising 344 patients, 114 patients were non-responders[14].

The overall sustained response rate of all patients (IFN non-responders receiving IFN–ribavirin combination) was 10%. The genotype 1 subgroup appears to be the least responsive, whereas the presence of cirrhosis was no longer a significant predictive factor of response. These results have been confirmed in several recent randomized controlled trials.

The data indicate that combining ribavirin with IFN markedly increases the sustained response in non-responders. The absolute response of 6 months of IFN–ribavirin combination therapy for non-responders is now in the range of standard interferon monotherapy for untreated patients. Retreatment of non-responders with standard IFN–ribavirin combination therapy leads to a clinically significant sustained response rate, irrespective of the presence of cirrhosis. An initial course of daily high dose IFN could further increase this response rate.

The combination of amantadine with IFN has been tested in several randomized controlled studies in non-responders. IFN plus amantadine appears to be less effective than IFN–ribavirin combination therapy[15–16].

Triple antiviral combination therapy (IFN, ribavirin and amantadine) has been evaluated in a small pilot study[16]. Triple therapy was generally well tolerated. In 10 patients fulfilling the criteria of non-responders to standard interferon, triple therapy induced a biochemical and virologic end-of-treatment response in 70% (7/10). Triple therapy therefore should be tested in a large randomized controlled trial.

THE ALTERNATIVE APPROACH: SUPPRESSIVE THERAPY WITH RIBAVIRIN MONOTHERAPY

Between 1992 and October 1995, we enrolled 95 patients (43 men and 52 women) with a mean age of 56 years (range 26–75 years). The known duration of hepatitis (raised ALT activity) was determined in 82 patients and ranged from 1 to 14 years (mean duration 4.4 years). The time from infection was known in 62 patients and ranged from 2 to 44 years (mean duration 12.9 years). Results of liver biopsy performed prior to ribavirin therapy showed chronic active hepatitis in 50 patients and liver cirrhosis in 45. Thirty-five patients had never received any previous antiviral therapy and 60 patients had been treated with a previous course of recombinant IFN without long-lasting beneficial effect. The minimum time interval between IFN therapy and ribavirin administration was 6 months. The mean cumulative dose of IFN was 309 million units (MU) over a mean period of 8 months. Before treatment, HCV RNA was detected in the serum of all patients by PCR.

Thirty-eight patients (40%) normalized serum ALT activity during therapy and were referred to as complete responders. The decrease in ALT levels occurred after a mean duration of 3.5 months and the levels remained constant thereafter. Serum ALT activity decreased by more than 50% without normalization in 20 patients (21%), who were considered as non-responders for statistical analysis. HCV RNA clearance from serum was observed in seven patients (8%). All were complete biochemical responders.

Before therapy, there was no statistical difference between responders and non-responders with respect to mean age, known duration of infection, the mode of contamination and ferritin levels. Females (26/52) were better responders than men (12/43) ($p < 0.05$) as were patients with normal γ-GT levels by comparison with those with elevated γ-GT levels ($p < 0.02$). Pretreatment ALT levels were lower in responders (2.7 times the upper limit of normal (ULN)) than in non-responders (3.6 $\times$ ULN) ($p < 0.05$). Among the 42 patients who were non-responders to a previous course of IFN, a complete response was observed in 11 (26%) and one (2.5%) patient became negative for HCV RNA in serum. In the group of 45 patients with contraindications to IFN therapy, ALT levels returned to normal in 48% and HCV RNA became negative in serum in 3%. responders. An improvement in the Knodell score was observed in eight (80%) responders, and in four (57%) non-responders. When all 17 patients were taken into account, the mean HAI decreased significantly during ribavirin therapy ($p <0.005$). In responders, the decrease of the HAI was still significant ($p = 0.018$), while in non-responders there was a trend towards a decrease of the HAI, which did not reach statistical significance (Friedman test, with Montecarlo modification, $p > 0.05$). However, the difference of evolution of the HAI in responders and non-responders was not statistically significant (Kruskall-Wallis test, Montecarlo modification, $p = 0.49$). The fibrosis score improved in only one responder.

The improvements in aminotransferases induced by ribavirin could be sustained for up to 24 months and this improvement was maintained even with a decrease in dosage from 1200 to 1000 mg/day[15]. Improvements in liver histology also occurred and in some cases the improvements were marked. The average decrease in HAI scores in patients treated for 2 years was 5.3 (from 11.7 to 6.4), which can be compared with the minimal change in average IIAI scores among these same patients during a prior period of placebo therapy, the decrease being 0.8 (from 12.5 to 11.7). The improvements can also be compared with those reported among patients treated with ribavirin for one year (among responders who had equivalent improvements in aminotransferases) of 4.3 (12.0 to 7.7) and with those reported among patients treated with IFN-α for 6 months of –3,6 (11.6 to 8.0). As might be expected, hepatic fibrosis did not improve with ribavirin therapy, but periportal and lobular necrosis decreased markedly. Interestingly, portal inflammation was unaffected. This pattern of improvement contrasts to that occurring with interferon therapy where portal and lobular necrosis improve.

Despite improvements in serum biochemical tests and histology with prolonged ribavirin therapy, HCV RNA levels did not change. Furthermore, no patient became HCV RNA negative and despite normal aminotransferase levels, no patient had completely normal hepatic histology at the end of therapy. Probably for these reasons most patients relapsed once therapy was stopped. Therefore, in this study[15] as well as in previous trials[17–22], ribavirin therapy led to amelioration of the disease. The reasons for the discrepancy between biochemical and virological responses during ribavirin therapy are unknown. However they are another illustration of the elusive immune mechanisms involved in the pathogenesis of hepatitis C with which ribavirin does interfere beneficially.

DISCUSSION

The data presented from major centres are similar and do confirm several pilot and placebo-controlled studies suggesting that ribavirin has a transient effect in chronic hepatitis C. In these studies, ribavirin was generally administered for 6 months (range 3–12 months). Ribavirin did not induce a marked and sustained antiviral effect but did improve serum ALT activity in half of the patients[17–22]. The time required for the return of ALT levels to normal values was longer (3–6 months) than with IFN therapy (1–3 months)[1]. When ribavirin was given for 6 months, there was no improvement in liver histology; however, continuation of therapy for 9–12 months may be associated with a statistically significant improvement in liver histology (especially lobular injury)[18,20–22]. The aim of our study was to address the question of the clinical utility of ribavirin monotherapy for more than 6 months, particularly in patients who were non-responders to IFN or who had contraindications for this therapy.

In the Lyon study, prolonged administration of ribavirin in a large cohort of 95 patients with chronic hepatitis C was associated with a normalization of serum ALT levels in 40% and with a partial response in 21% more. These results are in agreement with those of placebo-controlled trials published by other groups[17–22]. Interestingly, a sustained disappearance of HCV RNA from serum was observed in 8% of the patients, all biochemical responders, which suggests that in some patients, ribavirin may trigger a direct or host-mediated antiviral effect. A low rate of HCV RNA clearance has been reported in some studies[21–23] but was not statistically different from the one observed among placebo patients. Other groups have not observed HCV RNA clearance during the study period[10–12,18]. A decrease in viral titres has also been observed in some reports[23–33] but not in others[20–22]. Although this study is retrospective and uncontrolled, bearing in mind the natural history of chronic hepatitis C[1–6] it is probable that this beneficial effect is related to ribavirin administration.

Pretreatment serum ALT levels were lower in complete responders than in non-responders, and patients with high γ-GT levels prior to therapy had a lower response rate. Interestingly, the biochemical response rate was significantly higher in patients without cirrhosis (54%) compared with cirrhotic patients (24%). Moreover, in responders, the time required for the return of ALT levels to normal values was longer in patients with cirrhosis, indicating that prolonged administration of ribavirin is required to obtain a biochemical response. Taken together, these results suggest that patients with advanced liver disease are less likely to respond to ribavirin therapy. Ribavirin administration was associated with normalization of ALT levels in 48% of patients with contraindications to IFN and in 26% of non-responders to a previous course of IFN therapy. Although the clearance rate of HCV RNA from serum was low (< 5%) in these patients, these results suggest that ribavirin therapy may have a beneficial effect in controlling the progression of liver disease in these particular groups, as also suggested by other studies[15,25–33].

Paired liver biopsy specimens could be obtained during therapy in some patients. The results of liver histology showed a statistically significant decrease overall in hepatic inflammation and necrosis in both responder and non-responder patient groups. The decrease of the HAI reached statistical significance in responders but not in non-responders. This histological study confirms others who already observed an improvement of liver histology (lobular injury) in ribavirin responders, which was independent of viral clearance[15,25–33]. These findings are also consistent with those of Hoofnagle et al. who observe an improvement of HAI in five of six patients treated with ribavirin for 24 months[34].

Ribavirin was generally well tolerated. However, dose tapering was required in five patients because of haemolysis, as already described in other clinical trials[18,20–22]. Therapy had to be stopped in some patients because of side-effects, such as a flu-like syndrome, allergy and peripheral neuropathy. A greater number of patients with cirrhosis (16%) had to stop therapy than patients without cirrhosis (8%), but this difference did not reach statistical significance. However, these findings could indicate that ribavirin may not be as well tolerated in cirrhotic patients and that special care should be provided to these patients who experienced side effects (a total of 35%).

Although this is an uncontrolled retrospective study, our results, obtained in a large cohort of patients, suggest that long-term administration of ribavirin is generally well tolerated and may be beneficial in controlling the progression of chronic hepatitis C. This may represent an alternative therapy in patients with a primary or secondary contraindication to IFN use or a second line therapy in non-responders to IFN. In both instances the purpose of this prolonged therapy is to suppress or slow down the progression of the liver disease.

Suppressive therapy would be even more successful if not only carried out with monotherapy by ribavirin or IFN alone[34], but by double combination with ribavirin or triple association including amantadine, the surrogate end-points of the treatments being improvement or stabilization of histology and quality of life. This will make it possible for patients to wait under acceptable living conditions without progressive HCC, cirrhosis HCC or transplantation until the new generation of more active anti-HCV compounds comes of age.

REFERENCES

1. Hoofnagle JH, Di Bisceglie AM. The treatment of chronic viral hepatitis. N Engl J Med. 1997;336:347–56.
2. Poynard T, Bedossa P, Chevallier M, Mathurin P, Lemmonier C, Trépe C et al. A comparison of three interferon alfa-2b regimens for the long-term treatment of chronic non-A, non-B hepatitis. N Engl J Med. 1995;332:1457–62.
3. Fattovich G, Giustina G, Favarato S, Ruol A. A survey of adverse events in 11241 patients with chronic viral hepatitis treated with alfa interferon. J Hepatol. 1996;24:38–47.
4. Tong MJ, El Farra NS, Reikes AR et al. Clinical outcomes after transfusion associated hepatitis C. N Engl J Med. 1995;332:1463–6.
5. Poynard T, Bedossa P, Opolon P. Natural history of liver fibrosis progression in patients with chronic hepatitis C. Lancet. 1997;349:825–8232.
6. Tsukuma H, Hiyama T, Tanaka S, Nakao M, Yabuuchi T, Kitamura T et al. Risk factors for hepatocellular carcinoma among patients with chronic liver disease. N Engl J Med. 1993;328:1797–1801.
7. Patterson JL, Fernandez-Larsson R. Molecular mechanisms of action of ribavirin. Rev Infect Dis. 1990;12:1139–46.
8. Zoulim F, Trépo C. Nucleoside analogs in the treatment of chronic viral hepatitis. Efficiency and complications. J Hepatol. 1994;21:142–4.
9. Reichard O, Andersson J, Schvarcz R, Weiland O. Ribavirin treatment for chronic hepatitis C. Lancet. 1991;337:1058–61.
10. Di Bisceglie AM, Shindo M, Fong TL, Fried MW, Swain MG, Bergasa NV et al. A pilot study of ribavirin therapy for chronic hepatitis C. Hepatology. 1992;16:649–54.
11. Camps J, Garcia N, Riezu-Boj JI, Civeira MP, Prieto J. Ribavirin in the treatment of chronic hepatitis C unresponsive to alfa interferon. J Hepatol. 1993;19:408–12.
12. Di Bisceglie AM, Conjeevaram HS, Fried MW, Sallie R, Park Y, Yurdayin C et al. Ribavirin as therapy for chronic hepatitis C. Ann Intern Med. 1995;12:897–903.
13. Smith JP. Treatment of chronic hepatitis C with amantadine. Dig Dis Sci. 1997;42:1681–7.
14. Brillanti S, Garson J, Foli M, Whitby K, Deaville R, Masci C et al. A pilot study of combination therapy with Ribavirine plus Interferon alpha for alpha-interferon resistant chronic hepatitis C. Gastroenterology. 1994;107:812–17.
15. Younossi ZM, Mullen KD, Zakko X, Brandt E, Hodnick S, Easley K et al. Interferon alfa 2b and Ribavirine vs interferon alfa 2b and amantadine for chronic hepatitis C (non-responder): a multicenter, randomized, double-blind trial. Hepatology. 1998;28:284A.
16. Brillanti S, Foli M, Gramantieri L, Di Tomaso M, Masci C, Bolondi L. Triple antiviral therapy for chronic hepatitis C in interferon alpha non-responders: a pilot randomized controlled study. Hepatology. 1997;26:367A.
17. Dusheiko G, Main J, Thomas H, Reichard O, Lee C, Dhillon A et al. Ribavirin treatment for patients with chronic hepatitis C: results of a placebo-controlled study. J Hepatol. 1996;25:591–8.
18. Bodenheimer HC, Lindsay KL, Davis GL, Lewis JH, Thung SN, Seeff LB. Tolerance and efficacy of oral ribavirin treatment of chronic hepatitis C: a multicenter trial. Hepatology. 1997;26:473–7.
19. Ljungman P, Andersson J, Aschan J, Björkstrand B, Hägglund H, Lönnqvist B et al. Oral ribavirin for prevention of severe liver disease caused by hepatitis C virus during allogeneic bone marrow transplantation. Clin Infect Dis. 1996;23:167–9.
20. Brillanti S, Garson J, Foli M, Whitby K, Deaville R, Masci C et al. A pilot study of combination therapy with ribavirin plus interferon alfa for interferon alfa-resistant chronic hepatitis C. Gastroenterology. 1994;107:812–17.

21. Lai M-Y, Kao J-H, Yang P-M, Wang J-T, Chen PJ, Chan KW et al. Long-term efficacy of ribavirin plus interferon alfa in the treatment of chronic hepatitis C. Gastroenterology. 1996;111:1307–12.
22. Schalm SW, Hansen EH, Chemello L, Bellobuono A, Brouwer JT, Weiland O et al. Ribavirin enhances the efficacy but not the adverse effects of interferon in chronic hepatitis C. Meta-analysis of individual patient data from European centers. J Hepatol. 1997;26:961–6.
23. Heathcote EJL, Keeffe EB, Lee SS, Feinman SV, Tong MJ, Reddy KR et al. Re-treatment of chronic hepatitis C with consensus interferon. Hepatology. 1998;27:1136–43.
24. Bekkering FC, Brouwer JT, Leroux-Roels G, Vlierberghe H van, Elewaut A, Schalm SW. Ultrarapid hepatitis C virus clearance by daily high dose interferon in non-responders to standard therapy. J Hepatol. 1998;28:960–4.
25. Bekkering FC, Brouwer JT, Elewaut A, Schalm SW. Hepatitis C: viral kinetics. Hepatology. 1997;26:1691–2.
26. McCarthy ME, Ganger D, Flamm S, Lam NP, Wiley TE, Layden TJ. Early viral response to high dose interferon alpha-2b (IFN) predicts viral response in prior non-responders (NR) and relapsers (R) to IFN. Hepatology. 1998:28(suppl):287A.
27. Lam NP, Neumann AU, Gretch DR, Wiley TE, Perelson AS, Layden TJ. Dose-dependant acute clearance of hepatitis C genotype 1 virus with interferon alpha. Hepatology. 1997;26:226–31.
28. Brouwer JT, Nevens F, Michielsen P, Hautekeete ML, Chamuleau RAFM, Adler M et al. What opinions are left when hepatitis C does not respond to interferon? Placebo controlled Benelux multicentre retreatment trial on ribavirine monotherapy versus combination with interferon. J Hepatol. 1994:21(suppl 1):S17.
29. El- Zayadi A, Selim O, Shawky S, Moustapha H, El-Taxeel A. A controlled study of amantadine monotherapy vs. amantadine combined with interferon alpha. Hepatology. 1998;28:473A.
30. Sostegni R, Ghisetti V, Pittaluga F, Marchiaro G, Rocca G, Borghesio E et al. Sequential versus concombinant administration of ribavirine and interferon alpha-n3 in patients with chronic hepatitis C not responding to interferon alone: results of a randomized, controlled trial. In press.
31. Poynard T, Marcellin P, Lee S, Niederau C, Minuk GS, Ideo G et al. Randomised trial of interferon alpha-2b plus ribavirine for 48 weeks or for 24 weeks versus interferon alpha 2b plus placebo for 48 weeks for treatment of chronic infection with hepatitis C virus. Lancet. 1998;352:1426–32.
32. McHutchison JG, Gordon SC, Schiff ER, Schiffman ML, Lee WM, Rustgi VK et al. Interferon alpha-2b alone or in combination with ribavirine as initial treatment for chronic hepatitis C. N Engl J Med. 1998;339:1485–92.
33. Hoofnagle JH, Lau D, Conjeevaram H, Kleiner D, Di Bisceglie AM. Prolonged therapy of chronic hepatitis C with ribavirin. J Virol Hepatol. 1996;3:247–52.
34. Long term administration of interferon alpha in non responder patients with chronic hepatitis C: follow up liver fibrosis over five years. J Virol Hepat. 1999;6:125–133.

13
Hepatitis C – evolving therapeutic strategies

A. M. DI BISCEGLIE

INTRODUCTION

The hepatitis C virus (HCV) was identified in 1989 and a reliable serological test for its diagnosis developed shortly thereafter. This has resulted in the identification of large numbers of patients with chronic hepatitis C who appear to be candidates for therapy because of their risk of progressive liver disease, liver failure and hepatocellular carcinoma. The NIH Consensus Conference in 1997 codified the use of interferon (IFN) as the standard form of therapy[1]. The introduction of ribavirin as an adjunct to IFN was similarly established as being the standard of therapy in an EASL Consensus Conference held in 1999[2]. Even with these innovations, however, no more than 40% of treated patients can expect to achieve a sustained response. Thus, the majority of patients with chronic hepatitis C remain at risk of progressive liver disease and the complications of chronic HCV infection. Given this relative lack of efficacy and the known side effects of both IFN and ribavirin, new approaches to therapy are clearly needed.

NEW WAYS OF USING INTERFERON

Although IFN has been used in therapy of non-A, non-B hepatitis or hepatitis since the mid-1980s, the optimal use of IFN may not yet be clarified. It has become clear that longer therapy is better and that 12 months is superior to 6 months' treatment[3]. Recent studies of viral kinetics have suggested that alternate-day therapy (or three times a week) may be less effective than daily. Lam and colleagues observed that levels of HCV RNA begin to rise rapidly (within 24 hours) of a single dose of IFN[4]. Thus if interferon is used daily this may be more effective than alternate-day regimens. Similarly, studies of viral kinetics have also shown a greater degree of acute suppression in HCV RNA levels with higher doses of IFN (5 or 10 million units) than the standard dose of 3 million units.

These observations have led to the study of induction therapy, in which high doses of IFN are administered daily to begin with, and then decreased later to allow better tolerability. Several such studies have demonstrated improved virological responses while the patients are on treatment, but no clear benefit on sustained response has yet been observed, although many of these studies are still under way[5]. The use of long acting forms of IFN may also address the issue of daily dosing and rising viral titres during treatments. The addition of polyethylene glycol (PEG) to the IFN molecule has produced sustained levels of IFN in serum, as much as a week after a single injection. These PEGylated interferons have undergone extensive testing and preliminary results are very promising, although definitive studies are not yet complete. Shiffmann and colleagues observed a sustained virological response in as many as 35% of patients with chronic hepatitis C treated with PEGylated IFN-α2a (PEG-Roferon) compared to less than 10% among those treated with the conventional form of IFN-α 2a[6].

THERAPIES AIMED AT MINIMIZING LIVER DISEASE ACTIVITY AND FIBROSIS

Elimination of HCV infection as marked by sustained clearance of HCV RNA from serum is associated with marked clinical improvement in liver disease. However, patients who do not achieve this form of sustained response may be candidates for treatments which suppress the inflammatory activity and the progression of fibrosis with the hope of delaying or preventing the development of liver failure and hepatocellular carcinoma. Even in the absence of a sustained response, IFN itself has been shown to markedly improve the degree of necroinflammatory activity observed in liver biopsies[7]. The degree of fibrosis may also improve, although to a lesser extent. These beneficial effects are probably short-lived when IFN is stopped after only 6 or 12 months of therapy and very prolonged therapy may be needed to realize significant clinical benefits. Retrospective analyses have suggested that interferon therapy is associated with a significant decrease in the risk of hepatocellular carcinoma (HCC)[8,9]. However, prospective studies will be required to confirm this effect. One such study (the HALT-C [hepatitis antiviral long-term treatment to prevent cirrhosis] study) is currently under way and will examine the impact of IFN given for 4 years to patients with advanced hepatic fibrosis who have not responded previously to IFN.

Ribavirin is now established as an adjunct to IFN. Ribavirin monotherapy had no appreciable effect on levels of HCV RNA in serum[10,11]; however, in about one-third of patients receiving ribavirin serum aminotransferases decreased to normal, and in this group of patients significant improvement could be observed in necroinflammatory activity on liver biopsy, suggesting that ribavirin may have a role in long-term therapy to prevent disease progression[12].

Several studies have now demonstrated that iron reduction therapy by phlebotomy is associated with a consistent decrease in serum aminotransferase activities, often into the normal range[13–15]. This improvement is matched by a decrease in necroinflammatory activity seen on liver biopsy, raising the question of whether iron reduction has a role to play in minimizing disease activity and progression of hepatitis C.

SPECIFIC VIRAL INHIBITORS

The genome of HCV has been well characterized, and based on this structure, HCV has been classified as a member of the flaviviridae family[16]. Its proteins consist of structural and non-structural proteins, the latter playing important roles in the replication of HCV. They include an HCV protease derived from the NS3 portion of the genome, which is responsible for post-translational cleavage of viral proteins, a helicase responsible for unwinding of viral RNA during replication and an RNA-dependent RNA polymerase (RdRp) activity responsible for replication of the viral genome itself during replication. These viral proteins make obvious targets for antiviral therapy. Unfortunately, efforts are hindered by the lack of a suitable cell culture system to study the replication of HCV, so that these proteins must be studied in vitro. The three-dimensional crystalline structure of the protease, helicase and polymerase have been elucidated allowing the design of compounds to bind specifically and inhibit these proteins[17,18]. Although several candidate compounds have apparently been identified, none have made it to clinical use yet. The RdRp has been throughly studied by being cloned and expressed in various systems, allowing the production of functionally active enzyme[19,20]. Compounds which inhibit this enzyme are currently being sought.

It is very likely that specific inhibitors of these viral enzymes will be found and developed. If this occurs, they will probably have potent antiviral effects against HCV if the experience parallels that with HIV. As occurs with HIV, drug resistance is a very likely prospect and should be guarded against by using combination therapies wherever possible from the beginning.

IMMUNOTHERAPY OF HEPATITIS C

The immune response to HCV consists of both antibody production and cellular responses[21]. Neutralizing antibody reactivity may occur but appears to be very weak and not clinically applicable. However, attempts are under way to assess the value of hyperimmune C immunoglobulin (HCIg) as treatment of hepatitis C. HCIg has been manufactured from sterilized serum of patients with chronic HCV infection. Repeated infusions of HCIg into chimpanzees with chronic HCV infection has been associated with a reduction in the expression of HCV antigens within the liver and a steady and progressive decrease in serum aminotransferases[22]. When this preparation is used during acute infection it appears to minimize disease activity and perhaps prevent the development of chronicity.

Vaccines have also been suggested as possible therapy for chronic hepatitis C. These may take the form of peptide vaccines, recombinant proteins and DNA vaccines. Experience with recombinant E1 proteins in chimpanzees with chronic HCV infection has shown an effect similar to that observed with HCIg: multiple vaccination with these proteins has resulted in decreased expression of HCV antigens within the liver and a decrease in liver disease activity (Maertens G, personal communication, 1998). The mechanism of action of such vaccines is not clear, but they may be able to stimulate the host's own immune system to clear HCV by breaking tolerance for this virus.

PROSPECTS FOR NEW ANTIVIRAL TARGETS IN THE FUTURE

Given the large impact of HCV and the likelihood of resistance to specific antivirals, there will remain a need for other new treatments even in the future. HCV offers several potential viral targets which include the internal ribosomal entry site (IRES), the structural proteins themselves (core and surface) and the 3′ untranslated region of the genome. These viral genes or their gene products may be targeted by antisense oligonucleotides or other molecular approaches such as the use of ribozymes[23]. Antisense oligonucleotides have been shown in vitro to decrease the translation of HCV proteins, but before they can be clinically used, issues such as their delivery to hepatocytes and stability in serum must be addressed and overcome. Ribozymes act by an enzyme-like activity of RNA which results in degradation of RNA itself. Again, delivery and stability are issues for this form of therapy but clinical trials are under way already using this approach.

The recent description of CD81 as a possible receptor for HCV raises the prospect of this being adapted therapeutically[24]. CD81 is a ubiquitously expressed transmembrane protein of the tetraspanin family. The function of CD81 is not entirely known but it does play a role in the activation of B lymphocytes. HCV envelope proteins have been shown to bind specifically to CD81, which is found on the surface of hepatocytes, and this has led to speculation that it may function as a receptor for HCV[25]. If this is indeed the case, molecules that interfere with the binding of HCV to this receptor could have some therapeutic benefit.

SUMMARY

The therapy of chronic hepatitis is in a state of rapid evolution built on initial success with IFN and now its combination with ribavirin. Over the next few years we may come to optimize the use of IFN and explore its long-term use in reducing the impact of HCV-related liver disease. This may be considerably aided by the introduction of PEGylated IFNs, which appear to be very promising. The next major step is likely to be the introduction of specific inhibitors of HCV enzymes such as protease, helicase and RdRp, thus inhibiting the replication of this virus. Finally, new additional viral targets are being sought and new therapies developed, largely based on the molecular biology of HCV.

REFERENCES

1. National Institutes of Health Consensus Development Conference Panel Statement: Management of hepatitis C. Hepatology. 1997:26 (suppl 1):2S–10S.
2. EASL International Consensus Conference on Hepatitis C: Consensus Statement. J Hepatol. 1999;30:956–61.

3. Poynard T, Leroy V, Cohard M et al. Meta-analysis of interferon randomized trials in the treatment of viral hepatitis C: Effects of dose and duration. Hepatology. 1996;24:778–89.
4. Lam NP, Neumann AU, Gretch DR, Wiley TE, Perelson AS, Layden TJ. Dose-dependent acute clearance of hepatitis C genotype 1 virus with interferon alfa. Hepatology. 1997;26:226–31.
5. Shiffmann ML. Use of high-dose interferon in the treatment of chronic hepatitis C. Semin Liver Dis. 1999;19 (suppl. 1):25–34.
6. Shiffmann M, Pockros PJ, Reddy RK et al. A controlled, randomized, multicenter, descending dose phase II trial of Pegylated interferon alfa-2a (PEG) vs standard interferon alfa-2a (IFN) for treatment of chronic hepatitis C. Gastroenterology. 1999;A1275 (abstract).
7. Sobesky R, Mathurin P, Charlotte F et al. Modeling the impact of interferon alfa treatment on liver fibrosis progression in chronic hepatitis C: a dynamic view. Gastroenterology. 1999;116:378–86.
8. Imai Y, Kawata S, Tamura S, Yabuuchi I, Noda S, Inada M et al., for the Osaka Hepatocellular Carcinoma Prevention Study Group. Relation of interferon therapy and hepatocellular carcinoma in patients with chronic hepatitis C. Ann Intern Med. 1998;129:94–9.
9. Kasahara A, Hayashi N, Mochizuki K, Takayanagi M, Yoshioka K, Kakumu S et al., and the Osaka Liver Disease Study Group. Risk factors for hepatocellular carcinoma and its incidence after interferon treatment in patients with chronic hepatitis C. Hepatology. 1998;27:1394–402.
10. Di Bisceglie AM, Conjeevaram HS, Fried MW, Sallie R, Park Y, Yurdaydin C et al. Ribavirin as therapy for chronic hepatitis C: A randomized, double-blind, placebo-controlled trial. Ann Intern Med. 1996;123:897–903.
11. Bodenheimer HC, Lindsay KL, Davis GL et al. Tolerance and efficacy of oral ribavirin treatment of chronic hepatitis C: a multicenter trial. Hepatology. 1997;26:473–7.
12. Hoofnagle JH, Lau D, Conjeevaram H, Kleiner D, Di Bisceglie AM. Prolonged therapy of chronic hepatitis C with ribavirin. J Virol Hepatol. 1996;3:247–52.
13. Fong T, Han SH, Tsai NC, Morgan TR, Mizokami M, Qian D et al. A pilot randomized, controlled trial of the effect of iron depletion on long-term response to α-interferon in patients with chronic hepatitis C. J Hepatol. 1998;28:369–74.
14. Di Bisceglie AM, Bonkovsky H, Krawitt E, Grace N, Killenberg P, Hunt C et al. Iron reduction therapy in chronic hepatitis C. Hepatology. 1977;26:151A.
15. Van Thiel DH, Friedlander L, Molloy PJ, Kania RJ, Fagiuoli S, Wright HI et al. Retreatment of Hepatitis C interferon non-responders with larger doses of interferon with and without phlebotomy. Hepato-Gastroenterology. 1996;43:1557–61.
16. Reed KE, Rice CM. Molecular characterization of the hepatitis C virus. In: Reesink HW, ed. Hepatitis C virus, 2nd edn. Basel: Karger, 1998;1–37.
17. Love RA, Parge HE, Wiskersham JA et al. The crystal structure of hepatitis C virus NS3 proteinase reveals a trypsin-like fold and a structural zinc binding site. Cell. 1996;87:331–42.
18. Yao N, Hesson T, Cable M, Hong Z, Kwong AD, Le HV, Weber PC. Structure of the hepatitis C virus RNA helicase domain. Nature Struct Biol. 1997;4:463–7.
19. Hong Z, Ferrari E, Wright-Minogue J et al. Direct antiviral activity of ribavirin: hepatitis C virus NS5B polymerase incorporates ribavirin triphosphate into nasectin RNA products (abstract). Hepatology. 1999;30:345A.
20. Lesburg CA, Cable MB, Ferrari E, Hong Z, Mannarino AF, Weber PC. Crystal structure of the RNA-dependent RNA polymerase from hepatitis C virus reveals a fully encircled active site. Nature Struct Biol. 1999;6:937–43.
21. Nelson DR, Lau JYN. Host immune response in hepatitis C virus infection. Viral Hepatitis Rev. 1996;2:37–48.
22. Krawczynski K, Fattom A, Culver D et al. Passive transfer of anti-HCV in chronic and acute HCV infection in chimpanzees – trials of experimental immune treatment. Hepatology. 1999;30:423A (abstract).
23. Zu Putlitz J, Encke J, Wands JR. The use of antisense and other molecular approaches to therapy of chronic viral hepatitis. Viral Hepatitis Rev. 1998;4:207–28.
24. Pileri PY, Uematsu S, Campagnoli G et al. Binding of hepatitis C virus to CD81. Science. 1998;282:938–41.
25. Flint M, Maidens C, Loomis-Price LD et al. Characterization of hepatitis C virus E2 glycoprotein interaction with a putative cellular receptor, CD81. J Virol. 1999;73:6235–44.

Section III
Alcoholic liver diseases, NASH, drugs and toxins

14
Pathogenesis of alcoholic liver disease

H. DENK, C. STUMPTNER and K. ZATLOUKAL

Alcoholic liver disease may be expressed in three major clinicopathological settings: steatosis, alcoholic hepatitis, fibrosis and finally cirrhosis. Fibrosis and cirrhosis are most often the consequences of alcoholic (steato-)hepatitis, but may also develop directly as the result of stimulation of collagen producing cells[1–7].

Steatosis develops in most alcoholics and is the earliest light microscopically recognizable alcohol-induced lesion. In most cases alcoholic steatosis is benign and resolves within 3–4 weeks of abstinence. However, it may also progress to more advanced and chronic liver disease with worse prognosis; it has been shown in clinical as well as experimental studies that the risk of development of more aggressive disease correlates with severity of steatosis. In addition to toxicity of alcohol and its metabolites, genetic as well as environmental (e.g. high fat diet, drugs, viruses) factors may determine the final outcome of chronic alcohol abuse and account for the inter-individual variation in incidence and severity of disease[1,2,6–8].

Two major types of hepatic steatosis can be recognized at the light microscopic level: the common macrovesicular form, where hepatocytes contain a single large fat vacuole, and the microvesicular form. In liver biopsy specimens of alcoholics a mixture of macro- and microvesicular steatosis may be present suggesting that these different patterns represent sequential stages in the evolution of steatosis, the microvesicular form being the acute and the macrovesicular form the chronic manifestation[3–5].

Steatosis mainly results from an interference with several steps of lipid metabolism in the hepatocyte caused by the shift in the hepatocellular redox state, i.e. increase of the NADH/NAD ratio, as the consequence of ethanol metabolism by alcohol and aldehyde dehydrogenases. However, in the course of chronic alcohol intoxication the redox state of the hepatocyte returns to normal despite persistence of steatosis suggesting that other or additional factors may be involved in perpetuation and progression of alcoholic liver disease[7,9,10].

One or a combination of the following mechanisms are responsible for the development of fatty liver[7,9,10].

1. increased supply of free fatty acids and glycerol-3-phosphate as substrates for triacylglycerol synthesis by increased uptake of fatty acids from the blood, inhibition of fatty acid oxidation and increased endogenous fatty acid synthesis;
2. increased esterification of fatty acids to triacylglycerol; in response to excessive alcohol intake a metabolic stress response is initiated which is characterized by an increased corticosteroid-glucagon to insulin ratio leading to an increased capacity of the liver for fatty acid esterification;
3. decreased export of triacylglycerol, packaged together with phospholipids and apolipoproteins as very low density lipoprotein (VLDL) particles. The defect in VLDL secretion has been localized to the Golgi apparatus and may be related to acetaldehyde-mediated impairment of microtubule assembly.

Approximately 20–40% of heavy drinkers develop severe chronic liver disease, namely alcoholic hepatitis, which rapidly progresses to liver cirrhosis in most of the affected patients.

Alcoholic hepatitis is morphologically characterized by hepatocyte injury with ballooning, necrosis and apoptosis, development of Mallory bodies (MBs), cholestasis, inflammation consisting predominantly of neutrophils, cholestasis and pericellular and perivenular fibrosis. These alterations vary in severity in individual patients and neither clearly correlate with amount and duration of alcohol abuse nor with clinical or laboratory findings. Liver biopsy is, therefore, a valuable tool in the assessment of the disease[3–5].

What can we learn from morphology about the pathogenesis of alcoholic hepatitis and its morphological manifestations (Fig. 1)?

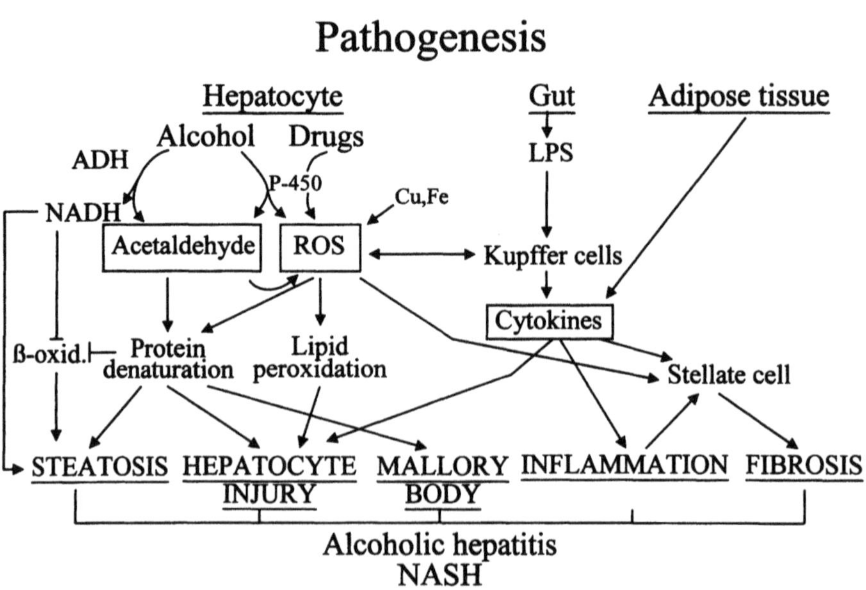

Figure 1 Schematic (and simplified) representation of pathogenetic principles involved in alcoholic and non-alcoholic steatohepatitis (NASH).

Ballooning degeneration of hepatocytes may result from microtubule failure with protein, lipid and fluid retention within the liver cell, as well as from disturbance of cytoskeleton architecture and function with adverse influence on cell stability[7,9–12]. Several factors, alone and in combination, are responsible for liver cell injury, including effects of cytokines, acetaldehyde and reactive oxygen species on membranes of mitochondria and cytoskeletal structures[13–20]. There is ample evidence on the basis of clinical and experimental studies that oxidative stress resulting from an imbalance between pro- and antioxidative processes plays a crucial role in alcoholic liver injury. Free radicals and reactive oxygen species (ROS) arise in hepatocytes from microsomal, mitochondrial and peroxisomal sources and interact with vital cellular molecules, like proteins, lipids and nucleic acids. Structural modifications and functional impairment induced by lipid peroxidation or protein denaturation and unfolding ensue[21]. The microsomal ethanol oxidizing system with cytochrome P450 2E1 is an important source of free radicals in the course of ethanol or drug metabolism and this process may be stimulated by dietary conditions, e.g. polyunsaturated fat, heavy metals and other factors. The inflammatory infiltrate is related to the generation of cytokines and chemokines, such as interleukin-8, mainly by Kupffer cells[15,22]. Inflammation in alcoholic liver disease results from an imbalance of pro- and anti-inflammatory cytokines. The activated Kupffer cell is a major player in chronic alcoholic liver damage by releasing pro-inflammatory cytokines and chemokines, proteolytic enzymes and reactive oxygen intermediates upon stimulation by ROS of hepatocellular origin and endotoxin (lipopolysaccharides; LPS) derived from a leaky gut[23,24]. Increased expression of adhesion molecules on endothelial cells promotes local binding and permeation of leukocytes. Fibrosis is a constant feature of alcoholic and other types of steatohepatitis. Stellate cells play a central role in the process of collagen production and deposition upon activation by cytokines but also ethanol metabolites[22,25].

Ballooned cells often contain irregular cytoplasmic inclusions with filamentous ultrastructure (Fig. 2) first described by F. B. Mallory in 1911 and called Mallory bodies (MBs) or alcoholic hyalin since then[26]. MB formation represents a special morphologic expression of chronic liver cell injury[1,2,26–30]. Although typical, they are not specific for alcoholic hepatitis and also associated with non-alcoholic steatohepatitis (NASH)[31], chronic cholestatic conditions, hepatocellular tumours, and certain metabolic diseases, including copper toxicosis. MBs are not primarily inducible in animal livers by ethanol administration but can easily be produced in mouse liver by chronic intoxication with the fungistatic antimicrotubular drug griseofulvin (GF) and the porphyrogenic agent 3,4-diethoxcarbonyl-1,4-dihydrocollidine (DDC)[27–32].

In our studies we have concentrated on structure, composition and pathogenesis of MBs in order to understand some of the complex mechanisms involved in alcoholic hepatitis and related liver disorders.

It has been shown many years ago that the cytokeratin (CK) intermediate filament (IF) cytoskeleton is severely affected in alcoholic hepatitis (but also in NASH)[1,12,27,28]. Immunofluorescence microscopy using antibodies to CKs and non-CK-MB components revealed that ballooned hepatocytes containing larger MBs are characterized by a deranged and sometimes even undetectable CK cytoskeleton (Fig. 2). Identical cytoskeleton alterations can be experimentally

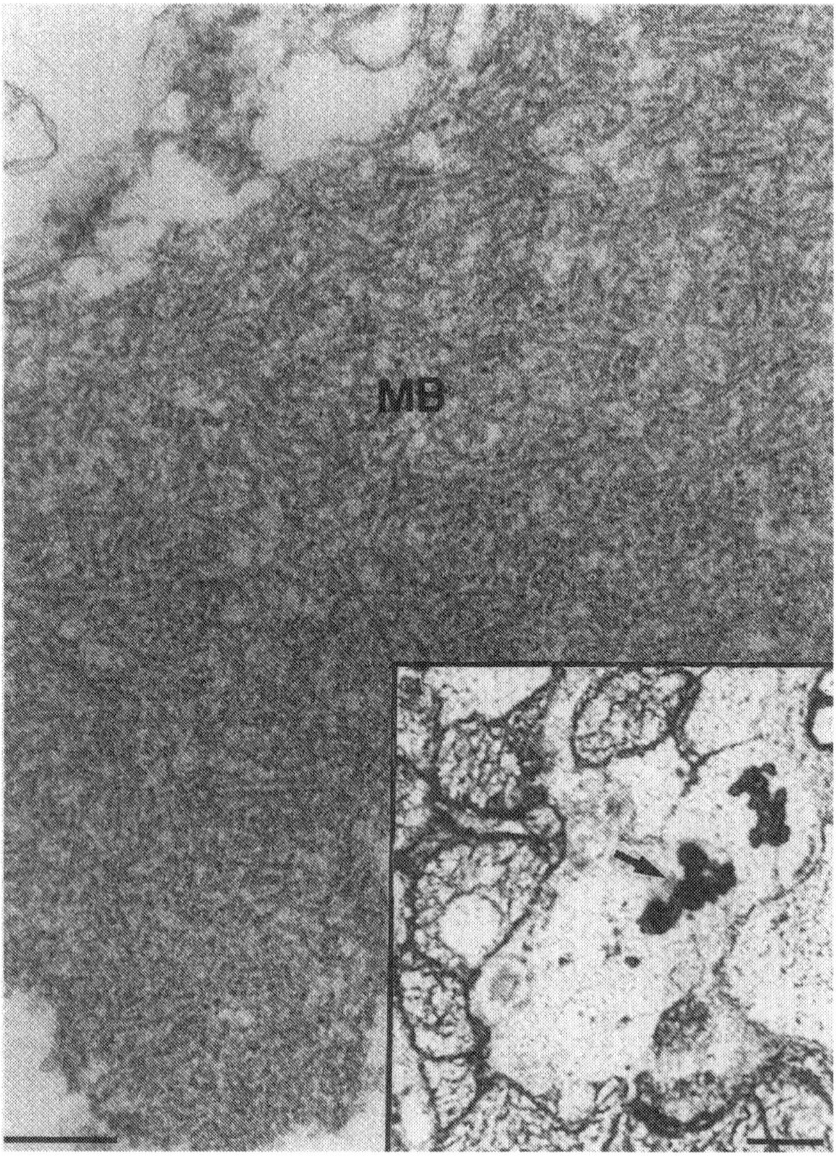

Figure 2 Ultrastructure of Mallory body: the Mallory body (MB) inclusion consists of haphazardly arranged filaments. Inset depicts Mallory bodies immunostained with a polyclonal cytokeratin antibody within an enlarged (ballooned) hepatocyte (arrow). The Mallory body-containing hepatocyte shows a highly diminished immunostainable cytokeratin cytoskeleton whereas the surrounding Mallory body-free hepatocytes display a regular cytokeratin filament network (immunogold-silver staining). Bar, 250 nm (in inset: 10 μm).

induced in mice by chronic intoxication with GF and DDC. Human as well as murine MBs contain CKs, predominantly CK8, the stress inducible M_M120-1 antigen, a novel component with a molecular weight around 62–65 kDa, which is phosphorylated as revealed by its reactivity with phosphoepitope antibodies (SMI31, MPM-2), heat shock proteins with low and high molecular weights (HSP 70 and HSP 25/28) and ubiquitin[28,30–40].

Further analyses of the 62–65 kDa component clearly identified this protein as p62 (Zatloukal et al., manuscript in preparation; ref. 41), a recently described stress-induced protein component of the signal transduction cascade, which binds ubiquitin, has kinase activity, and may play a role in the sequestration of proteins in the form of sequestosomes and in cell differentiation[42]. The function of this protein in the hepatocyte under physiologic and pathologic conditions needs further clarification.

As revealed by analysis of human MBs as well as by experiments with GF- and DDC-treated mice two major processes are essential for MB development: hyperphosphorylation of CKs and over-expression of predominantly CK8. Hyperphosphorylation is demonstrated by immunohistochemical, biochemical and ^{32}P-incorporation studies showing that phosphorylation of CKs is an early event followed by aggregation of phosphorylated CKs as MBs[43,44]. CK over-expression is revealed by quantitative RT-PCR and immunoblotting[45,46] as well as by *in situ* hybridization (Stumptner et al., manuscript in preparation). Analysis of early stages of MB development in intoxicated mice clearly revealed that the accumulation of CKs, M_M 120-1 antigen and p62 is the first step in MB formation followed by ubiquitination, association with low and high molecular weight heat shock proteins and cross-linking (Stumptner et al., manuscript in preparation).

What is the role of these different MB components and their posttranslational modifications in MB formation? To answer this question we studied mice in which the genes for CK8 and 18, respectively, had been deleted (CK knockout mice)[28,47–49]. Normal CK IFs of hepatocytes consist of equimolar amounts of the two CK (type II and type I) partners CK8 and CK18. In the absence of either CK8 or CK18 no CK filaments can be assembled. DDC feeding resulted in higher toxicity in CK8 knockout (–/–) mice than in CK wild type (+/+) animals. After 3 months of intoxication seven of 12 CK8–/– mice had died whereas all CK8+/+ survived. Thus, it is clear from these results that CK8 deficiency increases the sensitivity of hepatocytes to intoxication. Moreover, MBs did not form under CK8–/– conditions and neither CKs nor non-CK components accumulated in the hepatocytes. This proves that CK8 is the core component in MB formation to which the other components attach. DDC intoxication of CK8 heterozygous mice with only one inactivated CK8 allele (+/–) neither led to alterations of the CK cytoskeleton nor to the appearance of MBs, despite the presence of signs of DDC intoxication, such as development of porphyria. The different behaviour of CK8 +/+ and CK18 +/– mice has, therefore, to be attributed to the loss of one CK8 allele and the resulting imbalance between CKs 8 and 18. As revealed by quantitative RT-PCR, DDC intoxication led to an approximately 5-fold over-expression of both CK8 and CK18 mRNAs in CK8 +/+ and to a similar increase in the concentration of CK18 mRNA in CK8 +/– animals. The concentration of CK8 mRNA, however, only reached about 50% of CK18 mRNA level. This suggests that a certain threshold of CK8 over-expression in relation to CK18 has to be exceeded to provoke CK cytoskeleton alterations and MB formation.

These findings provided strong evidence that over-expression of CK8 enables hepatocytes to better tolerate toxic insults. The clinical relevance of this finding is supported by the recent observation of a patient with idiopathic liver cirrhosis who showed a mutation in the CK8 gene[50]. The question remained whether the increased tolerance to toxins is related to an intact cytoskeleton and resulting increased stability of hepatocytes, or due to novel non-skeletal functions of CK8. To clarify this issue we analysed mice in which the CK18 gene had been deleted (CK18 –/–)(ref. 49; Zatloukal et al., manuscript in preparation). These mice, like the CK8 –/– animals, were also unable to form an IF cytoskeleton. However, in contrast to CK8 –/– animals, CK18 –/– mice did not show increased sensitivity to DDC intoxication. Moreover, they developed classical MBs consisting of CK8 and the other non-CK components. From these experiments it not only became clear that CK8 is indeed the nucleating MB component and that the other non-CK components bind to or co-assemble with CK8 in the course of MB formation, but also that the increased sensitivity of CK8 –/– mice to intoxication is not due to the loss of the CK cytoskeleton but can be attributed to their inability to over-express CK8.

These data also shed light on the biologic significance of MBs in alcoholic hepatitis and related liver disease. Since, on the one hand, mice which did not form MBs showed increased sensitivity to the toxin, and, on the other, MBs formation was accompanied by increased tolerance, a detrimental effect of MBs on the hepatocyte can be ruled out. In contrast, MBs seem to be the cellular manifestation of a defence response against chronic stress.

At the present time we do not know how this putative defence process works. Since CKs are phosphoproteins, CK8 could act as phosphate sink protecting other cellular components, e.g. of the signal transduction system, from stress-induced hyperphosphorylation and consecutive dysfunction.

MB formation seems to reflect the fate of abnormally folded or denatured proteins. Every nascent protein consists of a long linear string of amino acids that normally folds up into a specific three-dimensional shape, determined by its amino acid sequence. Various chaperones are engaged in this folding process. Misfolding of proteins may result from mutation, influence of ROS, transcriptional and post-transcriptional modifications, unbalanced synthesis of subunits, or other insults. Under various stress conditions with related protein damage increased chaperone function is needed, and consequently, chaperones, i.e. heat shock or stress proteins, are induced as rescue response[21,51,52].

The cell has several options to deal with abnormally folded or unfolded proteins (refs. 49,51–54; Fig. 3):

1. refolding with the help of chaperones.
2. degradation by the proteasome system after polyubiquitination.
3. aggregation and sequestration with the help of p62[42]. Aggregation is promoted by the exposure of hydrophobic protein sequences which are normally buried in the folds of the mature and correctly folded protein.

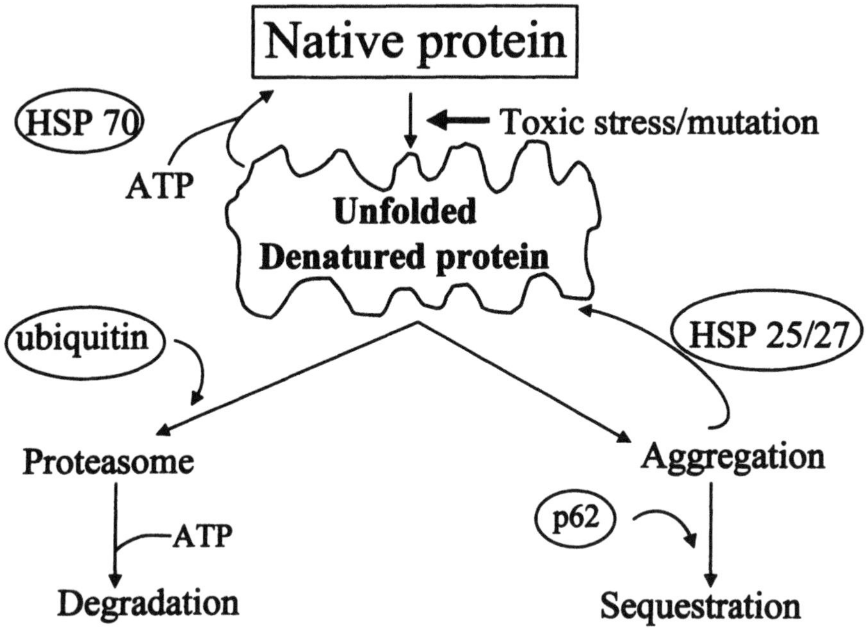

Figure 3 Fate of denatured (unfolded) proteins.

The latter scenario seems to apply to MB formation, suggesting that functional impairment of the chaperone and/or the protease systems[54,55] leads to aggregation of over-expressed, abnormally phosphorylated and in the quantitative type I to type II relationship altered CKs together with other proteins. These aggregates are finally cross-linked by the action of transglutaminase[56]. ROS generated by a diversity of mechanisms are possibly involved in the early stages of this process and may even be its initiators by inducing kinases and CK8 (type II) over-expression (Fig. 4).

Similar pathogenetic principles seem to play a role in the development of inclusion bodies of amyloid type associated with a diversity of diseases, including neurodegenerative disorders, prion diseases, motor neuron disease[52], but also of the cytoplasmic globules in α_1-antitrypsin deficiency[57]. It is, therefore, a new aspect of our work (and that of other authors) to include alcoholic hepatitis and other MB-associated liver disorders into the group of diseases based on abnormal protein folding (Fig. 5) and this opens an avenue for novel therapeutic strategies.

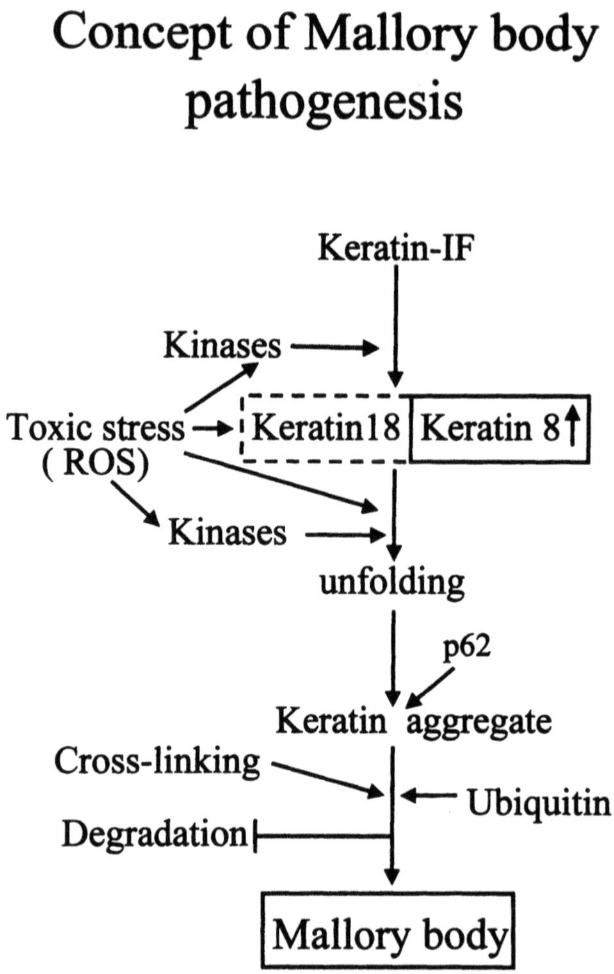

Figure 4 Concept of Mallory body pathogenesis based on studies of human alcoholic hepatitis and related animal models.

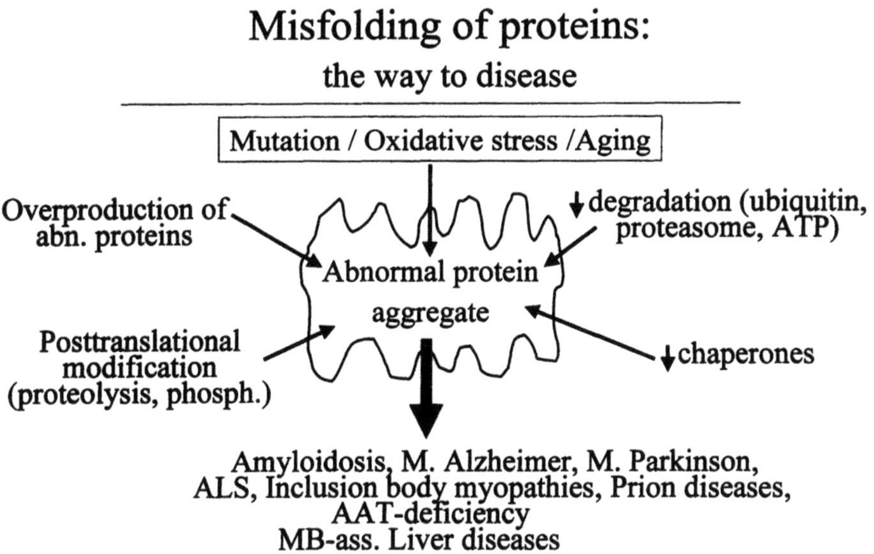

Figure 5 Pathogenetic principles involved in the appearance of abnormal protein aggregates associated with a variety of diseases, including liver disorders associated with Mallory body formation.

REFERENCES

1. Jensen K, Gluud C. The Mallory body: morphological, clinical and experimental studies (part 1 of a literature survey). Hepatology. 1994;20:1061–77.
2. Jensen K, Gluud C. The Mallory body: theories on development and pathological significance (part 2 of a literature survey). Hepatology. 1994;20:1330–42.
3. Ishak KG, Zimmerman HJ, Ray MB. Alcoholic liver disease: pathologic, pathogenetic and clinical aspects. Alcoholism: Clin Exp Res. 1991;15:45–66.
4. French SW, Nash J, Shitabata P, Kachi K, Hara C, Chedid A, Mendenhall CL, VA Cooperative Study Group 119. Pathology of alcoholic liver disease. Sem Liver Dis. 1993;13:154–69.
5. Burt AD, Mutton A, Day CP. Diagnosis and interpretation of steatosis and steatohepatitis. Semin Diagn Pathol. 1998;15:246–58.
6. Lindros KO. Alcoholic liver disease: pathobiological aspects. J Hepatol. 1995;23 (Suppl):7–15.
7. Lieber CS. Biochemical factors in alcoholic liver disease. Semin Liver Dis. 1993;13:136–53.
8. Bosron WF, Ehrig T, Li TK. Genetic factors in alcohol metabolism and alcoholism. Semin. Liver Dis. 1993;13:126–35.
9. Eaton S, Record CO, Bartlett K. Multiple biochemical effects in the pathogenesis of alcoholic fatty liver. Eur J Clin Invest. 1997;27:719–22.
10. Day CP, Yeaman SJ. The biochemistry of alcohol-induced fatty liver. Biochim Biophys Acta. 1994;1215:33–48.
11. Zatloukal K, Spurej G, Rainer I, Lackinger E, Denk H. Fate of Mallory body-containing hepatocytes: disappearance of Mallory bodies and restoration of the hepatocytic intermediate filament cytoskeleton after drug withdrawal in the griseofulvin-treated mouse. Hepatology. 1990;11:652–61.
12. Denk H, Lackinger E. Cytoskeleton in liver diseases. Semin Liver Dis. 1986;6:199–211.
13. Tuma DJ, Sorrell MF. The role of acetaldehyde adducts in liver injury. In: Hall P, ed. Alcoholic Liver Disease. Pathology and Pathogenesis. London: Edward Arnold; 1995: pp. 89–99.

14. Adachi Y, Bradford BU, Gao W, Bojes HK, Thurman RG. Inactivation of Kupffer cells prevents early alcohol-induced liver injury. Hepatology. 1994;20:453–60.
15. Deaciuc IV. Alcohol and cytokine networks. Alcohol. 1997;14:421–30.
16. Dilger K, Metzler J, Bode JC, Klotz V. CYP 2E1 activity in patients with alcoholic liver disease. J Hepatol. 1997;27:1009–14.
17. Ingelman-Sundberg M, Johansson I. Mechanisms of hydroxyl radical formation and ethanol oxidation by ethanol-inducible and other forms of rabbit liver microsomal cytochrome P-450. J Biol Chem. 1984;259:6447–58.
18. Lauterburg BH, DeQuay B. Radicals and oxidants in ethanol induced liver injury. In: Moslen MT, Smith CV, eds. Free Radical Mechanisms of Tissue Injury. London: CRC Press, 1992: pp. 33–43.
19. Weltman MD, Farrell GC, Hall P, Ingelman-Sundberg M, Liddle C. Hepatic cytochrome P450 2E1 is increased in patients with non-alcoholic steatohepatitis. Hepatology. 1998;27:128–33.
20. Nanji AA. Apoptosis and alcoholic liver disease. Semin Liv Dis. 1998;18:187–90.
21. Stadtman ER, Berlett BS. Free-radical-mediated modification of proteins. In: Wallace KB, ed. Free Radical Toxicity. Washington DC: Taylor and Francis. 1997: pp. 71–87.
22. McClain CJ, Barve S, Deacine I, Kugelmas M, Hill D. Cytokines in alcoholic liver disease. Semin Liver Dis. 1999;19:205–19.
23. Bjarnson I, Peters TJ, Wise RJ. The leaky gut of alcoholism: possible route of entry for toxic compounds. Lancet. 1984;1:179–82.
24. Bode C, Kugler V, Bode JC. Endotoxemia in patients with alcoholic and non-alcoholic cirrhosis and in subjects with no evidence of chronic liver disease following acute ethanol excess. J Hepatol. 1987;4:8–14.
25. Tsukamoto H, Cheng S, Blander WS. Effects of dietary polyunsaturated fat on ethanol-induced Ito cell activation. Am J Physiol. 1996;270: (Gastrointest Liver Physiol 33):G581–6.
26. Mallory FB. Cirrhosis of the liver: five different lesions from which it may arise. Bull Johns Hopkins Hosp. 1911;22:69–75.
27. Denk H, Franke WW, Kerjaschki D, Eckersdorfer R. Mallory bodies in experimental animals and man. Int Rev Exp Pathol. 1979;20:77–121.
28. Denk H, Stumptner C, Zatloukal K. Mallory bodies-revisited. J Hepatol. in press.
29. Denk H, Gschnait F, Wolff K. Hepatocellular hyalin (Mallory bodies) in long term griseofulvin-treated mice: a new experimental model for the study of hyalin formation. Lab Invest. 1975;32:773–6.
30. Denk H, Zatloukal K, Stumptner C. Alcoholic hepatitis. In: Sherman D, Preedy V, Watson R, eds. Ethanol and the Liver. Harwood Academic Publications. In press.
31. James OFW, Day CP. Non-alcoholic steatohepatitis (NASH): a disease of emerging identity and importance. J Hepatol. 1998;20:495–501.
32. Tsunoo C, Harwood TR, Arak S, Yokoo H. Cytoskeletal alterations leading to Mallory body formation in livers of mice fed 3,5-diethoxycarbonyl-1,4-dihydrocollidine. J Hepatol. 1987;5:85–97.
33. Denk H, Franke WW, Eckerstorfer R, Schmid E, Kerjaschki D. Formation and involution of Mallory bodies (alcoholic hyalin) in murine and human livers revealed by immunofluorescence microscopy with antibodies to prekeratins. Proc Natl Acad Sci USA. 1979;76:4112–16.
34. Hazan R, Denk H, Franke WW, Lackinger E, Schiller DL. Change of cytokeratin organization during development of Mallory bodies as revealed by a monoclonal antibody. Lab Invest. 1986;54:543–53.
35. Denk H, Franke WW, Dragosics B, Zeiler I. Pathology of cytoskeleton of liver cells: Demonstration of Mallory bodies (alcoholic hyalin) in murine and human hepatocytes by immunofluorescence microscopy using antibodies to cytokeratin polypeptides from hepatocytes. Hepatology. 1981;1:9–20.
36. Zatloukal K, Denk H, Spurej G, Lackinger E, Preisegger KH, Franke WW. High molecular weight component of Mallory bodies detected by a monoclonal antibody. Lab Invest. 1990;62:427–34.
37. Preisegger KH, Zatloukal K, Spurej G, Riegelnegg D, Denk H. Common epitopes of human and murine Mallory bodies and Lewy bodies as revealed by a neurofilament antibody. Lab Invest. 1992;66:193–9.

38. Lichtenberg-Kraag B, Mandelkow EM, Biernat J, Steiner B, Schröter C, Gustke N. Phosphorylation – dependent epitopes of neurofilament antibodies on tau protein and relationship with Alzheimer tau. Proc Natl Acad Sci USA. 1992;89:5384–8.
39. Westendorf JM, Rao PN, Gerace L. Cloning of cDNAs for M-phase phosphoproteins recognized by the MPM2 monoclonal antibody and determination of the phosphorylated epitope. Proc Natl Acad Sci USA. 1994;91:714–18.
40. Lowe J, Mayer RJ, Landon M. Ubiquitin in neurodegenerative diseases. Brain Pathol. 1993;3:55–65.
41. Stumptner C, Zatloukal K, Fickert P, Denk H. P62/A 170- a novel component of Mallory bodies associated with alcoholic hepatitis. Hepatology. 1999;30:412A.
42. Shin J. P62 and the sequestosome, a novel mechanism for protein metabolism. Arch Pharmacol. 1998;21:629–33.
43. Salmhofer H, Rainer I, Zatloukal K, Denk H. Posttranslational events involved in griseofulvin-induced keratin cytoskeleton alterations. Hepatology. 1994;20:731–40.
44. Stumptner C, Omary MB, Fickert P, Denk H, Zatloukal K. Hepatocyte cytokeratins are hyperphosphorylated at multiple sites in human alcoholic hepatitis and in a Mallory body mouse model. Am J Pathol, in press.
45. Hutter H, Zatloukal K, Winter G, Stumptner C, Denk H. Disturbance of keratin homeostasis in griseofulvin-intoxicated mouse liver. Lab Invest. 1993;69:576–82.
46. Stumptner C, Fuchsbichler A, Denk H, Zatloukal K. Overexpression of cytokeratin induces accumulation of the Mallory body-specific component M_M 120-1 in vitro. Hepatology. 1996;24:129A.
47. Baribault H, Penner J, Iozzo RV, Wilson-Heiner M. Colorectal hyperplasia and inflammation in keratin 8-deficient FVB/N mice. Genes Dev. 1994;8:2964–74.
48. Zatloukal K, Stumptner C, Lechner M, Fuchsbichler A, Eshkind LG, Baribault H et al. Cytokeratin protects hepatocytes from intoxication: a possible new function of intermediate filaments revealed by cytokeratin 8 knock-out mice. Hepatology. 1997;26:182A.
49. Magin TM, Schröder R, Leitgeb S, Wanninger F, Zatloukal K, Grund C, Melton DW. Lessons from keratin 18 knockout mice; formation of novel keratin filaments, secondary loss of keratin 7 and accumulation of liver specific keratin 8-positive aggregates. J Cell Biol. 1998;140:1441–51.
50. Ku NO, Wright TL, Terrault NA, Gish R, Omary MB. Mutation of human keratin 18 in association with cryptogenic cirrhosis. J Clin Invest. 1997;99:19–23.
51. Hartl FU. Molecular chaperones in cellular protein folding. Nature. 1996;381:571–80.
52. Taubes G. Misfolding the way to disease. Science. 1996;271:1493–6.
53. Grune T, Reinheckel T, Davies KJA. Degradation of oxidized proteins in mammalian cells. FASEB J. 1997;11:526–34.
54. Lee DH, Goldberg AL. Proteasome inhibitors: valuable new tools for cell biologists. Trends Cell Biol. 1998;8:397–403.
55. Fataccioli V, Andrand E, Gentil M, French SW, Rouach H. Effects of chronic ethanol administration on rat liver proteasome activities: relationship with oxidative stress. Hepatology. 1999;29:14–20.
56. Zatloukal K, Fesus L, Denk H, Tarcsa E, Spurej G, Böck G. High amount of ε – (γ-glutamyl) lysine cross-links in Mallory bodies. Lab Invest. 1992;66:774–7.
57. Perlmutter DH. Alpha-1-antitrypsin deficiency. Semin Liver Dis. 1998;18:217–25.

15 Alcoholic liver disease: natural course, mechanisms and therapeutic strategies

C. S. LIEBER

NATURAL COURSE OF THE DISEASE

Fatty liver

Fat accumulation in the liver cells is the earliest and most common response to alcohol[1,2] (Fig. 1). In massive steatosis, the hepatocytes are uniformly filled by large fat droplets, the cell nucleus may be eccentrically placed and, when the cell membranes between adjacent hepatocytes rupture, fatty cysts are formed. Ultrastructural changes reveal enlarged and distorted mitochondria with shortened cristae containing crystalline inclusions[3]. The endoplasmic reticulum shows vacuolar dilatation and proliferation. Despite adequate nutrition, alcohol

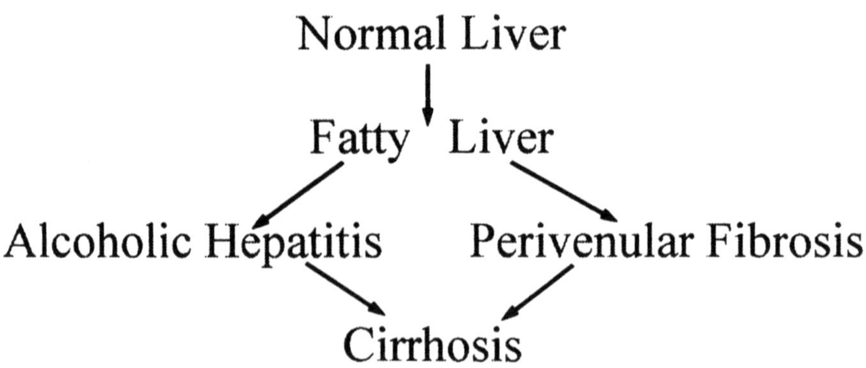

Figure 1 Progression of alcoholic liver disease. Experiments in animals and judicious clinical trials indicate that alcohol can lead to fatty liver, independent of nutritional deficiencies. A more severe consequence of hepatotoxicity is alcoholic hepatitis, a precursor of cirrhosis. Cirrhosis may also result more directly (via perivenular fibrosis) from toxicity of ethanol, mediated, in part, by aldehydes (acetaldehyde and products of lipid peroxidation)[433].

has been shown to induce these alterations in rats, baboons and in both alcoholic and non-alcoholic human volunteers[4,5].

The clinical spectrum of alcoholic fatty liver may extend from silent non-symptomatic hepatomegaly to severe hepatocellular failure with cholestasis and portal hypertension[6,7]. Most of the patients with pure fatty liver are virtually asymptomatic. Hepatomegaly is the commonest clinical sign, present on physical examination in 75% of patients[6]. In more advanced cases, hepatic tenderness, anorexia, nausea, emesis, jaundice, fluid accumulation and even spider angiomas are present. Severe forms of fatty liver may present a clinical picture mimicking extrahepatic obstructive jaundice, especially if associated with dark urine and acholic stools[7,8]. Typical abnormalities in laboratory tests are slightly or moderately elevated γ-glutamyltransferase (GGT) and serum transaminases (AST and ALT). In contrast to more advanced alcoholic liver injury, all the abnormalities in laboratory tests tend to return to normal rapidly within the first days of hospitalization.

Perivenular fibrosis

Although it can occur anywhere in the hepatic acinus, the earliest deposition of fibrous tissue is generally seen around the central veins and venules, now called terminal hepatic venules. Such perivenular fibrosis has been described in alcoholic hepatitis.

It is important to note that perivenular fibrosis can also be seen in the absence of widespread inflammation and necrosis, in association with what most pathologists would label as 'simple' fatty liver. Of 75 hospitalized alcoholic subjects in whom the diagnosis of simple fatty liver had been made on the basis of liver biopsy, 40% were found to have perivenular fibrosis upon review of the histology. There was no evidence of diffuse alcoholic hepatitis. Once perivenular fibrosis has developed, it indicates that the patient already entered the fibrotic process and that, upon continuation of drinking, he or she will rapidly develop more severe stages, including cirrhosis[9]. Thus this lesion can be considered a marker of vulnerability to the development of subsequent cirrhosis and can be used as an indication for active intervention. Although fibrosis as a result of necrosis and inflammation is thought to be the underlying mechanism of alcoholic cirrhosis (Fig. 1), cirrhosis commonly develops without an apparent intermediate stage of alcoholic hepatitis, both in alcoholics[9,10] and in baboons given alcohol[11–13]. Indeed, independently of necrosis and inflammation, alcohol (via acetaldehyde) directly affects stellate cells (also called cells Ito or lipocytes) in the liver. Long-term alcohol consumption transforms stellate cells into collagen-producing myofibroblast-like cells[14–17], and acetaldehyde stimulates collagen synthesis in these cells[18] causing the deposition of collagen, the characteristic protein of the fibrous tissue.

Alcoholic hepatitis

This stage is characterized by the appearance of necrosis with an inflammatory reaction, including polymorphonuclear cells. From either clinical or pathological signs, this inflammatory response of the liver to alcohol has been called florid cirrhosis, acute hepatic insufficiency, progressive alcoholic cirrhosis, or steatonecrosis Mallory body type. The term alcoholic hepatitis, used by Beckett and co-workers[19], is now widely accepted by most pathologists and clinicians. While the incidence of fatty liver in alcoholics is very common, alcoholic hepatitis develops in only a fraction of heavy drinkers, even after decades of abuse[20,21]. The long-term incidence of cirrhosis in patients with alcoholic hepatitis is nine times higher than in those with fatty liver[22]. Thus, traditionally, alcoholic hepatitis has been viewed as the precursor lesion of alcoholic cirrhosis (Fig. 1) but, as mentioned above, alcoholic cirrhosis can also develop in the absence of overt alcoholic hepatitis.

Histological characteristics of alcoholic hepatitis are ballooning and great disarray of hepatocytes, predominantly in perivenular areas, parenchymal and portal infiltration with polymorphonuclear leukocytes, varying degrees of steatosis, necrosis, fibrosis, and cholestasis. Lymphocytes are seen in perivenular zones or within the parenchyma. Mallory's alcoholic hyaline irregular cytoplasmic bodies can be considered as a diagnostic hallmark[23–28] but it is not always present. Ultrastructural changes in alcoholic hepatitis are similar to those seen in fatty liver, but more severe[3]. Collagenous material may be found in the space of Disse and associated with loss of microvilli that normally project from the hepatocyte[29,30].

The depression of serum albumin and prolongation of the prothrombin time has been shown to correlate with the severity of the histological lesion[31].

Cirrhosis

Microscopically, scar tissue distorts the normal architecture of the liver by forming bands of connective tissue joining portal and central zones. At first, nodules are regular in size and shape[32]. In more advanced cirrhosis nodules become larger and frequently irregular in size and shape.

One of the most characteristic features of cirrhosis is the change in the hepatic blood circulation. Endophlebitis[33] and perivenular fibrosis[34] may impair outflow from the sinusoids and the regenerative nodules may compress the hepatic veins, resulting in post sinusoidal portal hypertension. The total as well as the effective blood flow in the liver decreases in cirrhosis[35]. The total blood flow is reduced by extrahepatic portasystemic shunts and the effective circulation is limited by neovascularization of connective tissue septa which form anastomoses between the afferent branches of the portal vein and hepatic artery and the efferent tributaries of the hepatic veins[36]. Collagen deposits in the space of Disse[29,30] and reduction in the number of patent fenestrations[16] may further increase the resistance to blood flow and isolate the hepatocyte from its blood supply. As a result of these changes, marked deterioration in residual hepatic function may occur, especially if either the cardiac output or the circulating blood volume changes.

In addition to fibrosis, various admixtures of fat, inflammatory reactions, and cholestasis may be seen. Histologically stainable iron deposits are common in cirrhotic livers, especially in alcoholic subjects[37,38]. However, total iron stores are very seldom increased and never exceed 179 mmol (10 g). The differentiation from primary haemochromatosis is possible by measuring the total hepatic iron content from liver biopsies.

Hepatocellular carcinoma (HCC) has become a relatively frequent finding in liver cirrhosis, presumably because of improved management and prolonged survival[39,40]. Pathogenetically it has been traditionally related to cirrhosis, but possible carcinogenic properties of alcohol must also be considered, since primary hepatocellular carcinoma can complicate non-cirrhotic alcoholic liver disease[41]. Furthermore, there appears to be a significant interaction between alcohol and viral hepatitis, especially hepatitis C, in hepatocarcinogenesis.

Low-grade and continuous fever is also common in decompensated cirrhosis[42]. Jaundice and hepatomegaly are typical primary physical signs of cirrhosis. Secondary phenomena include portal hypertension with splenomegaly, oedema and ascites, encephalopathy, gastrointestinal haemorrhage from oesophageal or gastric varices and bleeding tendencies due to clotting factor abnormalities. Tertiary complications include spontaneous peritonitis caused by anaerobic bacteria[43].

Typically, serum electrophoresis reveals a decrease in serum albumin and prealbumin and a broad elevation of the beta- and gammaglobulins[44]. Frequently, IgA and also IgG and IgM are elevated[45–48]. Serum transaminases and alkaline phosphatases are usually only mildly elevated.

Alcoholic liver disease is commonly diagnosed at this late stage, when complications of portal hypertension become obvious. Although these can be alleviated by corresponding treatments, the underlying liver pathology is usually not reversible at that stage. Earlier diagnosis can be achieved with liver biopsy through the recognition of pre-cirrhotic lesions such as perivenular fibrosis (*vide supra*). At that stage, further progression of liver disease can be slowed or even stopped through control of alcohol consumption, facilitated by the use of agents that oppose craving, such as naltrexone[49,50]. Additional benefits can be obtained through replenishment of nutritional deficiencies, when present. It is important to recognize, however, that because of the alcohol-induced disease process, several of the nutritional requirements change and more specific therapy is now available (*vide infra*).

Outlook

The clinical course and ultimate outcome of alcoholic liver disease is dismal. Indeed, in a prospective survey of 280 subjects with alcoholic liver injury[51] within 48 months of follow-up, more than half of those with cirrhosis, and two-thirds of those with cirrhosis plus alcoholic hepatitis had died. This disastrous outcome is more severe than that of many cancers, yet it is attracting much less concern, both among the public and the medical profession. This may be due, at least in part, to the general perception that not much can be done about this major public health issue. One purpose of this review is to analyse how concepts about alcoholic liver disease have evolved and how elucidation of the biochemical effects of ethanol allows for a more optimistic outlook in terms of diagnosis and treatment.

PATHOGENESIS

Respective role of alcohol and nutrition

Ethanol is not only a psychoactive drug. Besides ethanol's pharmacological action, it has a considerable energy value (7.1 kcal/g). Therefore, in many societies alcoholic beverages are considered part of the basic food supply,

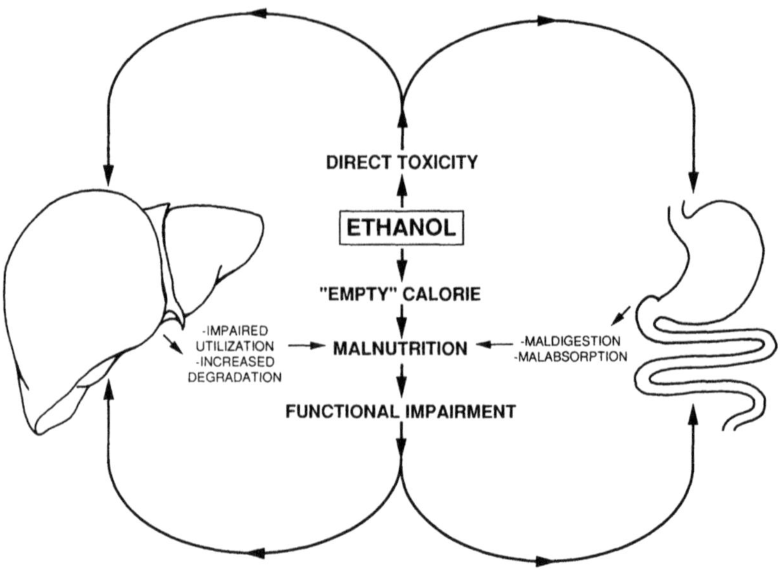

Figure 2 Interaction of direct toxicity of ethanol with malnutrition due to primary or secondary deficiencies. Secondary malnutrition may be caused by either maldigestion and malabsorption or impaired utilization (decreased activation and/or increased inactivation) of nutrients. Both direct toxicity of ethanol and malnutrition (whether primary or secondary) may affect function and structure of liver and gut[434].

whereas in others alcohol is consumed mainly for its mood-altering effects. Under both circumstances, a substantial use of alcohol has profound effects on nutritional status[52]. Such consumption may cause primary malnutrition by displacing other nutrients in the diet because of the high energy content of the alcoholic beverages (Fig. 2) or because of associated socioeconomic and medical disorders. Secondary malnutrition may result from either maldigestion or malabsorption of nutrients caused by gastrointestinal complications associated with alcoholism, involving especially the pancreas and the small intestine. Alcohol also promotes nutrient degradation or impaired activation. Such primary and secondary malnutrition can affect virtually all nutrients (*vide infra*). At the tissue level, alcohol replaces various normal substrates, with the liver being the most seriously affected organ and malnutrition being incriminated as a primary etiologic factor of liver dysfunction.

Theories of the exclusively nutritional origin of alcoholic liver disease were supported very strongly by Best, the prominent codiscoverer of insulin who wrote that 'there is no more evidence of a specific toxic effect of pure ethyl alcohol upon liver cells than there is for one due to sugar'[53]. This notion was based largely on experimental work in rats given ethanol in drinking water[52]. Under these conditions no liver lesions developed, unless the diet was deficient in proteins, methionine, or choline. Deficiency alone sufficed to produce the liver lesions. However, with the technique of alcohol administration in drinking water, ethanol consumption usually does not exceed 10–25% of the total energy intake of the animal, because rats have an aversion for alcohol. A comparable amount of alcohol resulted in negligible ethanol concentrations in the blood[53]. Thus, administration of alcohol in drinking water to rodents is not a suitable model for the human disease. When ethanol was incorporated into a totally liquid diet[53,54], the aversion for alcohol was overcome because, in order to eat or drink, the animals had no choice but to take the alcohol along with whatever diet was given. With this technique, the quantity of ethanol consumed was increased to 36% of total energy, an amount relevant to alcohol intake in man. The introduction of the liquid diet model represented a turning point in alcohol research, not only by producing meaningful blood alcohol concentrations, but also by allowing for better dietary control and strict pair-feeding techniques. In that way, it was found that even with nutritionally adequate diets, isoenergetic replacement of sucrose or other carbohydrates by ethanol consistently produced a 5- to 10-fold increase in hepatic triglycerides[53–55]. Furthermore, isoenergetic replacement of carbohydrate by fat instead of ethanol did not produce steatosis[53]. With this liquid diet technique, alcohol was also shown to be capable of producing cirrhosis in non-human primates, even when there was an adequate diet[56]. In addition, the hepatotoxicity of ethanol was established by controlled clinical investigations which showed that even in the absence of dietary deficiencies, alcohol can produce fatty liver and ultrastructural lesions in humans[53,54].

Some dietary deficiencies were found to exacerbate the effects of alcohol, whereas judicious supplementations were shown to have beneficial effects. When protein deficiency is present, the deficiency may potentiate the effect of ethanol. In rats, a combination of ethanol and a diet deficient in both protein and lipotropic factors leads to more pronounced hepatic steatosis than with either factor alone[57]. Indeed, protein deficiency impairs lipoprotein secretion, which can be expected to markedly potentiate hepatic lipid accumulation secondary to the direct effects of alcohol resulting from its metabolism in the liver. However, the effect of protein deficiency has not been clearly delineated in human adults. In children, protein deficiency leads to hepatic steatosis, one of the manifestations of kwashiorkor, but this condition does not progress to cirrhosis. In adolescent baboons, protein restriction to 7% of total energy did not result in conspicuous liver injury (even after 19 months) either by biochemical analysis or by light and electron microscopic examination. Significant steatosis was observed only when the protein intake was reduced to 4% of total energy[58]. On the other hand, an excess of protein (25% of total energy or 2.5 times the recommended amount) did not prevent alcohol from producing fat accumulation in human volunteers[59]. Thus, in humans, ethanol is capable of producing striking changes in liver lipids even in the presence of a protein-enriched diet, an effect linked to the metabolism of ethanol.

The hepatocyte contains three main pathways for ethanol metabolism, each located in a different subcellular compartment: (1) the alcohol dehydrogenase (ADH) pathway of the cytosol or the soluble fraction of the cell, (2) the microsomal ethanol oxidizing system located in the endoplasmic reticulum, and (3) catalase located in the peroxisomes[52]. Each of these pathways produces specific metabolic and toxic disturbance and all three result in the production of acetaldehyde, a highly toxic metabolite.

The alcohol dehydrogenase (ADH) pathway and associated metabolic disorders

ADH isozymes

ADH is the liver's major pathway for ethanol disposition. One *raison d'être* of ADH might be to rid the body of the small amounts of alcohol produced by fermentation in the gut[60]. ADH has a broad substrate specificity, which includes dehydrogenation of steroids, oxidation of the intermediary alcohols of the shunt pathway of mevalonate metabolism and ω-oxidation of fatty acids[61]; these processes may act as the physiological substrates for ADH.

Human liver ADH is a zinc metalloenzyme with 5 classes of multiple molecular forms which arise from the association of eight different types of subunits, $\alpha, \beta 1, \beta 2, \beta 3, \gamma 1, \gamma 2$, π and χ, into active dimeric molecules. A genetic model accounts for this multiplicity as products of five gene loci, ADH1 through ADH5[62]. There are three types of subunit, α, β and γ in class I. Polymorphism occurs at two loci, ADH2 and ADH3, which encode the β and γ subunits. Class II isozymes migrate more anodically than class I isozymes and, unlike the latter which generally have low K_m values for ethanol, class II (or π) ADH has a relatively high K_m (34 mM) and a relative insensitivity to 4-methylpyrazole inhibition. Class III (χADH) does not participate in the oxidation of ethanol in the liver because of its very low affinity for that substrate. More recently, a new isoenzyme of ADH has been purified from human stomach, so-called σ- or μ-ADH (Class IV).

Metabolic effects of excessive ADH-mediated hepatic NADH generation

The oxidation of ethanol via the ADH pathway results in the production of acetaldehyde with loss of H which reduces NAD to NADH. The large amounts of reducing equivalents generated overwhelm the hepatocyte's ability to maintain redox homeostasis and a number of metabolic disorders ensue (Fig. 3)[52], including hypoglycaemia and hyperlactacidaemia. The latter contributes to the acidosis and also reduces the capacity of the kidney to excrete uric acid, leading to secondary hyperuricaemia, which is aggravated by the alcohol-induced ketosis and acetate-mediated enhanced ATP breakdown and purine generation[63]. Hyperuricaemia explains, at least in part, the common clinical observation that excessive consumption of alcoholic beverages commonly aggravates or precipitates gouty attacks. The increased NADH also promotes fatty acid synthesis and opposes lipid oxidation with, as a net result, fat accumulation[64].

The effects of ethanol were reproduced in vitro by an alternate NADH generating system (sorbitol–fructose) and were blocked by a H+ acceptor (methylene blue)[64,65]. The preventive effect of methylene blue against ethanol-induced fat accumulation was recently confirmed[66].

Hepatic steatosis and other zonal effects in the liver

One of the earliest pathological manifestations of alcohol abuse is the development of a fatty liver. Fatty acids of different origins can accumulate as triglycerides in the liver because of different metabolic disturbances: decreased hepatic release of lipoproteins, increased mobilization of peripheral fat,

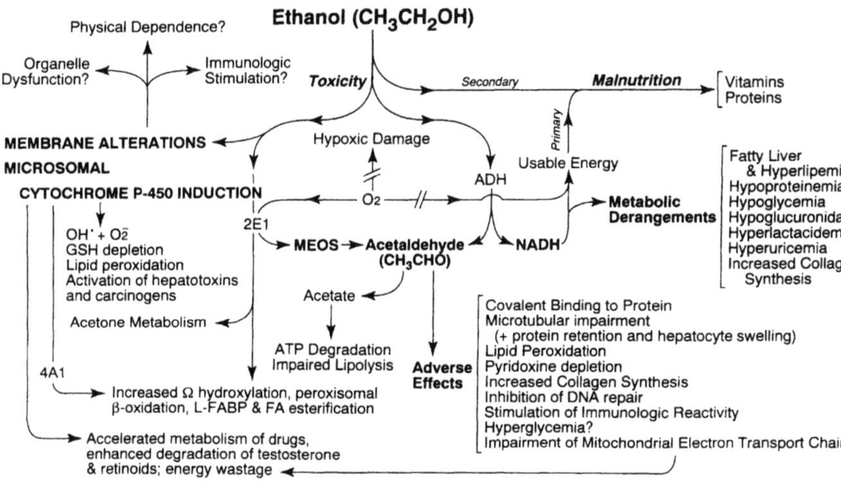

Figure 3 Hepatic, nutritional and metabolic abnormalities after ethanol abuse. Malnutrition, whether primary or secondary, can be differentiated from metabolic changes or direct toxicity, resulting partly from ADH mediated redox changes, or effects secondary to microsomal induction, or acetaldehyde production (from ref. 435).

enhanced hepatic uptake of circulating lipids, enhanced hepatic lipogenesis (*vide supra*) and, most importantly, decreased fatty acid oxidation, whether as a function of the reduced citric acid cycle activity secondary to the altered redox potential (*vide supra*) or as a consequence of permanent changes in mitochondrial structure and functions[4,51,52].

A characteristic feature of liver injury in the alcoholic is the predominance of steatosis and other lesions in the perivenular (also called centrilobular zone or zone 3) of the hepatic acinus. The mechanism for this zonal selectivity of the toxic effects has been postulated to involve a relative lack of oxygen[67]. The low oxygen tensions (normally prevailing in perivenular zones) exaggerate the redox shift produced by ethanol[68]: ethanol increased the lactate/pyruvate ratio and decreased pyruvate more in hepatic venous blood than in total liver. In isolated rat hepatocytes, the ethanol-induced redox shift was markedly exaggerated by lowering the oxygen to a tension similar to those found in centrilobular zones. The process was also assessed in isolated perfused rat livers by varying the oxygen supply to produce the oxygen tensions prevailing in vivo along the sinusoid[69]. Hypoxia increased NADH which in turn inhibited the activity of NAD^+-dependent xanthine dehydrogenase, thereby favouring that of oxygen-dependent xanthine oxidase (XO)[70]. It has been postulated that, due to the acetate derived from ethanol, purine metabolites accumulate and could be metabolized via XO. This process leads to the production of oxygen radicals which may mediate toxic effects towards liver cells, including peroxidation. Physiological substrates for XO, hypoxanthine and xanthine, as well as AMP, significantly increased in the liver after ethanol, together with an enhanced urinary output of allantoin (a final product of xanthine metabolism). Allopurinol pretreatment resulted in 90% inhibition of XO activity, and also significantly decreased ethanol induced lipid peroxidation[70]. Zonal distribution of some enzymes can influence the selective perivenular toxicity. Proliferation of the smooth endoplasmic reticulum after chronic ethanol consumption is maximal in the perivenular zone, with associated microsomal enzyme induction and related effects (*vide infra*). Furthermore, by means of immunohistochemical techniques, human ADH has also been demonstrated to be present mainly in hepatocytes around the terminal hepatic venule[71]. Thus, a presumably higher level of ethanol metabolism in the perivenular zone could contribute to the increased hepatotoxicity of ethanol in that area.

Pathogenic role of ADH polymorphism

Individual differences in the rate of ethanol metabolism may be genetically controlled. Furthermore, genetic factors influence the severity of alcohol-induced liver disease. Indeed, the frequency of an alcohol dehydrogenase 3 allele has been found to differ in patients with alcohol-related end-organ damage (including cirrhosis) and matched controls, suggesting that genetically determined differences in alcohol metabolism may explain differences in the susceptibility to alcohol-related disease (possibly through the enhanced generation of toxic metabolites)[72], but this hypothesis has been questioned[73].

Microsomal ethanol oxidizing system (MEOS)

This new pathway has been the subject of extensive research, reviewed in detail elsewhere[74,75]. The first indication of an interaction of ethanol with the microsomal fraction of the hepatocyte was provided by the morphological observation that alcohol consumption results in a proliferation of the smooth endoplasmic reticulum (SER)[4]. This increase in SER resembles that seen after the administration of a wide variety of hepatotoxins[76], therapeutic agents[77] and some food additives[78]. Since most of the substances that induce a proliferation of the SER are metabolized, at least in part, by the cytochrome P-450 enzyme system that is located on the SER, the possibility that alcohol may also be metabolized by similar enzymes was raised. Such a system was indeed demonstrated in liver microsomes in vitro and found to be inducible by chronic alcohol feeding in vivo[79] and was named the microsomal ethanol oxidizing system (MEOS)[79,80].

That a distinct cytochrome P-450 enzyme system is involved was shown by (a) isolation of a P-450-containing fraction from liver microsomes which, although devoid of any ADH or catalase activity, could still oxidize ethanol as well as higher aliphatic alcohols (e.g. butanol, which is not a substrate for catalase)[81,82] and (b) reconstitution of ethanol-oxidizing activity using NADPH-cytochrome P-450 reductase, phospholipids, and either partially-purified or highly-purified microsomal P-450 from untreated[83] or phenobarbital-treated[84] rats. That chronic ethanol consumption results in the induction of a unique P-450 was also shown by Ohnishi and Lieber[83] using a liver microsomal P-450 fraction isolated from ethanol-treated rats. An ethanol-inducible form of P-450, purified from rabbit liver microsomes[84], catalysed ethanol oxidation at rates much higher than other P-450 isozymes. The purified human protein (now called CYP2E1) was obtained in a catalytically active form, with a high turnover rate for ethanol and other specific substrates[85]. Contrasting with hepatic ADH, which is not inducible in primates as well as most other animal species, a fourfold induction of CYP2E1 was found in biopsies of recently drinking subjects, using the Western blot technique with specific antibodies against this CYP2E1[86], accompanied by a corresponding rise in mRNA[87]. Other cytochromes P-450 (1A2, 3A4) are also involved[88].

The induction of CYP2E1 contributes to the metabolic tolerance to ethanol that develops in chronic and heavy drinkers[89]. In addition to this tolerance to ethanol, alcoholics tend to display tolerance to various other drugs. Indeed, it has been shown that the rate of drug clearance from the blood is enhanced in alcoholics[90,91]. Of course, this could be caused by a variety of factors other than ethanol, such as the congeners and the use of other drugs so commonly associated with alcoholism. Controlled studies showed, however, that administration of pure ethanol with non-deficient diets either to rats or man (under metabolic ward conditions) resulted in a striking increase in the rate of blood clearance of meprobamate and pentobarbital[92] and propranolol[93]. The metabolic tolerance persists several days to weeks after cessation of alcohol abuse, and the duration of recovery varies depending on the drug considered[94]. Similarly, increases in the metabolism of antipyrine[95], tolbutamide[90,91,96], warfarin[91], propranolol[97], diazepam[98] and rifamycin[99] were found. Furthermore, the capacity of liver slices from animals fed ethanol to metabolize drugs such as meprobamate was increased[92], which clearly showed that ethanol consumption affects drug metabolism in the liver itself, independent of changes in drug excretion or distribution or hepatic blood flow.

Experimentally, this effect of chronic ethanol consumption is modulated, in part, by the dietary content in carbohydrates[100], lipids[101], and proteins[102].

It is now recognized that CYP2E1, in addition to its ethanol oxidizing activity, catalyzes fatty acid ω-1 and ω-2 hydroxylations[103–105]. Furthermore, acetone is both an inducer and a substrate of CYP2E1[106–108] (Fig. 4). Excess ketones and fatty acid commonly accompany diabetes and morbid obesity, conditions associated with non-alcoholic steatohepatitis (NASH). Experimentally obese, overfed

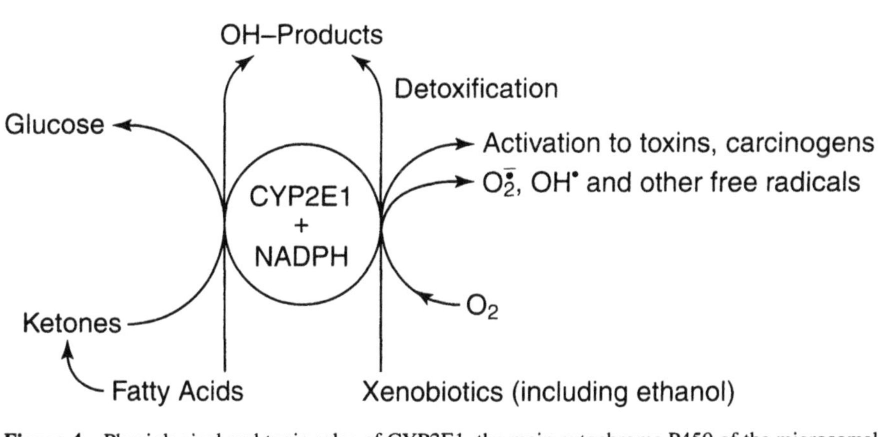

Figure 4 Physiological and toxic roles of CYP2E1, the main cytochrome P450 of the microsomal ethanol oxidizing system (MEOS). Many endogenous and xenobiotic compounds are substrates for CYP2E1 and induce its activity through various mechanisms, resulting in an array of beneficial as well as harmful effects[75].

rats also exhibit substantially higher microsomal ethanol oxidation, acetaminophen activation, and p-nitrophenol hydroxylation (monooxygenase activities catalyzed by CYP2E1)[109]. These diabetic rats are experimental models relevant to NASH, and indeed, the hepatopathology of NASH appears to be due, at least in part, to excess CYP2E1 induction[110].

Clinically, a most important feature of CYP2E1 is not only ethanol oxidation, but also its extraordinary capacity to convert many xenobiotics to highly toxic metabolites, thereby explaining the increased vulnerability of the alcoholic. These agents include *industrial solvents* (e.g., bromobenzene and vinylidene chloride), anaesthetic *agents* (e.g., enflurane[111] and methoxyflurane), commonly used medications (e.g., isoniazid, phenylbutazone), illicit drugs (e.g., cocaine) and over-the-counter analgesics (e.g., acetaminophen)[112], all of which are substrates for, and/or inducers of, CYP2E1. The effects of acetaminophen, ethanol, and fasting are synergistic[113], because all three deplete the level of reduced glutathione, a scavenger of toxic free radicals. Rats fed ethanol chronically have increased rates of GSH turnover[114] and ethanol produces an enhanced loss from the liver[115]. The selective loss of the compound from liver mitochondria[116] contributes to the striking alcohol-induced oxidant stress and impairment of this organelle.

CYP2E1 also generates several species of active oxygen (Figs 3, 4) which, in concert with a decrease in the level of GSH, promote injury by inactivation of enzymes and peroxidation of lipids. In patients with cirrhosis, hepatic depletion of α-tocopherol[117], a major antioxidant, potentiates this effect. GSH offers one of the mechanisms for the scavenging of toxic free radicals. Replenishment of GSH can be achieved by administration of precursors of cysteine (one of the amino acids of this tripeptide) such as acetylcysteine or S-adenosyl-L-methionine (SAMe)[118,119]. Experimentally, CYP2E1 has also been down-regulated by PPC[120], a potentially beneficial therapeutic approach.

Nutritional status of alcoholics

Overall assessment

Alcoholics hospitalized for medical complications of alcohol intoxication (such as states of acute intoxication and withdrawal) have the most severe malnutrition. These alcoholics have inadequate dietary protein[121], signs of protein malnutrition[122,123] and anthropomorphic measurements indicative of impaired nutrition: their height-to-weight ratio is lower[124], muscle mass estimated by the creatinine-height index is reduced[123,124] and triceps skin folds are thinner[123–125]. Continued drinking results in weight loss, whereas abstinence results in weight gain[126,127] in patients with and without liver disease[126].

Many patients who drink to excess are either not malnourished or are less malnourished than the hospitalized group. Women drinking one or more drinks per day weigh on average 2.3 kg less than nondrinkers, and they and their male counterparts continued on a more stable weight over the next ten years than the nondrinkers whose weight rose[127]. Other surveys, however, found that alcohol intake, especially when accompanied by high fat intake and sedentary behavior[128] favors truncal obesity, particularly in women[129]. Those with moderate alcohol intake[130], even those admitted to hospital for alcohol rehabilitation rather than for medical problems[131], often hardly differ nutritionally from controls (matched for socioeconomic status and health history), except that females have a lower level of thiamin excretion than control patients following a thiamin load test[131].

The wide range in nutritional status of our alcoholic population surely reflects, in part, differences in what they eat. Moderate alcohol intake with alcohol accounting for 16% of total calories (alcohol included) is associated with slightly increased total energy intake[132].

Although ethanol is rich in energy (7.1 cal/g), chronic consumption does not produce the expected gain in body weight[133]. This energy deficit can be attributed, in part, to damaged mitochondria and the resulting poor coupling of oxidation of fat with energy production, as well as to microsomal pathways that oxidize ethanol without conserving chemical energy (Fig. 3). Thus, perhaps because of these energy considerations, this group with higher total caloric intake has no weight gain despite physical activity levels comparable to those of the non-alcohol consuming population. This level of alcohol intake, and even slightly higher levels (23%)[134], is associated with a substitution of alcohol for carbohydrate in the diet. In those individuals consuming more than 30% of total calories as alcohol, significant decreases in protein and fat intake occur too, and the consumption of vitamins A, C, and thiamin may descend below the recommended daily allowances[132]. Calcium, iron, and fibre intake are also lowered[134].

The mechanisms underlying the altered pattern of food intake are under debate. Suppression of appetite has been postulated[135]. Depressed consciousness during inebriation, hangover, and gastroduodenitis due to ethanol, partly explain the decreased food intake. The contribution of subtle nutritional alterations produced by ethanol to the pathogenesis of ethanol-induced or other disease states, including alcoholism, is largely unchartered.

Specific nutrients

The vitamin C status of alcoholic patients admitted to a hospital is lower than that of non-alcoholics as measured by serum ascorbic acid, peripheral leukocyte ascorbic acid, or urinary ascorbic acid after an oral challenge[136]. In addition to a lower mean ascorbic acid level, some 25% of patients with Laennec's cirrhosis had serum ascorbic acid levels below the range of healthy controls[136]. Ascorbic acid status is low in alcoholic patients with and without liver disease. When alcohol intake exceeds 30% of total calories, vitamin C generally falls below recommended dietary allowances[137]. The clinical significance is unknown for patients who have low ascorbic acid levels but who are not clearly scorbutic.

Alcoholics have illness related to abnormalities of calcium, phosphorus, and vitamin D homeostasis. They have decreases in bone density[138] and bone mass[139], increased susceptibility to fractures[140] and increased osteonecrosis[141]. Low blood calcium, phosphorus, magnesium, and low, normal, or high vitamin D_3 levels have been reported, indicating disturbed calcium metabolism[139]. In patients with alcoholic liver disease, vitamin D deficiency probably derives from too little vitamin D substrate, which results from poor dietary intake, malabsorption due to cholestasis or pancreatic insufficiency, and insufficient sunlight.

Vitamin K deficiency in alcoholism may arise when there is an interruption of fat absorption due to pancreatic insufficiency, biliary obstruction, or intestinal mucosal abnormality secondary to folic acid deficiency. Dietary vitamin K inadequacy is not a likely cause of clinical deficiency unless there is concomitant sterilization of the large gut, a reliable source of the vitamin.

Alcoholics tend to have low folic acid status when they are drinking heavily and their folic acid intake is reduced. For example, a group of unselected alcoholics showed a 37.5% incidence of low serum folate levels and a 17.6% incidence of low red blood cell folate levels[126].

In pigs fed ethanol for 11 months, folic acid absorption was normal, but jejunal folate hydrolase, an early enzyme of folate polyglutamate breakdown, was decreased[142,143]. In vitro preparations of rat intestine absorb folate less well when exposed to a variety of alcohols[144]. Malnourished alcoholics without liver disease also absorb folic acid less well compared to their better-nourished counterparts[145]. Folic acid absorption, usually increased by partial starvation, is less increased in rats when alcohol is ingested[146]. It has not been clearly shown, however, that either protein deficiency or alcohol[141,146] decrease folate absorption in vivo. Thus, it is still unclear what aspects of malnutrition adversely affect folate absorption and under what clinical circumstances alcohol may interfere with folate absorption.

Alcohol accelerates the production of megaloblastic anemia in patients with depleted folate stores[147] and suppresses the hematologic response to folic acid in folic acid-depleted patients[148]. Alcohol also has other effects on folate metabolism but their significance is not clear: alcohol given acutely causes a decrease in serum folate, which is partly explained by increased urinary excretion[149]; alcohol administered chronically to monkeys decreased hepatic folate levels, partly because of the inability of the liver to retain folate[150], and perhaps partly because of increased urinary and faecal losses[151].

Alcoholics do not commonly develop vitamin B_{12} deficiency[152]. Their serum levels are usually normal even when they are deficient in folate, whether they have cirrhosis[153,154] or not[145,146]. This is probably due to large body stores of vitamin B_{12}. Pancreatic insufficiency, however, results in decreased vitamin B_{12} absorption as measured by the Schilling test. In this circumstance there is insufficient luminal protease activity and alkalinity, which normally serve to release vitamin B_{12} from the 'r' protein that is secreted by salivary glands, intestines, and possibly the stomach[155]. Alcohol ingestion has also been shown to decrease vitamin B_{12} absorption in volunteers after several weeks of intake[156]. The alcohol effect may be in the ileum because co-administration of intrinsic factor or pancreatin does not correct the Schilling test results. It had been suggested but not proven that the binding of intrinsic factor-vitamin B_{12} complex to ileal sites is abnormal[157,158].

When there is a general lack of B vitamin intake, riboflavin deficiency may be encountered[159]. In one study, deficiency was found in 50% of a small group of patients with medical complications severe enough to warrant hospital admission[160]. Although none of the patients exhibited classic signs of riboflavin deficiency, they had an abnormal activity coefficient (AC) that returned to normal 2–7 days after intramuscular replacement with 5 mg riboflavin daily. Activity coefficient is measured as the ratio of erythrocyte glutathione reductase activity upon addition of flavin adenine dinucleotide to the activity with no additions. Riboflavin deficiency could be induced readily by alcohol feeding to the Syrian hamster; the most severe deficiency was seen in animals also restricted in riboflavin intake[161]. Riboflavin and pyridoxine storage in the liver is adversely affected by alcohol, at least in experimental animals.

Vitamin E deficiency is not a recognized complication of alcoholism, although patients with chronic alcoholic pancreatitis have a lower vitamin E to total plasma lipid ratio[162].

When rodents were fed ethanol repeatedly in one study, their hepatic vitamin E levels, measured as α-tocopherol, were low[163]; this was accompanied by increased hepatic lipid peroxidation when alcohol was combined with a low-vitamin E diet[164]. The mechanism of hepatic vitamin E depletion by ethanol is probably enhanced oxidation of α-tocopherol to α-tocopherol quinone in liver microsomes[164]. Alcohol-induced liver injury may be mediated, in part, by stress on cellular antioxidant mechanisms interrelated with vitamin E and selenium. Considering the findings in humans with fat malabsorption or severe cholestasis, and the evidence of vitamin E depletion by chronic alcohol feeding of experimental animals, it would seem that there is great potential for vitamin E deficiency in chronic alcoholics who combine low vitamin E intake with steatorrhea from chronic pancreatitis or prolonged cholestasis, or who have low E because of cirrhosis (*vide infra*).

Acute doses of ethanol cause magnesium loss in the urine[165] and alcoholism is associated with magnesium deficiency[166]. Alcoholics have low blood magnesium and low body exchangeable magnesium; symptoms in alcoholics resemble those in patients with magnesium deficiency of other causes; upon withdrawal from alcohol, magnesium balance is positive. Hypocalcaemia in alcoholics in the setting of magnesium deficiency has been ascribed, in part, to impaired parathyroid hormone (PTH) secretion as well as renal and skeletal resistance to PTH[167], and the hypocalcaemia may only be responsive to magnesium repletion. Hospitalized alcoholics with normal serum total magnesium had significantly lower serum ionized magnesium[168].

There may be either deficiency or excess of iron in the body. Alcoholics may be iron-deficient as a result of the several gastrointestinal lesions to which they are prone and that may bleed. Hepatic iron content was found to be increased in autopsy studies of most patients with early alcoholic cirrhosis[169]. In most alcoholics however, the iron content of the liver is normal or only modestly elevated, although there may be stainable iron in reticuloendothelial cells, possibly because of bouts of haemolysis. It is unclear whether increased intestinal absorption of iron because of alcohol[170] or hepatic uptake of iron from serum in established alcoholic liver disease[171] contributes significantly to increased hepatic iron levels. There is usually little difficulty in distinguishing the hepatic iron increases of alcoholic liver disease from the much higher amounts characteristic of genetic haemochromatosis, using a measure of absolute iron content/gr liver with upward adjustments for age[172]. The contribution hepatic iron may make to liver damage via its role in lipid peroxidation[173] (in conjunction with the effects of alcohol) and its possible role in promoting fibrogenesis[174] are of great potential significance.

Patients have low plasma zinc[175], low liver zinc[176], and increased urinary zinc levels[176,177]. Acute ethanol ingestion, however, does not cause zincuria[178]. The low zinc content of chronic alcoholics with cirrhosis is attributed to decreased intake and absorption as well as increased urinary excretion. Many Americans have a diet marginal in zinc[179]. Alcoholics fall into several of those groups with marginal intake. It is interesting that zinc absorption has been shown to be low in alcoholic cirrhotics but not in patients with cirrhosis of other causes[180], although cirrhosis of varied aetiologies is characterized by low serum zinc[181]. Currently, the therapeutic use of zinc in alcoholism is restricted to the treatment of night blindness not responsive to vitamin A.

Hepatic copper content is increased in advanced alcoholic cirrhosis[169]. Serum copper content has been reported to be elevated in alcoholics independent of the stage of liver disease[182], but others have reported normal levels[183].

Nickel levels are consistently high in alcoholic liver disease; manganese and chromium are unchanged[169]. Intracellular shifts in trace metals have been described upon acute administration of alcohol[184]. Versieck et al. reported increased serum molybdenum in patients with acute liver disease[185]; increased levels were not seen in those patients with cirrhosis. The clinical significance of trace metal changes is still obscure, except for the cardiotoxicity ascribed to alcoholic beverages with high cobalt content.

Effects of ethanol on digestion and absorption

Diarrhoea frequently occurs in alcoholics. In the heavy drinker, diarrhoea may occur for a variety of reasons, including ethanol-exacerbated lactase deficiency, especially in Blacks[186]. Another major complication is alcoholic pancreatitis.

Intestinal malabsorption may also be secondary to folic acid deficiency (*vide supra*).

Steatorrhoea is commonly due to folic acid deficiency and luminal bile salt deficiency. Intraluminal bile salts are decreased by acute ethanol administration[187]. In rodents, long-term ethanol administration delays the half-time excretion of cholic and chenodeoxycholic acids by decreasing the daily excretion and expanding the pool size slightly[188]. Alcoholic cirrhotic patients may have bile low in deoxycholic acid, possibly due to impaired conversion of cholate to deoxycholate by bacteria[189].

Hospitalized alcoholics were reported to have impaired thiamine absorption compared to control patients when tested by radioactive thiamine excretion[190], a test also affected by steps not related to absorption. However, folic acid deficiency was not adequately excluded as a cause of thiamine malabsorption in these studies. Refined testing revealed reduced thiamine absorption due to alcohol in a minority of subjects[191]. Jejunal perfusion studies did not show an effect of 5% alcohol on thiamine absorption in man[192]. Thus, whereas human thiamine absorption may not be affected by alcohol, it is clearly impaired in rodents. Alcohol also interferes with riboflavin absorption in rodents, but this has not been studied in humans. Alcohol impairs folic acid absorption in malnourished humans, but the mechanism is unclear (*vide supra*).

Effect of alcohol on nutrient activation

Thiamine and pyridoxine

Thiamine deficiency in alcoholics causes Wernicke–Korsakoff syndrome and beriberi heart disease, and probably contributes to polyneuropathy. There has been no confirmation of an inborn error of transketolase affinity for its co-factor thiamine pyrophosphate in Wernicke–Korsakoff syndrome as was once claimed.

Neurological, haematological, and dermatological disorders can be caused in part by pyridoxine deficiency. Pyridoxine deficiency, as measured by low plasma pyridoxal-5′-phosphate (PLP), was reported in over 50% of alcoholics without hematologic findings or abnormal liver function tests[193,194]. Inadequate intake may partly explain low PLP, but increased destruction and reduced formation may also contribute. PLP is more rapidly destroyed in erythrocytes in the presence of acetaldehyde, the product of ethanol oxidation, perhaps by displacement of PLP from protein and consequent exposure to phosphatase[193,195]. Studies showed that chronic ethanol feeding lowered hepatic content of PLP by decreasing net synthesis from pyridoxine[196–198]. The acetaldehyde produced on alcohol oxidation was thought to enhance hydrolysis of PLP by cellular phosphatases[193].

Methionine and S-adenosylmethionine (SAMe)

Methionine deficiency has been described and its supplementation has been considered for the treatment of liver diseases, especially the alcoholic variety, but excess methionine was shown to have some adverse effects[199], including a decrease in hepatic ATP[200]. Furthermore, whereas in some patients with alcoholic liver disease, circulating methionine levels are normal[201], in others elevated levels were observed[202–204]. Kinsell et al.[205] found a delay in the

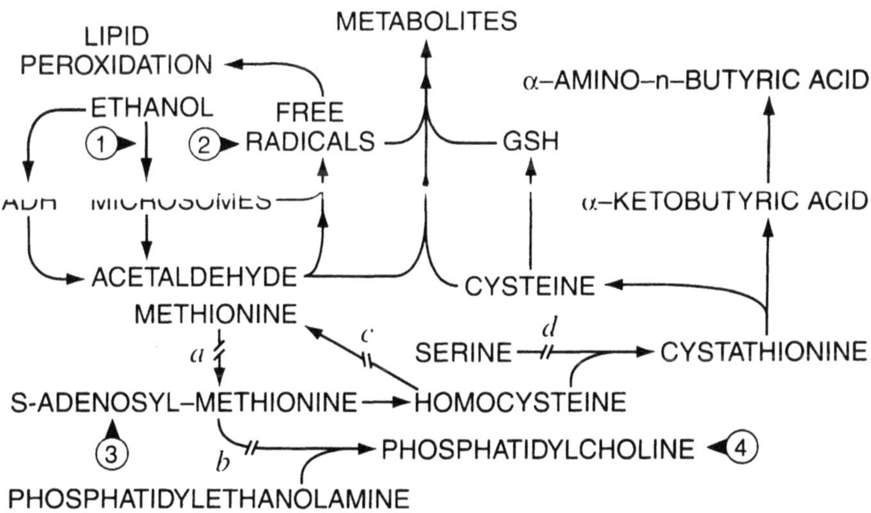

Figure 5 Lipid peroxidation and other consequences of alcoholic liver disease and/or increased free radical generation and acetaldehyde production by ethanol-induced microsomes, with sites of possible therapeutic interventions. Metabolic blocks caused by liver disease (a,b), folate (c), B_{12} (c) or B_6 (d) deficiencies are illustrated, with corresponding depletions in S-adenosylmethionine, phosphatidylcholine and glutathione (GSH). New therapeutic approaches include (1) down-regulation of microsomal enzyme induction especially of CYP2E1, (2) decrease of free radicals, with antioxidants (3) replenishment of S-adenosylmethionine and of (4) phosphatidylcholine[348].

clearance of plasma methionine after its systemic administration to patients with liver damage. Similarly, Horowitz et al.[206] reported that the blood clearance of methionine after an oral load of this amino acid was slowed. Since about half the methionine is metabolized by the liver, these observations suggested impaired hepatic metabolism of this amino acid in patients with alcoholic liver disease. Indeed, for most of its functions, methionine must be activated to S-adenosylmethionine (SAMe) and in cirrhotic livers, Duce et al.[207] reported a decrease in the activity of SAMe synthetase, the enzyme involved, also called methionine adenosyltransferase (Fig. 5).

Various mechanisms of inactivation of SAMe synthetase have been reviewed recently[208]. One factor that may have contributed to the defect is relative hypoxia, with nitric oxide mediated inactivation and transcriptional arrest[209]. In addition, long-term alcohol consumption was found to be associated with enhanced methionine utilization and depletion[210]. As a consequence, SAMe depletion as well as its decreased availability could be expected and, indeed, long term ethanol consumption under controlled conditions by non-human primates was associated with a significant depletion of hepatic SAMe[118]. Potentially, such SAMe depletion may have a number of adverse effects. SAMe is the principal methylating agent in various transmethylation reactions which are important to nucleic acid and protein synthesis. Hirata and Axelrod[211] and Hirata et al.[212] also demonstrated the importance of methylation to cell membrane function with regard to membrane fluidity and the transport of metabolites and transmission of signals across membranes. Thus, depletion of SAMe, by impairing methyltransferase activity, may promote the membrane injury which has been documented in alcohol-induced liver damage[213]. Furthermore, SAMe plays a key role in the synthesis of polyamines and provides a source of cysteine for glutathione production (Fig. 5). Thus, the deficiency in methionine activation and in SAMe production resulting from the decrease in the activity of the corresponding synthetase results in a number of adverse effects, including inadequate cysteine and GSH production, especially when aggravated by associated folate, B_6 or B_{12} deficiencies (Fig. 5). The consequences of this enzymic defect can be alleviated by providing SAMe, the product of the reaction. SAMe is unstable, but the synthesis of a stable salt allowed for replenishment of SAMe through ingestion of this compound: blood levels of SAMe increased after oral administration in rodents[214] and in man[215]. Although it has been claimed that the liver does not take up SAMe from the bloodstream[216], other results indicated uptake of SAMe by isolated hepatocytes either at pharmacological[217] or at physiological[218,219] extracellular levels. Results in baboons[118] also clearly showed hepatic uptake of exogenous SAMe in vivo. The effective use of SAMe for transmethylation and trans-sulfuration has been demonstrated in vivo[220].

Clinical trials revealed that SAMe treatment is beneficial in intrahepatic cholestasis[221], including recurrent intrahepatic cholestasis and jaundice caused by androgens or oestrogens. Given either orally or parenterally, SAMe improved both the pruritus and the biochemical parameters of cholestasis such as serum bilirubin, alkaline phosphatase and γ-glutamyl transferase. It was also used successfully in severe cholestasis of pregnancy[222] with few, if any, untoward effects. Especially noteworthy is a prospective, multicenter, double-blind, placebo-controlled trial[223] performed in 220 inpatients with chronic liver disease (chronic active hepatitis and cirrhosis, including primary biliary cirrhosis) in whom serum markers of cholestasis and subjective symptoms significantly improved after SAMe. Oral administration of 1200 mg/day SAMe for 6 months also resulted in a significant increase of hepatic GSH in patients with alcoholic as well as non-alcoholic liver disease[224].

The most impressive therapeutic success was achieved in a recent long-term randomized, placebo-controlled, double-blind, multicenter clinical trial of SAMe in patients with alcoholic liver cirrhosis in whom SAMe improved survival or delayed liver transplantation[225]. One-hundred and twenty-three patients with Child class A, B, or C cirrhosis were studied for 2 years. The overall mortality or liver transplantation at the end of the trial was 30% in the placebo group and only 16% in the SAMe group, but the difference was not statistically significant ($p = 0.077$). However, when patients in Child C class where excluded, the overall mortality/liver transplantation was significantly greater in the placebo group (29% vs. 12%, $P = 0.025$), and differences between both groups in the 2-year survival curves were also significant. A compliance rate of greater than 75% in about 68 or 69% of patients was achieved, which is remarkable indeed considering the nature of the population studied. An additional positive feature of this study is the confirmation of a virtually total lack of side effects of SAMe. Thus, despite a relatively modest number of subjects, the study of Mato et al.[225] provides the first clinical demonstration of such a significant successful therapy of alcoholic cirrhosis in man.

Phosphatidylcholine (PC)

In the presence of liver disease, the activity of phosphatidylethanolamine methyltransferase is depressed[207], with significant pathologic effects. This enzymatic block can again be bypassed through the administration of the product of that reaction, in this case phosphatidylcholine (PC)[13] (Fig. 5). This is emerging as potentially important approach to the treatment of liver disease. Characteristic features of alcoholic liver injury include scarring or fibrosis and striking membrane alterations with associated phospholipid changes[52]. In an attempt to offset some of these abnormalities, polyunsaturated lecithin (extracted from soybeans) was fed to baboons given ethanol for up to 8 years[12]. Whereas fibrosis or cirrhosis ensued in most of the baboons fed the diet with ethanol alone, no cirrhosis or septal fibrosis developed in the animals fed ethanol with the lecithin. The soybean lecithin extract used was rich in polyunsaturated phospholipids, with 55–60% phosphatidylcholine (PC). To assess whether PC was the active agent, a more purified extract was fed comprising 94–96% PC. The feeding of this mixture rich in polyunsaturated PCs (PPC), especially dilinoleoylphosphatidylcholine (DLPC), which has a high bioavailability, exerted a remarkable protection against alcohol-induced fibrosis and cirrhosis[226] (Fig. 6).

PPC contains choline, but choline, in amounts present in PPC, had no protective action against the fibrogenic effects of ethanol in the baboon[227]. In primates in general, choline plays a lesser role as a dietary nutrient than in rodents, because of lesser choline oxidase activity. In fact, as reviewed elsewhere[228], choline becomes essential for human nutrition only in severely restricted feeding situations.

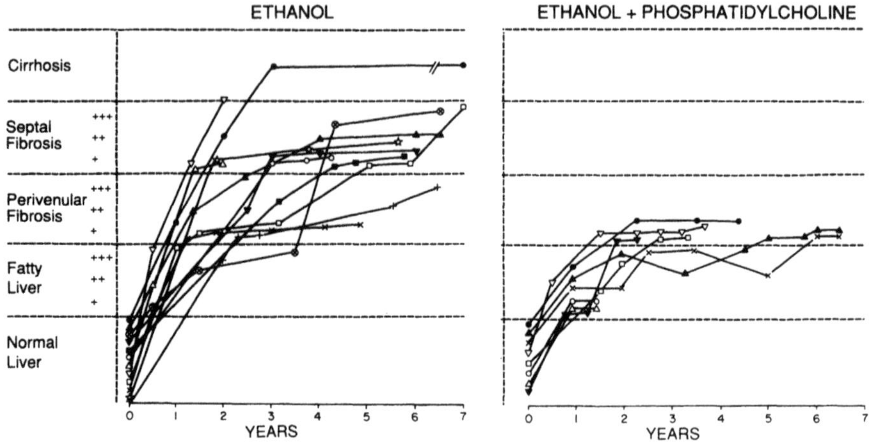

Figure 6 Sequential development of alcoholic liver injury in baboons fed ethanol with an adequate diet (left panel) and prevention of septal fibrosis and cirrhosis by supplementation with phenyl-phosphatidylcholine (PPC) (right panel). Liver morphology in animals pair-fed control diets (with or without PPC) remained normal (not shown) (data from Ref. 226).

PPC is rich in linoleic acid, but this fatty acid *per se* is probably not responsible for the protective effect because the basic diet was supplemented with linoleate and contained large amounts of corn oil which is rich in linoleic acid. Furthermore, this fatty acid has been incriminated as a permissive rather than as a protective factor in alcoholic liver injury[229]. Thus the polyunsaturated phospholipids themselves appear to be responsible for protection, perhaps because of their high bioavailability and selective incorporation into liver membranes[230], where they may act as a 'sink' for free radicals, thereby attenuating their adverse effects (*vide infra*) and when they may also be required for the optimal functions of key enzymes (*vide infra*).

In baboons given ethanol that developed significant fibrosis, type I procollagen mRNA content was significantly enhanced[231]. The number of stellate cells was also found to increase strikingly in alcohol-fed baboons, contributing to the progression of fibrosis[16]. PPC not only corrected the ethanol-induced PC depletion, but it also totally prevented the associated septal fibrosis and cirrhosis in baboons fed adequate diets[226], with an associated reduction in the number of activated stellate cells. A similar transformation of the stellate cells was observed in patients with alcoholic liver disease[15]. More recently, an attenuation of the transformation of stellate cells to myofibroblast-like cells was also observed in vitro[232]. In addition, the activity of membrane-bound enzymes was normalized: cytochrome C oxidase, a key enzyme of the mitochondrial electron-transport chain, which requires a normal phospholipid milieu for optimal activity and is severely depressed by chronic ethanol consumption[233], was restored to normal by addition of PC in vitro[234] or by PPC supplementation in vivo[235] with improvement of hepatic mitochondrial respiration, assessed by the respiratory control (determined by the ratio between the ADP-stimulated and nonstimulated O_2 consumption), with glutamate, succinate or palmitoyl-1-carnitine used as substrates.

The decreased phospholipid methyltransferase activity (Fig. 5), described in cirrhotic livers[207], is not simply secondary to the cirrhosis, but may in fact be a primary defect related to alcohol, as suggested by the observation that the enzyme activity is already decreased prior to the development of cirrhosis[13].

Another mechanism whereby ethanol may affect phospholipids is via formation of phosphatidylethanol, with possible impact on signal transduction, as shown in isolated rat hepatocytes[236]. A third mechanism is increased lipid peroxidation, as reflected by increased F_2-isoprostanes[227] which could explain the associated decrease of arachidonic acid in phospholipids[234]. However, beneficial effects of PPC were not limited to a correction of oxidative stress. Indeed, in an experimental model devoid of oxidative stress, namely fibrosis and cirrhosis induced by the injection of heterologous albumin in rats, PPC was nevertheless protective[237]. This may reflect, at least in part, the fact that both PPC[238] and DLPC[226] stimulate collagenase production in stellate cells, resulting in a decrease of collagen accumulation.

One concern was that PPC and DLPC, because of their polyunsaturated nature, may aggravate the oxidative stress, but the opposite was found, both in vitro and in vivo. In alcohol-fed baboons, PPC not only prevented septal fibrosis and cirrhosis[226], but it also resulted in a total protection against oxidative stress, as determined by normalization of 4-hydroxynonenal, F_2-isoprostanes and GSH levels[239].

In patients with hepatitis C, PPC improved the transaminase levels but the effect on liver fibrosis was not assessed[240]. However, a clinical trial on alcoholic fibrosis is presently ongoing in the USA.

Toxic interaction of alcohol with nutrients

Adverse interaction with retinol

In addition to the classic aspects of vitamin A deficiency due to either poor dietary intake or severe liver disease, direct effects of alcohol on vitamin A metabolism, and resulting alterations in hepatic vitamin A levels, have been elucidated[241].

Depletion of hepatic vitamin A by ethanol, its mechanism and pathological consequences Alcoholic liver disease is associated with severely decreased hepatic vitamin A levels (Fig. 7), even when liver injury is moderate (fatty liver) and when blood values of vitamin A, RBP and prealbumin are still unaffected[243]. It is noteworthy that serum RBP, which has been considered as a good index of vitamin A deficiency and more sensitive even than dark adaptation[242] was in fact still normal in these subjects with alcoholic fatty liver.

Malnutrition, when present, can of course contribute to hepatic vitamin A depletion but the patients with low liver vitamin A in the study of Leo and Lieber[243] appeared well nourished, which suggested a more direct effect of alcohol. Under strictly controlled conditions, chronic ethanol consumption was found to decrease hepatic vitamin A in baboons pair-fed a nutritionally adequate liquid diet containing 50% of total energy either as ethanol or isocaloric carbohydrate. In these baboons, fatty liver developed after 4 months of ethanol

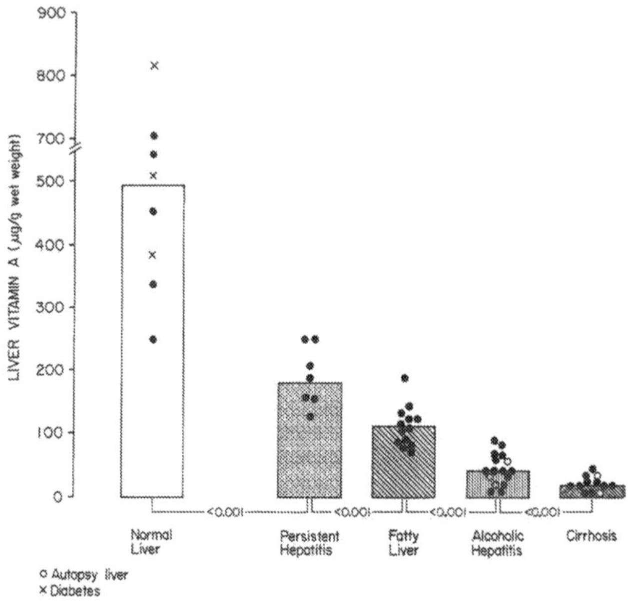

Figure 7 Hepatic vitamin A levels in subjects with normal livers, chronic persistent hepatitis, and various stages of alcoholic injury (data from Ref. 243).

feeding, with a 59% decrease in hepatic vitamin A levels, and fibrosis or cirrhosis appeared after 24–84 months with a 95% decrease in hepatic vitamin A concentrations[112]. Similarly, hepatic vitamin A levels of rats fed ethanol (36% of total energy) were decreased after 3 weeks (by 42%) and continued to decline up to 9 weeks. In contrast, serum vitamin A and RBP levels were not significantly changed. When dietary vitamin A was increased 5-fold, hepatic vitamin A nevertheless decreased in ethanol-fed rats relative to the corresponding controls, and sometimes even compared to the rats given five times less vitamin A (without ethanol)[112]. To avoid the confounding effect of dietary vitamin A, it was virtually eliminated in some experiments. Under those conditions, the depletion rate of vitamin A from endogenous hepatic storage was 2.5 times faster in ethanol-fed rats than in controls.

When dietary vitamin A intake was virtually eliminated, the difference in hepatic storage between ethanol-fed rats and controls was much greater than could be accounted for by the total vitamin A intake. Thus, malabsorption was not the only reason for the depletion of hepatic vitamin A. Two possible mechanisms other than malabsorption can be invoked: increased mobilization of vitamin A from the liver, and enhanced catabolism of vitamin A in the liver or in other organs. There is experimental evidence for both[244,245].

The various pathways involved in hepatic vitamin A metabolism are shown schematically in Fig. 8 and have been reviewed recently[246]. Drugs that induce the cytochromes P-450 in liver microsomes were shown to result in a depletion of hepatic vitamin A[247]. A similar effect was observed after administration of

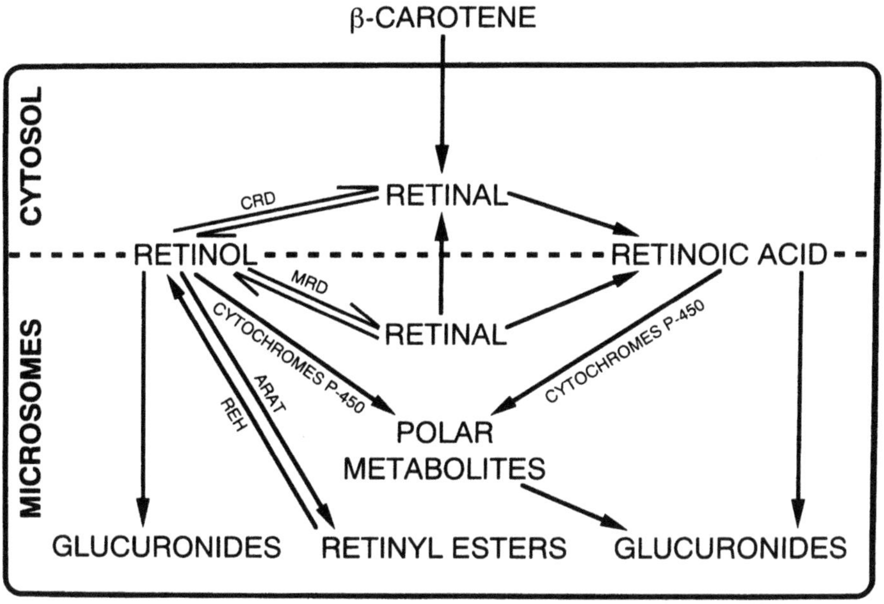

Figure 8 Simplified schematic representation of the putative role of cytosolic and microsomal systems in the hepatic metabolism of retinol. CRD: cytosolic retinol dehydrogenase; MRD: microsomal retinol dehydrogenase; ARAT: acyl CoA retinol acyltransferase; REH: retinyl esters hydrolase (from Ref. 241).

ethanol[112,243] and other xenobiotics that are known to interact with liver microsomes, including carcinogens[248]. The hepatic depletion was strikingly exacerbated when ethanol and drugs were combined[249], which mimicks a common clinical occurrence.

Retinoic acid has been shown to be degraded in microsomes of either hamsters[250] or rats[245,251]. In both species, the reported activity was very low compared to the degree of hepatic vitamin A depletion. These observations prompted the search for alternate pathways of retinol metabolism and two new pathways of retinol metabolism in liver microsomes were described: rat liver microsomes, when fortified with NADPH, converted retinol to polar metabolites, including 4-hydroxyretinol[252]. This activity was also demonstrated in a reconstituted monooxygenase system containing purified forms of rat cytochromes P-450[252], including P-4502B1 (a phenobarbital-inducible isozyme). More recently, it has been shown that other cytochromes (such as P-450 CYP 1A1) also catalyse the conversion of retinal to retinoic acid[253]. In addition, a new microsomal NAD^+-dependent retinol dehydrogenase was described (Fig. 8)[254]. The classic pathway for the conversion of retinol to retinal in the liver involves a cytosolic NAD-dependent retinol dehydrogenase (CRD), believed to be similar, if not identical, to the liver cytosolic alcohol dehydrogenase (ADH, alcohol: NAD^- oxidoreductase, EC 1.1.1.1)[255,256]. The observation that a strain of deermice lacks this enzyme without apparent adverse effects[257] prompted a search for an alternate pathway for the production of retinal, the precursor of retinoic acid. Evidence was obtained for the existence of an NAD-dependent microsomal retinol dehydrogenase (MRD)[254] which can convert retinol to retinal using NAD, and retinal to retinol using NADH as co-factors. The activity of the retinol[254a] as well as of the retinal[254b] dehydrogenases is inducible by chronic alcohol consumption, thereby contributing to hepatic vitamin A depletion. Finally, metabolism of retinol and retinoic acid was also demonstrated with human liver microsomes and purified cytochrome P-4502C8[258].

In patients with severe as well as moderate depletion of hepatic vitamin A, multivesicular lysosome-like organelles were detected in increased numbers[259]. That a low hepatic vitamin A concentration contributes to these lesions was also verified experimentally in rats[260].

Hepatic vitamin A depletion plays a key role in hepatic fibrosis, and both hepatocytes and stellate cells are involved. Hepatic stellate cells are the principal storage site of vitamin A. The activation of stellate cells into myofibroblast-like cells, which then synthesize collagen, is associated with a decrease in vitamin A storage in these cells[261]. Retinoic acid, and to a lesser extent retinol, were shown to reduce stellate cell proliferation and collagen production in culture[261–263]. Conversely, lack of retinoids could promote fibrosis in these tissues, especially in the liver, consistent with the associated activation of stellate cells[261]. Paradoxically, however, vitamin A excess may also promote fibrosis (*vide infra*).

A place for vitamin A in both cancer therapy and prevention has been proposed[262]. Indeed, increasing evidence for a role of vitamin A in the proliferation and differentiation of a variety of human cells makes it apparent that reduction in vitamin A levels may be significant in the development of tumors. In fact, vitamin A deficiency has been associated with the formation of various types of tumors[263]. Epidemiological studies in the UK[264–266] and in the USA[267] revealed an increased risk of bronchogenic carcinoma in association with low serum vitamin A levels and, in experimental animals, deficiency of vitamin A is known to lead to the development of squamous metaplasia. Such changes in the respiratory epithelium are frequently found to precede, or to be associated with, tumour development[268–278].

Concomitant ethanol consumption and vitamin A deficiency resulted in an increased severity of squamous metaplasia of the trachea[16,279]. This potentiation of vitamin A deficiency by alcohol may predispose the tracheal epithelium to neoplastic transformation.

A relatively high risk of squamous cell carcinoma of the lung was found in a Norwegian population that drank large amounts of alcohol and had a low dietary intake of vitamin A[280]. Furthermore, a positive association of alcohol consumption with lung cancer has been reported in Japanese men in Hawaii[281]. In addition, ethanol-induced vitamin A depletion is associated with decreased detoxification of xenobiotics, including carcinogens such as nitrosodimethylamine[282], thereby playing a role in chemical carcinogenesis (*vide supra*). Recent data also suggest that functional down-regulation of retinoic acid receptors, by inhibiting biosynthesis of retinoic acid and up-regulating activator protein-1 (c-Jun and c-Fos) gene expression, may be important mechanisms for causing malignant transformation by ethanol[283].

In addition to promoting vitamin A depletion, ethanol may interfere more directly with retinoic acid synthesis since both were shown in vitro to serve as substrates for the same enzymes[284]. Specifically, one of the mechanisms by which ethanol induces gastrointestinal cancer may be an inhibition of ADH-catalysed gastrointestinal retinoic acid synthesis which is needed for epithelial differentiation. Indeed, class I ADH (ADH-I) and class IV ADH (ADH-IV) function as retinol dehydrogenases in vitro are abundantly distributed along the GI tract[285]. Deficiency of retinoic acids can produce birth defects and, as discussed before, ethanol promotes deficiency of retinoids. Duester[284,286] and Pullarkat[287] implicated competitive inhibition, by ethanol, of the biosynthesis of retinoic acid from retinol since class I alcohol dehydrogenase (E.C. 1.1.1.1) can contribute to the biosynthesis of retinoic acid from retinol. Indeed, this group identified one human ADH isozyme that exists in the affected embryonic tissues to act as a retinol dehydrogenase catalysing the synthesis of retinoic acid. Ethanol did, in fact, reduce retinoic acid levels in cultured mouse embryos[288]. However, other results[289] failed to verify, in conceptual tissues, that competitive inhibition of the conversion of retinol to retinoic acid is a significant factor in ethanol-induced embryotoxicity. More recently, Kedishvili et al.[290] characterized an ADH enzyme (ADH-F) that oxidize all-*trans*-retinol and steroid alcohols in fetal tissues. In any event, deficiency in vitamin A, especially when exacerbated by ethanol, is associated with various extra-hepatic complications.

Abnormalities associated with excess vitamin A

Vitamin A deficiency promotes carcinogenesis (*vide supra*), but paradoxically, vitamin A excess may have a similar effect: Tuyns et al.[291] and DeCarli et al.[292] noted that foods providing large amounts of retinol increase the risk of cancer of the oesophagus and, in an epidemiological study, the increased cancer risk associated with the use of cigarettes and alcohol was enhanced upon ingestion of foods containing retinol[293]. Other food constituents could also play a role in that regard.

The teratogenic potential of excessive intake of retinoid has been clearly demonstrated in experimental animals[294], with corresponding data evolving in humans: teratogenicity of 13-*cis*-retinoic acid, used to treat cystic acne, has been established in epidemiological studies[295]. In addition, among babies born to women who took more than 10 000 IU of preformed vitamin A per day as supplements, about one infant in 57 had a malformation[296]. However, some caution in the interpretation of these data is still indicated[297]. Furthermore, acetaldehyde can cross the placenta[298] and may also contribute to the development of the fetal alcohol syndrome, the most prevalent cause of preventable congenital abnormality[299]. Therefore, in addition to potentiating the teratogenicity of vitamin A deficiency, alcohol can be expected to aggravate that of vitamin A excess, and this was indeed verified experimentally[300].

An excess of vitamin A is also known to be hepatotoxic[301,302]. The smallest daily supplement of vitamin A reported to be associated with liver cirrhosis is 7500 μg RE (25 000 IU) taken for 6 years[303]. These supplements fall well within common therapeutic dosages and amounts used prophylactically with over-the-counter preparations by the population at large.

Potentiation of vitamin A hepatotoxicity by ethanol was first demonstrated in rats fed diets for 2 months with either normal or 5-fold increased vitamin A content, both with or without ethanol[304]. Whereas under these conditions ethanol alone produced only modest changes, and vitamin A supplementation at the dose used had no adverse effect, the combination resulted in striking lesions, with giant mitochondria containing paracrystalline filamentous inclusions and depression of oxygen consumption in state 3 respiration with five different substrates. The potentiation of vitamin A toxicity by ethanol was also seen in patients treated with 10 000 IU vitamin A/day for sexual dysfunction attributable to excess alcohol consumption[305]. In addition to giant mitochondria, filamentous or crystalline-like inclusions were seen in the liver mitochondria of patients with hypervitaminosis A[306,307]. The potentiation of vitamin A toxicity by ethanol was most dramatically documented in another study, in which rats were given a combination of vitamin A supplementation and ethanol up to 9 months[308]. There was striking hepatic inflammation and necrosis, accompanied by a rise in the serum level of liver enzymes (glutamic dehydrogenase and AST).

Since retinol, retinal and retinoic acid can be further metabolized by liver microsomes, particularly when the latter system is induced by chronic ethanol consumption[245,251,252,254] one can postulate that some of these metabolites produced in increased amounts (possibly by some specific forms of cytochrome P-450) might also participate in the enhanced toxicity, but at the present time direct experimental evidence to support such a hypothesis is lacking.

Adverse interactions of ethanol with β-carotene

In contrast to retinoids, carotenoids were not known to produce toxic manifestations even when ingested chronically in large amounts[309,310]. Therefore, it made sense to assess whether carotenoids may serve as effective (but less toxic) substitutes for retinol, especially in alcoholic liver injury which has been attributed, in part, to oxidative stress and since β-carotene is an antioxidant. It was not known, however, whether β-carotene can actually offset alcohol-induced lipid peroxidation.

Effects of alcohol on β-carotene concentrations Studies in man revealed that for a given β-carotene intake, there is a correlation between alcohol consumption and plasma β-carotene concentration[311]. Thus, whereas in general, alcoholics have low plasma β-carotene levels[311,312], presumably reflecting low intake, alcohol *per se* might in fact increase blood levels in man[311]. There was also an increase in women with a dose as low as two drinks a day[313]. Furthermore, there was an increase in non-human primates studied under strictly controlled conditions[314]. Indeed, in baboons fed ethanol chronically, liver β-carotene was increased, in contrast to vitamin A, which was depleted. Similarly, plasma β-carotene levels were elevated in these ethanol-fed baboons, with a striking delay in the clearance from the blood after a β-carotene load. Furthermore, whereas β-carotene administration increased hepatic vitamin A in control baboons, this effect was much less evident in alcohol-fed animals. The combination of an increase in β-carotene and a relative lack of a corresponding rise in vitamin A suggests a blockage in the conversion of β-carotene to vitamin A by ethanol.

β-Carotene, alcohol, oxidative stress and liver injury

In the baboon, the administration of ethanol together with β-carotene resulted in a more striking hepatic injury than with either compound alone[314], with increased leakage of liver enzymes in the plasma, an inflammatory response in the liver and, at the ultrastructural level, striking autophagic vacuoles and alterations of the endoplasmic reticulum and the mitochondria[315]. The ethanol-induced oxidative stress, assessed by an increase in hepatic 4-hydroxynonenal and F_2-isoprostanes (measured by gas chromatography-mass spectrometry), was not improved despite a concomitant rise in hepatic antioxidants (β-carotene and vitamin E).

Extra-hepatic side effects

Cardiovascular complications There was no evidence of lower mortality from cardiovascular disease or other causes following β-carotene supplementation[316]. Similarly, the study of Hennekens et al.[317] ruled out the possibility that there was even a slight reduction in the incidence of mortality from cardiovascular disease with supplementation of 50 mg β-carotene on every other day, for an average of 12 years. Recent results even suggest that β-carotene participates as a pro-oxidant in the oxidative degradation of LDL and that increased LDL β-carotene may cancel the protective qualities of α-tocopherol[318].

In the α-tocopherol, β-carotene and Cancer (ATBC) Prevention Study[319] and in the CARET Trial[320], it was noted that, in smokers, β-carotene supplementation increased death from coronary heart disease.

Interaction with cancer Two epidemiological investigations[319,320] revealed that β-carotene supplementation increases the incidence of pulmonary cancer in smokers. Because heavy smokers are commonly heavy drinkers, we raised the possibility that alcohol abuse was contributory[321], since alcohol is known to act as a carcinogen and to exacerbate the carcinogenicity of other xenobiotics, especially those of tobacco smoke[322]. Why this should be aggravated by β-carotene is not clear, but β-carotene was found in rat lung to produce a powerful booster effect on phase I carcinogen-bioactivating enzymes, including activators of polycyclic aromatic hydrocarbons (PAHs)[323,324]. In addition, since pulmonary cells are exposed to relative high oxygen pressures, and because β-carotene loses its anti-oxidant activity and shows an autocatalytic, pro-oxidant effect at these higher pressures[325], such an interaction is at least plausible and deserves further study, especially since recent studies showed that β-carotene protects against oxidative damage in HT29 cells at low concentrations but rapidly lose this capacity at higher doses[326] and that β-carotene enhances hydrogen peroxide-induced DNA damage in human hepatocellular HepG2 cells[327]. Furthermore, the more recent publications of the ATBC and CARET studies showed that the increased incidence of pulmonary cancer was related to the amount of alcohol consumed by the participants[328–330].

Concentrations of carotenoids, retinoids and tocopherols were also determined in the homogenate of macroscopically normal appearing oropharyngeal mucosa from chronic alcoholics and from control patients. All the alcoholics except one had oropharyngeal cancer. No significant difference was found in tissue levels of carotenoids and tocopherols between alcoholics and controls. Furthermore, in seven of 11 controls, retinol was undetectable in the oropharyngeal mucosa, while in the alcoholics only two out of 10 had unmeasurable retinol levels[331]. These results did not support the concept that ethanol-associated oropharyngeal carcinogenesis is due, at least in part, to local deficiencies in retinoids, carotenoids or α-tocopherol.

Contrasting with the investigations showing a lack of beneficial effects of β-carotene supplementation (reviewed above), β-carotene was found to inhibit rat liver chromosomal aberrations and DNA chain break after a single injection of diethylnitrosamine[332]. Furthermore, a study of non-melanocytic skin cancer showed that a high intake of vegetables and other β-carotene containing foods is protective for non-melanocytic skin cancers[333]. Conversely, Menkes et al.[334] showed an association between low levels of serum beta-carotene and the risk of squamous-cell carcinoma of the lung. However, the latter two observations do not necessarily prove a causal link since the beneficial effects may be associated with active nutrients other than β-carotene.

Therapeutic window of retinoids and carotenoids

As already mentioned, vitamin A deficiency aggravates alcohol-induced liver injury, the fetal-alcohol syndrome and carcinogenesis. Vitamin A deficiency results not only from a poor dietary intake, but may also derive from direct effects of ethanol on the breakdown of retinol in the liver. Supplementation of vitamin A in the heavy drinker may thus be indicated, but it is complicated by the intrinsic hepatotoxicity of large amounts of vitamin A, which is strikingly potentiated by concomitant alcohol use. β-Carotene is a precursor and a non-toxic substitute for retinol, but ethanol interferes with its conversion to vitamin A, and even moderate alcohol intake can result in increased levels of β-carotene when the latter is given in commonly used dosage for supplementation. Side effects observed under these conditions include hepatotoxicity, promotion of pulmonary cancer and possibly cardiovascular complications. Thus, detrimental effects result from deficiency as well as from excess of retinoids and carotenoids and, paradoxically, both have similar adverse effects in terms of fibrosis, carcinogenesis and possibly embryotoxicity. Treatment efforts therefore must carefully respect the resulting narrow therapeutic window, especially in drinkers in whom alcohol narrows this therapeutic window even further by promoting the depletion of retinoids and by potentiating their toxicity.

Effects of dietary factors on ethanol metabolism

Low-protein diets reduce hepatic ADH in rats[335] and lower ethanol oxidation rates in rats[335] and in man[336]. Prolonged fasting also decreases ethanol oxidation rates as shown in isolated rat liver cells. A mechanism for lowered metabolism of ethanol during fasting is the lack of available metabolites to shuttle reducing equivalents from ethanol oxidation into mitochondria[337]. For a given alcohol intake, malnourished alcoholics may develop higher blood alcohol levels and sustain them longer than normally nourished individuals[338].

In rats, MEOS activity in the liver showed greater induction by alcohol on a normal than a low-fat diet, although induction of CYP2E1 was the same[339].

THERAPEUTIC STRATEGIES

Nutritional therapy in alcoholism

Individuals consuming over 30% of total calories as alcohol have a high probability of ingesting less than the recommended daily amounts of carbohydrate, protein, fat, vitamins A, C, and B (especially thiamine), and minerals such as calcium and iron (*vide supra*). It is sensible to recommend a complete diet comparable to that of non-alcoholics to forestall deficiency syndromes, although this does not suffice to prevent some organ damage due to the direct toxicity of alcohol (e.g., alcoholic liver disease).

Damage due to lack of thiamine is serious but treatable with a great margin of safety; therefore thiamine deficiency should be presumed and, if not definitely disproved, parenteral therapy with 50 mg thiamine per day should be given until similar doses can be taken by mouth. Riboflavin and pyridoxine should be routinely administered at the dosages usually contained in standard multivitamin preparations. Adequate folic acid replacement can be accomplished with the usual hospital diet. Additional replacement is optional unless deficiency is severe. Vitamin A replacement should only be given for well-documented deficiency, and to patients whose abstinence from alcohol is assured.

Zinc replacement is indicated only for night blindness unresponsive to vitamin A replacement. Magnesium replacement is recommended for symptomatic patients with low serum magnesium. Iron deficiency that has been clearly diagnosed may be corrected orally.

The nutritional management of acute and chronic liver disease due to alcoholism should include feeding programs to achieve protein replenishment without promoting hepatic encephalopathy, as reviewed elsewhere[52].

Acute pancreatitis may require withholding oral feeding for prolonged periods, during which time venous alimentation must be given. Chronic pancreatic exocrine insufficiency is treated by dietary manipulation (including decreases in fat) with oral pancreatic enzymes at mealtime. Thus, the nutritional management of acute and chronic liver disease due to alcoholism has the aim of defining feeding programs to reverse malnutrition, ameliorate liver disease, and decrease mortality, without promoting hepatic encephalopathy.

A pathogenic concept is emerging that is particularly useful therapeutically. Whereas it continues to be important to replenish nutritional deficiencies, when present, it is crucial to recognize that because of the alcohol-induced disease process, some of the nutritional requirements change. This is exemplified by methionine which normally is one of the essential amino acids for humans, but needs to be activated to S-adenosylmethionine (SAMe), a process impaired by the disease. Thus, SAMe rather than methionine is the compound that must be supplemented in the presence of significant liver disease[119]. Indeed, SAMe was found to attenuate mitochondrial lesions in baboons, replenish glutathione[118], and significantly reduce mortality in patients with Child A or B cirrhosis. Similarly, serious consequences of the decreased phosphatidylethanolamine methyltransferase activity associated with alcoholic liver disease can be offset by the administration of PPC which is rich in some of the products of the reaction such as DLPC, a PC species of high bioavailability. PPC (and/or DLPC) oppose oxidative stress, deactivate hepatic stellate cells and increase collagenase activity, resulting in prevention of ethanol-induced septal fibrosis and cirrhosis in the baboon (*vide infra*). Furthermore, PPC down-regulates CYP2E1 which, when excessively induced by alcohol, becomes toxic through free radical generation.

Redox shift, oxidative stress and antioxidant therapy, including CYP2E1 inhibition by PPC, bile acids and pharmacologic agents

The redox shift and oxidative stress related to the metabolism of ethanol have been shown to play a major role in the pathogenesis of alcoholic liver disease. Hence, corresponding therapy is taking an increasing role in treatment.

The focus on oxygen as a pathogenetic mechanism in alcoholic liver disease results, in part, from the observation that a characteristic feature of liver injury in the alcoholic is the predominance of steatosis and other lesions in the perivenular (also called centrilobular zone or zone 3) of the hepatic acinus (*vide supra*). The mechanism for this zonal selectivity of the toxic effects is multi factorial (*vide supra*) and has been postulated to involve, at least in part, a relative lack of oxygen supply. Accordingly, propylthiouracil treatment has been proposed to attenuate this deficit.

The hypoxia hypothesis originated from the observation that liver slices from rats fed alcohol chronically consume more oxygen than those of controls[67]. It was then postulated that the enhanced consumption of oxygen would increase the gradient of oxygen tensions along the sinusoids to the extent of producing anoxic injury of perivenular hepatocytes[340]. Indeed both in human alcoholics[341] and in animals fed alcohol chronically[68,342], decreases in either hepatic venous oxygen saturation[341] or PO_2[68] and in tissue oxygen tensions[342] have been found during the withdrawal state. However, these changes in hepatic oxygenation disappeared[68,343] or decreased[342] when alcohol was present in the blood. Acute ethanol administration increased splanchnic oxygen consumption in naive baboons, but the consequences of this effect on oxygenation in the perivenular zone were offset by increased blood flow resulting in unchanged hepatic venous oxygen tension[68]. Ethanol in fact induced an increase in portal hepatic blood flow[68,343–345]. In baboons fed alcohol chronically, defective O_2 utilization rather than lack of blood O_2 supply characterized liver injury produced by high concentration of ethanol[346].

The low oxygen tensions (normally prevailing in perivenular zones) exaggerate the redox shift produced by ethanol[68]. Indeed, ethanol increased the lactate/pyruvate ratio and decreased pyruvate more in hepatic venous blood than in total liver. In isolated rat hepatocytes, the ethanol-induced redox shift was markedly exaggerated by lowering the oxygen to a tension similar to those found in centrilobular zones. The process was also assessed in isolated perfused rat livers by varying the oxygen supply to produce the oxygen tensions prevailing in vivo along the sinusoid[69]. Hypoxia increased NADH which in turn inhibited the activity of NAD^+-dependent xanthine dehydrogenase, thereby favoring that of oxygen-dependent xanthine oxidase (XO)[70]. It has been postulated that, due to the acetate derived from ethanol, purine metabolites accumulate and could be metabolized via XO. This process may lead to the production of oxygen radicals which may mediate toxic effects towards liver cells, including peroxidation (Fig. 5). Physiological substrates for XO, namely hypoxanthine and xanthine, as well as AMP, significantly increased in the liver after ethanol, together with an enhanced urinary output of allantoin (a final product of xanthine metabolism). Allopurinol pretreatment resulted in 90% inhibition of XO activity, and also significantly decreased ethanol induced lipid peroxidation[70].

The ethanol-induced redox changes may also play a role in fibrogenesis. This was suggested by the observation that methylene blue, a scavenger of reducing equivalents, totally inhibits the stimulatory effect of acetaldehyde on $\alpha 1$ (I) procollagen and fibronectin gene expression in stellate cells[347]. These observations have not been exploited as yet for therapeutic purposes.

A major source of oxygen free radicals and meaningful to a therapeutic approach is the microsomal ethanol oxidizing system (MEOS). The induction of MEOS is associated with proliferation of the endoplasmic reticulum (*vide supra*), which is accompanied by increased oxidation of NADPH, with resulting H_2O_2 generation[348]. There is also increased superoxide radical production[349]. In addition, the CYP2E1 induction contributes to the well-known lipid peroxidation associated with alcoholic liver injury. Lipid peroxidation correlated with the amount of CYP2E1 in liver microsomal preparations, and it was inhibited by antibodies against CYP2E1 in control and ethanol-fed rats[350,351]. Indeed, CYP2E1 is rather leaky and its operation results in a significant release of free radicals, including 1-hydroxyethyl-free radical intermediates[352,353], confirmed by detecting the hydroxyethyl radicals in vivo[354]. The presence of CYP2E1 and its upregulation by ethanol was also shown in Kupffer cells[355].

The product of ethanol oxidation, namely acetaldehyde, promotes glutathione (GSH) depletion, resulting in free radical-mediated toxicity, and lipid peroxidation. Indeed, in isolated perfused livers, acetaldehyde was shown to cause lipid peroxidation[356,357]. In vitro, metabolism of acetaldehyde via xanthine oxidase or aldehyde oxidase may generate free radicals, but the concentration of acetaldehyde required is much too high for this mechanism to be of significance in vivo. However, another mechanism to promote lipid peroxidation is via GSH depletion. One of the three amino acids of this tripeptide is cysteine. Binding of acetaldehyde with cysteine and/or glutathione (GSH) may contribute to a depression of liver GSH[358] (Fig. 5). Rats fed ethanol chronically have significantly increased rates of GSH turnover[114]. Acute ethanol administration inhibits GSH synthesis and produces an increased loss from the liver[115]. GSH is selectively depleted in the mitochondria[359] and may contribute to the striking alcohol-induced alterations of that organelle since GSH offers one of the mechanisms for the scavenging of free radicals (Fig. 5).

Since the up-regulation of CYP2E1 activity by ethanol results in increased generation of reactive radicals and toxic metabolites, it has been suggested that CYP2E1 inhibitors may eventually provide useful tools for the prevention and treatment of the hepatotoxicity associated with heavy drinking. Several compounds were shown to exert some inhibiting effects on CYP2E1[74], including chlormethiazole[360–362]. Experimentally, a decrease in the inducibility of CYP2E1 was found to be associated with a reduction in associated liver injury[363,364] but when the liver pathology was semiquantitated, it was only partially ameliorated by CYP2E1 inhibitors[365,366]. Furthermore, CYP2E1 inhibition was incompletely effective in reducing induction of CYP2E1 by ethanol. Whereas CYP2E1 inhibitors completely blocked lipid peroxidation, they only partially prevented other lipid abnormalities[363]. More effective inhibitors are being developed[367] but there is still a need to obtain CYP2E1 inhibitors which are not only effective but

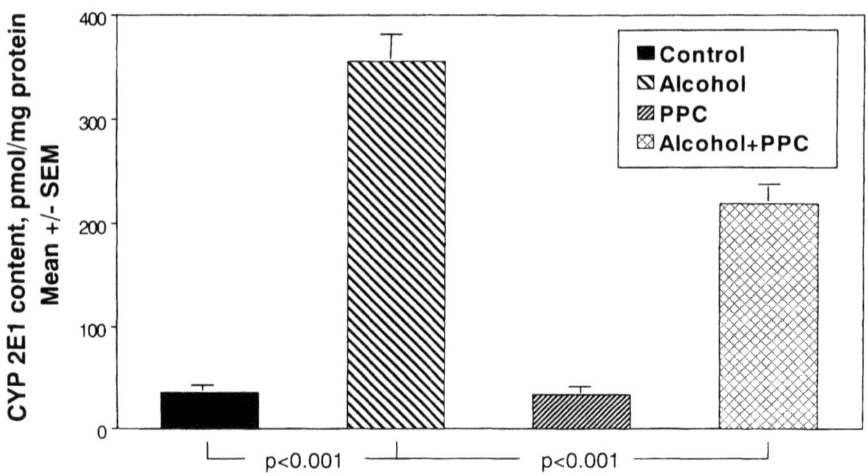

(A)

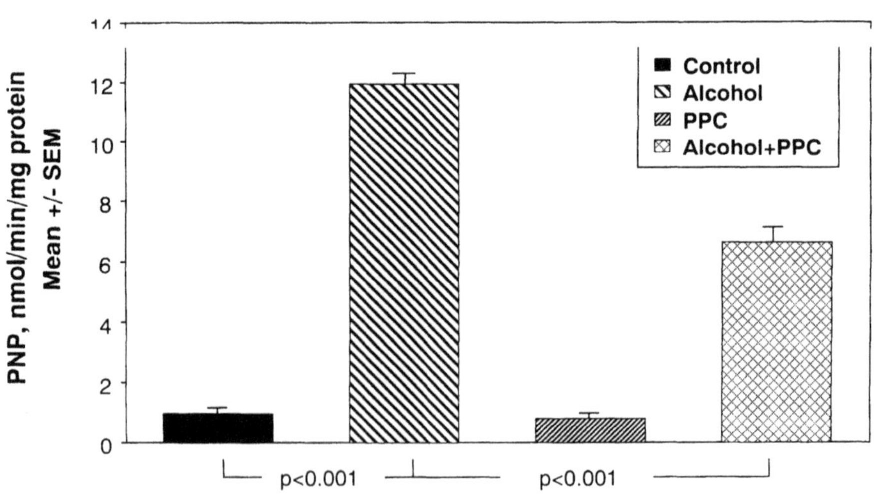

(B)

Figure 9 Inhibition of CYP2E1 content (A) and its activity (B) by PPC (data from Ref. 120).

also innocuous enough for prolonged use in humans. Polyenylphosphatidylcholine (PPC) a mixture of polyunsaturated phosphatidylcholine extracted from soybeans, may provide such a tool. PPC, and its main component DLPC, have a capacity to oppose both CCl_4- and alcohol-induced oxidative stress[239,368,369] (*vide supra*). PPC also corrects alcohol-induced abnormalities in lipid metabolism[235,370]. Furthermore, recent results revealed a significant reduction, by PPC feeding, of the CYP2E1 induction by ethanol[120] (Fig. 9). Unlike some of the experimental CYP2E1 inhibitors referred to above, PPC is innocuous; it is currently being tested in man.

Bile acids may also play an important role. That ethanol impairs bile acid excretion was already shown by Lefevre et al.[188] and Vendemiale et al.[371]. More recently, Vendemiale et al.[372] found that tauro-ursodeoxycholate administration protects proteins and lipids from ethanol-induced oxidative damage without influencing the glutathione content and compartmentalization. Furthermore, in a placebo-controlled, crossover study, administration of ursodeoxycholic acid for 4 weeks reduced both bilirubin and liver enzyme levels in patients with alcoholic cirrhosis who were actively drinking[373]. Bile acids such as taurine were found to have protective properties against ethanol-induced hepatic steatosis and lipid peroxidation during chronic ethanol consumption in rats[374], possibly again because of inhibition of the activity of CYP2E1, assessed indirectly by hepatic 4-nitrophenol hydroxylation. Similarly, ursodeoxycholate protected against ethanol-induced liver injury[375] by improving ATP synthesis and preserving liver mitochondrial morphology; it also attenuated alcoholic fatty liver in rats[376]. Finally, Neuman et al.[377] showed favourable effects of tauro-ursodeoxycholic and ursodeoxycholic acid on ethanol-induced cell injuries using a human Hep G2 cell line.

In patients with cirrhosis, diminished hepatic vitamin E levels have been observed[117], as also shown by von Herbay et al.[378]. However, in alcoholics without cirrhosis, hepatic vitamin E levels were generally within the normal range[117], raising the question of the usefulness of supplementation in that group of subjects. Moreover, even in baboons with normal vitamin E liver levels, alcohol administration resulted in the production of septal fibrosis in most, and full blown cirrhosis in some[226,239]. Thus, while vitamin E deficiency increases the hepatic vulnerability to ethanol, even in the presence of normal α-tocopherol, ethanol is hepatotoxic and causes fibrosis. Effectiveness of vitamin E supplementation in the prevention of alcoholic liver injury is presently being evaluated in humans.

Another antioxidant which has shown promising results in experimental animals is silymarin. Experimentally, silymarin exerts hepatoprotective actions through free-radical scavenging and immunomodulatory effects. In clinical trials, it appears to improve liver function test results and to decrease immunologic abnormalities in patients with ALD. However, both positive and negative effects on survival have been reported, and the role of silymarin in the treatment of ALD remains to be established[379,380]. The results of an ongoing double blind placebo controlled trial are presently awaited.

Iron overload may play a contributory role, as chronic alcohol consumption results in an increased iron uptake by hepatocytes[381] and as iron exposure accentuates the changes of lipid peroxidation and in the glutathione status of the liver cell induced by acute ethanol intoxication[382]. Hence iron chelation is being explored therapeutically.

Prevention and treatment of alcoholic fatty liver

A key pathogenic observation was the discovery that alcohol interferes with the oxidation of fatty acids[64,65]. As a result, alcohol was found to promote the deposition of dietary fat in the liver, both in rats[383] and in man[384]. Consequently, decreasing the amount of dietary fat resulted in a reduction in the severity of the alcoholic fatty liver[385]. Furthermore, replacement of the dietary long-chain triglycerides with medium-chain triglycerides (MCT) also significantly reduced the alcohol induced steatosis[386], most likely because medium-chain fatty acids have a much lesser propensity to undergo oxidation than the long-chain ones[387]. This protective effect of MCT has been more recently confirmed by others[388] and may be of therapeutic interest, particularly for relatively short term interventions in patients recovering from alcohol-induced liver injury.

Impairment of the mitochondrial function is exacerbated after chronic ethanol consumption[234] and includes a significant decrease in cytochrome oxidase activity, associated with a depletion in mitochondrial phosphatidylcholine due, in part, to increased phospholipase A2 activity[233]. Replenishment of phosphatidylcholine with PPC restored the cytochrome oxidase activity in vitro[233] and in vivo, with improvement of the capacity of the mitochondria for fatty acid oxidation and a corresponding reduction of hepatic fat accumulation[235] which supports the therapeutic use of PPC (*vide supra*).

Treatment of inflammation

The usefulness of steroids as an anti-inflammatory agent in severe alcoholic hepatitis and encephalopathy is now generally accepted (*vide infra*). Other approaches pertain to anti-endotoxin therapy (including antibiotic treatment) as well as inhibition of Kupffer cell activation with associated decreased production of tumor necrosis factor (TNF)-α and other cytokines. None of the latter approaches has yet been applied clinically. Of interest, again, are 2 CYP2E1 inhibitors. Indeed, a potent stimulant of Kupffer cell activation is the gut-derived endotoxin lipopolysaccharide[389–391], but an additional possible stimulator of Kupffer cells also is CYP2E1, shown to be increased after chronic alcohol consumption not only in hepatocytes (*vide supra*) but also in Kupffer cells[355]. In both acute and chronic liver diseases, Kupffer cells become activated to produce cytokines and reactive oxygen radicals[392–397], known mediators of hepatocellular injury. How and to what extent the induction of Kupffer cell CYP2E1 plays a role in these processes is now being investigated.

Experimentally, acute administration of alcohol enhanced endotoxin hepatotoxicity when the dose of endotoxin was small, but the effect of alcohol was masked when larger doses of endotoxin were given[398]. Circulating TNF-α and interleukin (IL)-1 remained elevated for up to 6 months after the diagnosis of alcoholic hepatitis, whereas interleukin-6 normalized in parallel with clinical recovery[399]. Concentrations of all three cytokines correlated with biochemical parameters of liver injury. Sheron et al.[400] also found that the cytokine IL-6 is activated in severe alcoholic hepatitis and postulated that this may mediate hepatic or extrahepatic tissue damage. On the one hand, TNF appears to be a proximal mediator of multiple types of experimental injury and TNF is elevated in alcoholic liver disease, as are the levels of certain other cytokines. However, on the other hand, low physiologic amounts of cytokines appear to be important for liver function and regeneration (and perhaps are beneficial to the organism as a whole). The challenge is to acquire sufficient knowledge to conserve the positive growth enhancing effects of cytokines while attenuating their cytotoxic effects. Sorting out the optimal amount of TNF is now required to exploit the experimental observation that antibodies to TNF-α attenuate hepatic necrosis and inflammation caused by chronic exposure to ethanol in the rat[401] or of prevention of carbon tetrachloride-induced rat liver injury by soluble tumor necrosis factor receptors[402] or the use of antisense oligonucleotides to target RNA transcripts for TNF-α, with inhibition of its synthesis[403].

Effective therapy should limit the catabolic processes underlying alcoholic hepatitis (AH) and promote anabolism. The inflammatory nature of AH and the possibility that immunological factors influence its perpetuation suggested that therapy with corticosteroids might reduce short-term mortality[404,405]. Furthermore, in experimental models of liver failure, corticosteroids lead to decreased ammonia levels through improved liver function[406]. These agents might, therefore, indirectly decrease hepatic encephalopathy. Initial investigations yielded conflicting results. Some placebo controlled studies demonstrated decreased short-term morbidity and more rapid biochemical improvement, whereas others were unable to document a beneficial effect[404,405,407]. The negative results have been attributed to the inclusion of two disparate groups, namely patients who had mild disease with good prognosis and little risk of dying suddenly, as well as those who had extremely advanced cirrhosis who were too moribund to benefit from potentially effective therapy. These included patients with active Gl bleeding or other co-morbid disorders for whom the outcome is more strongly influenced by those disorders than by AH[404,405,407].

A meta-analysis of the randomized trials concluded that corticosteroids do indeed reduce short-term (2-month) mortality in patients with severe AH, if patients with acute GI bleeding are excluded[407]. This conclusion was confirmed in a subsequent trial[408].

Good candidates for corticosteroid therapy are patients with severe disease with either spontaneous hepatic encephalopathy or high bilirubin and prothrombin time. It is strongly recommended that one performs a liver biopsy to confirm the diagnosis before initiating treatment, because a small but significant proportion (12%) of patients who fulfill the clinical and laboratory criteria for severe AH lack the appropriate histological findings[409].

Prednisolone, rather than prednisone, is recommended because hepatic metabolism of prednisone to its biologically active form may be incomplete in patients with liver disease[404]. The initial dosage is 40 mg/day prednisolone (orally or intravenously) or 32 mg/day methylprednisolone for 28 days, then a 2-week taper. Therapy is generally well tolerated.

Of potential therapeutic interest is the observation that DLPC selectively modulates the LPS-induced activation of Kupffer cells by decreasing the production of the cytotoxic TNF-α, while potentiating the release of the protective IL-1β[410]. This dual action of DLPC on cytokines may provide a potent mechanism against liver injury. In addition to the reduction in TNF-α, the enhanced release of IL-1β could oppose the hepatotoxicity of TNF-α, either directly and/or indirectly through an IL-1β related increase in the tolerance to TNF-α mediated toxicity[411].

Derangements of immune systems are also present in alcoholic liver disease[412], but there is still some debate whether they represent a consequence or a cause of the liver injury. Indeed, acetaldehyde is a very reactive compound that forms adducts with a variety of proteins. These, in turn, represent neoantigens and elicit an antibody response which may reflect, as well as contribute to, the pathogenesis of alcoholic liver injury.

Prevention and treatment of fibrosis

Individual susceptibility to the development of cirrhosis varies. Therefore recognition of those individuals prone to progress to cirrhosis at an early, and still reversible, stage is of practical importance for prevention and treatment. In that regard, recognition of perivenular fibrosis on liver biopsy is valuable (*vide supra*). This lesion has been described in association with full-blown alcoholic hepatitis[29], but it can occur at the fatty liver stage in the absence of hepatitis[34]. Experimental data suggested that perivenular fibrosis is a common and early warning sign of impending cirrhosis if drinking continues[34], and similar conclusions were derived from clinical studies in alcoholics[9] and, interestingly, in diabetics[413].

The accumulation of hepatic collagen during the development of cirrhosis could theoretically result from increased synthesis, decreased degradation, or both. The role of increased collagen synthesis was suggested by enhanced activity of hepatic peptidylproline hydroxylase in rats and primates and increased incorporation of proline ^{14}C into hepatic collagen in rat liver slices[414]. Increased hepatic peptidylproline hydroxylase activity was also found in patients with alcoholic cirrhosis[415] and hepatitis[416]. In baboons given ethanol who developed significant fibrosis, the hepatic type I procollagen mRNA content was significantly higher (per liver RNA) as determined by hybridization analysis[231]. Concerning the respective role of hepatocytes and stellate cells, a consensus has been reached that stellate cells, which are activated after chronic alcohol consumption[15,417], appear to play the major role in the production of collagen in the liver. Normal stellate cells, when isolated and cultured on plastic, undergo spontaneous transformation into transitional-like cells, thereby mimicking in vitro the condition that prevails in vivo after chronic alcohol consumption[18]. These cells in culture produce collagen[18]. When acetaldehyde, the active metabolite of ethanol, is added to these cells, they respond with a further increase in collagen accumulation[18] and synthesis, with increased mRNA for collagen[347] because collagen synthesis by liver stellate cells is released from feedback inhibition by the carboxy terminal propeptide of procollagen by adduct formation of acetaldehyde with the latter[418].

Collagen accumulation reflects not only enhanced synthesis, but it also results from an imbalance between collagen degradation and collagen production. Thus, cirrhosis might, in part, represent relative failure of collagen degradation to keep pace with synthesis. Interestingly, PPC may affect this balance. Indeed addition of PPC to transformed stellate cells was found to prevent the acetaldehyde-mediated increase in collagen accumulation, possibly by stimulation of collagenase activity[238] as well as by reduction of collagen production through a decrease in stellate cell activation demonstrated for the active component of PPC, namely DLPC[419]. Furthermore, since in vitro, the capacity to stimulate collagenase activity was found to reside exclusively with DLPC[226], it would make sense to switch from PPC to DLPC for the therapeutic uses in vivo as soon as an economical DLPC preparation becomes available. This would facilitate the administration of the compound and may thereby enhance its efficiency.

Finally, the aldehydic products of lipid peroxidation[420,421] may also play a role in fibrogenesis. As discussed under C1, PPC and DLPC exert remarkable antioxidant effects, both in vitro and in vivo. Thus, PPC may attenuate the development of cirrhosis after chronic alcohol administration in baboons[226] and CCl_4 in rats[237] through, at least in part, its antioxidative effects[239]. However, it should be pointed out that PPC is active as an antifibrotic agent even in the absence of oxidative stress, as demonstrated with the model of fibrosis and cirrhosis caused by heterologous albumin in the rat[237]. In that case, the other antifibrotic properties of PPC (*vide supra*) are obviously involved.

Colchicine attenuates the inflammatory response associated with alcohol injury to the liver and may also decrease collagen deposition. Kershenobich et al.[422] showed a significant reduction in mortality and reversal of fibrosis on serial biopsies but there was a difference in the severity of the liver disease in the treated vs. the placebo group, and there was a very high 19% dropout rate[423]. Therefore confirmatory studies are desirable and thus ongoing.

Viral hepatitis B or C commonly accompany chronic hepatitis in alcoholics. The association is particularly striking for hepatitis C. Indeed, in these patients, even in the absence of risk factors for the hepatitis C virus[424], portal or lobular inflammation (or both) are strongly associated with antibody to this virus, suggesting that alcohol may favour acquisition, replication or persistence of the virus. There may be potentiation of associated liver disorders, including fibrosis, but no satisfactory specific antiviral therapy is currently available, since α-interferon is relatively contraindicated in alcoholics, unless they stop drinking.

In summary, multiple agents have been proposed for the prevention and treatment of fibrosis. SAMe was reported to oppose CCl_4-induced fibrosis in the rat, to attenuate the consequences of the ethanol-induced oxidative stress and to decrease mortality in cirrhotics (*vide supra*). Anti-inflammatory medications and agents that interfere with collagen synthesis, such as inhibitors of prolyl-4-hydroxylase and antioxidants, are also being tested. In non-human primates, PPC, extracted from soybeans, protected against alcohol-induced fibrosis and cirrhosis and prevented the associated hepatic phosphatidylcholine (PC) depletion by increasing 18:2 containing PC species; it inhibits CYP2E1 activity and the associated oxidative stress also attenuated the transformation of stellate cells into collagen-producing transitional cells. Furthermore, it increased collagen breakdown, as shown in cultured stellate cells enriched with PPC or pure dilinoleoyl PC, the main PC species present in the extract. Since PPC and DLPC promote the breakdown of collagen, there is reasonable hope that this treatment may be useful for the management of fibrosis of alcoholic as well as non-alcoholic etiologies and that it may affect not only the progression of the disease, but may also reverse pre-existing fibrosis, as demonstrated for CCl_4-induced cirrhosis in the rat[237] and as presently tested in an ongoing clinical trial.

Transplantation

Orthotopic liver transplantation is an appropriate option for patients with alcoholic cirrhosis in whom liver failure progresses and life threatening complications develop despite abstinence from alcohol[425]. Most patients are compliant with therapy and resume a satisfactory degree of social and occupational function[426,427]. Between 10% and 20% of patients resume drinking; however, recidivism is frequently difficult to confirm[428,429]. There is no satisfactory solution to this problem as yet but the obvious answer would be a better control of relapse of drinking (*vide supra*).

CONCLUSIONS

As the papers of this symposium clearly show, much progress has been made in the understanding of the pathogenesis of alcoholic liver disease, resulting in improvement of prevention and therapy and promising prospects for even more effective treatments. The most successful approaches that one can expect to evolve are those that deal with the most fundamental cellular disturbances resulting from excessive alcohol consumption. It continues to be important to replenish nutrition deficiencies when present but it is crucial to recognize that, because of the alcohol-induced disease process, some of the nutritional requirements change. An excellent example is that of methionine. For many of its key functions, methionine, one of the essential amino acids for humans, must first be activated to SAMe but, in severe liver disease, the activity of the corresponding enzyme is depressed (Fig. 5). Therefore, the resulting deficiencies and associated pathology can be attenuated by the administration of SAMe, but not by methionine. Fundamentally, in healthy subjects, methionine is essential and must be provided in the diet, whereas its product SAMe can be synthesized endogenously. By contrast, in patients with severe alcoholic liver disease, the converse pertains: methionine is often plentiful because of the impairment in its utilization, whereas SAMe must be provided exogenously since the capacity for its synthesis is affected by the disease process. Similarly, phosphatidylethanolamine methyltransferase (PEMT) activity, which is important for hepatic phosphatidylcholine (PC) synthesis, is also depressed in alcoholic liver disease (Fig. 5), making it necessary to administer the products of the reaction, which not only replenishes PC in the membranes, but also restores the activity of PEMT[13,226]. Thus far, PPC and SAMe have been administered separately and, although they produce beneficial effects, the therapeutic results were incomplete. This is not surprising, since the deficiencies in SAMe and PC are interdependent (Fig. 5). SAMe alone cannot be expected to be fully corrective, since in its function of methylation of phosphatidylethanolamine to PC, it depends on the normal activity of the corresponding enzyme, namely PEMT, which is depressed by alcohol but can be reactivated by PPC[13]. Conversely, optimal activity of the enzyme requires ample supply of SAMe, which is depleted in alcoholic liver disease[118]. Thus, it would make sense to base the therapy on the administration of both compounds.

Similar combination therapies may also be beneficial for other compounds, particularly those that act on the fundamental pathogenetic mechanisms of the disease, such as oxidative stress. Since free radical generation by the ethanol-induced CYP2E1 plays a key role in the oxidative stress, inhibitors of this enzyme have great promise. Several have been investigated experimentally and PPC is particularly interesting in view of its innocuity. Therapeutic cocktails are now part of the armamentarium in infectious diseases and such an approach should also be considered for alcohol-induced liver injury. In view of the striking negative interaction between alcoholic liver injury and hepatitis C[424,430–432], an antiviral agent is eagerly awaited that, unlike Interferon, is not contraindicated in the alcoholic. Furthermore, since excess drinking is the crux of the issue, anticraving agents should be incorporated in any contemplated cocktail, in view of the recent promising results obtained with some of these agents such as naltrexone.

ACKNOWLEDGEMENTS

Original studies reviewed here were supported by NIH grants AA05934, AA11115, AA11160, AA07275, the Kingsbridge Research Foundation and the Department of Veterans Affairs. Skillful typing of the manuscript by Ms. D. Perez is gratefully acknowledged.

REFERENCES

1. Leevy CM. Fatty liver: a study of 270 patients with biopsy proven fatty liver and a review of the literature. Medicine. 1962;41:249–76.
2. Brunt PW, Kew MC, Scheuer PJ, Sherlock S. Studies in alcoholic liver disease in Britain. 1. Clinical and pathological patterns related to natural history. Gut. 1974;15:52–8.
3. Svoboda DJ, Manning RT. Chronic alcoholism with fatty metamorphosis of the liver. Am J Pathol. 1964;44:645–62.
4. Lane BP, Lieber CS. Ultrastructural alterations in human hepatocytes following ingestion of ethanol with adequate diets. Am J Pathol. 1966;49:593–603.
5. Rubin E, Lieber CS. Alcohol-induced hepatic injury in non-alcoholic volunteers. N Engl J Med. 1968;278:869–76.
6. Leevy CM, Zinke MR, White TJ, Grassi AM. Clinical observations on fatty liver. Arch Intern Med. 1953;72:527–41.
7. Ballard H, Bernstein M, Farrar JT. Fatty liver presenting as obstructive jaundice. Am J Med. 1961;30:196–201.
8. Phillips GB, Davidson CS. Liver disease of the chronic alcoholic simulating extrahepatic biliary obstruction. Gastroenterology. 1957;33:236–44.
9. Worner TM, Lieber CS. Perivenular fibrosis as precursor lesion of cirrhosis. JAMA. 1985;254:627–30.
10. Hasumura Y, Minato Y, Nishimura M et al. Hepatic fibrosis in alcoholics: Morphologic characteristics, clinical diagnosis, and natural course. Pathobiol Hepatic Fibrosis. 1985;7:13–24.
11. Lieber CS, DeCarli LM, Rubin E. Sequential production of fatty liver, hepatitis and cirrhosis in sub-human primates fed ethanol with adequate diets. Proc Natl Acad Sci USA. 1975;72:437–41.
12. Lieber CS, DeCarli LM, Mak KM, Kim C-I, Leo MA. Attenuation of alcohol-induced hepatic fibrosis by polyunsaturated lecithin. Hepatology. 1990;12:1390–8.
13. Lieber CS, Robins SJ, Leo MA. Hepatic phosphatidylethanolamine methyltransferase activity is decreased by ethanol and increased by phosphatidylcholine. Alcohol Clin Exp Res. 1994;18:592–5.
14. Mak KM, Lieber CS. Portal fibroblasts and myofibroblasts in baboons after long-term alcohol consumption. Arch Pathol Lab Med. 1986;110:513–16.

15. Mak KI, Lieber CS. Lipocytes and transitional cells in alcoholic liver disease: a morphometric study. Hepatology. 1988;8:1027–33.
16. Mak KM, Leo MA, Lieber CS. Alcoholic liver injury in baboons: transformation of lipocytes to transitional cells. Gastroenterology. 1984;87:188–200.
17. Friedman SL. The cellular basis of hepatic fibrosis: mechanisms and treatment strategies. N Engl J Med. 1993;328:1828–35.
18. Moshage H, Casini A, Lieber CS. Acetaldehyde selectively stimulates collagen production in cultured rat liver-storing cells but not in hepatocytes. Hepatology. 1990;12:511–18.
19. Beckett AG, Livingston AV, Hill KR. Acute alcoholic hepatitis. Br Med J. 1961;ii:1113–19.
20. Kyösola K, Salorinne Y. Liver biopsy and liver function tests in 28 consecutive long-term alcoholics. Ann Clin Res. 1975;7:80–4.
21. Lelbach WK. Cirrhosis in the alcoholic and its relation to the volume of alcohol abuse. Ann NY Acad Sci. 1975;252:85–105.
22. Sörensen TIA, Orholm M, Bentsen KD, Eghoje K, Christoffersen P. Prospective evaluation of alcohol abuse and alcoholic liver injury in man as predictors of development of cirrhosis. Lancet. 1984;ii:241–4.
23. Hall EM, Ophuls W. Progressive alcoholic cirrhosis. Report of four cases. Am J Pathol. 1925;477–93.
24. Phillips GB, Davidson CS. Acute hepatic insufficiency of the chronic alcoholic. Arch Intern Med. 1954;94:585–603.
25. Popper H, Szanto PB, Parthasarathy M. Florid cirrhosis. A review of 35 cases. Am J Clin Pathol. 1955;25:889–901.
26. Edmondson HA, Peters RL, Reynolds TB, Kuzma OT. Sclerosing hyaline necrosis of the liver. A recognizable clinical syndrome. Ann Intern Med. 1963;59:646–73.
27. Harinasuta U, Zimmerman HJ. Alcoholic steatonecrosis. I. Relationship between severity of hepatic disease and presence of Mallory bodies in the liver. Gastroenterology. 1971;60:1036–46.
28. Lischner MW, Alexander JF, Galambos JT. Natural history of alcoholic hepatitis. I. The acute disease. Am J Dig Dis. 1971;16:481–94.
29. Edmondson HA, Peters RL, Frankel HH, Borowsky S. The early stage of liver injury in the alcoholic. Medicine. 1967;46:119–29.
30. Klion FM, Schaffner F. Ultrastructural studies in alcoholic liver disease. Digestion. 1968;1:2–14.
31. Helman, RA, Temko MH, Nye SW, Fallon HJ. Alcoholic hepatitis: Natural history and evaluation of prednisolone therapy. Ann Intern Med. 1971;74:311–21.
32. Rubin E, Popper H. The evolution of human cirrhosis deduced from observations in experimental animals. Medicine. 1967;46:163–83.
33. Goodman ZD, Ishak KG. Occlusive venous lesions in alcoholic liver disease. A study of 200 cases. Gastroenterology. 1982;83:786–96.
34. Van Waes L, Lieber CS. Early perivenular sclerosis in alcoholic fatty liver: an index of progressive liver injury. Gastroenterology. 1977;73:646–50.
35. Bradley SE, Ingelfinger FJ, Bradley GP. Hepatic circulation in cirrhosis of the liver. Circulation. 1952;5:419–29.
36. Popper H. The pathogenesis of alcoholic cirrhosis. In: Fisher MM, Rankin JG, eds. Alcohol and the Liver. New York: Plenum Press, 1977; pp. 289–305.
37. Bell ET. Relation of portal cirrhosis to hemochromatosis and to diabetes mellitus. Diabetes. 1955;4:435–46.
38. Powell LW. The role of alcoholism in hepatic iron storage disease. Ann NY Acad Sci. 1975;252:124–34.
39. Gall EA. Primary and metastic carcinoma of liver – relationship to hepatic cirrhosis. Arch Pathol. 1960;70:226–32.
40. Lee FI. Cirrhosis and hepatoma in alcoholics. Gut. 1966;7:77–85.
41. Lieber CS, Seitz HK, Garro AJ, Worner TM. Alcohol related diseases and carcinogenesis. Cancer Res. 1979;39:2863–86.
42. Tisdale WA, Klatskin G. The fever of Laennec's cirrhosis. Yale J Biol Med. 1960;33:94–106.
43. Targan SR, Chow AW, Guze LB. Role of anaerobic bacteria in spontaneous peritonitis of cirrhosis. Report of two cases and review of the literature. Am J Med. 1977;62:397–403.
44. Skrede S, Blomhoff JP, Gjone E. Biochemical features of acute and chronic hepatitis. Ann Clin Res. 1976;8:182–99.

45. Agostoni A, Vergani C, Stabilini R, Marasini B. Determination of seven serum proteins in alcoholic cirrhosis. Clin Chim Acta. 1969;26:351–5.
46. Feizi T. Immunoglobulins in chronic liver disease. Gut. 1968;9:193–8.
47. Iturriaga H, Pereda T, Estevez A, Ugarte G. Serum immunoglobulin changes in alcoholic patients. Ann Clin Res. 1977;9:39–43.
48. Skrede S, Blomhoff JP, Elgjo K, Gjone E. Serum proteins in diseases of the liver. Scand J Clin Lab Invest. 1975;35:399–406.
49. Volpicelli JR, Alterman AI, Hayashida M, O'Brien CP. Naltrexone in the treatment of alcohol dependence. Arch Gen Psychiatry. 1992;49:876–80.
50. O'Malley SS, Jaffe AJ, Chang G, Schottenfeld RS, Meyer RE, Rounsaville B. Naltrexone and coping skills therapy for alcohol dependence. Arch Gen Psychiatry. 1992;49:881–7.
51. Chedid A, Mendenhall CL, Garside P, French SW, Chen T, Rabin L and the VA Cooperative Group. Prognostic factors in alcoholic liver disease. Am J Gastroenterol. 1991;82:210–16.
52. Best CH, Hartroft WS, Lucas CC, Ridout JH. Liver damage produced by feeding alcohol or sugar and its prevention by choline. Br Med J. 1949;2:1001–6.
53. Lieber CS. Medical and Nutritional Complications of Alcoholism: Mechanisms and Management. New York: Plenum Press, 1992: p. 579.
54. Lieber CS, Jones DP, Mendelson J, DeCarli LM. Fatty liver, hyperlipemia and hyperuricemia produced by prolonged alcohol consumption, despite adequate dietary intake. Trans Assoc Am Phys. 1963;76:289–300.
55. DeCarli LM, Lieber CS. Fatty liver in the rat after prolonged intake of ethanol with a nutritionally adequate new liquid diet. J Nutr. 1967;91:331–6.
56. Lieber CS, DeCarli LM. An experimental model of alcohol feeding and liver injury in the baboon. J Med Primatol. 1974;3:153–63.
57. Lieber CS, Spritz N, DeCarli LM. Fatty liver produced by dietary deficiencies: its pathogenesis and potentiation by ethanol. J Lipid Res. 1969;10:283–7.
58. Lieber CS, DeCarli LM, Gang H, Walker G, Rubin E. Hepatic effects of long term ethanol consumption in primates. In: Goldsmith EI, Moor-Jankowski J, eds. Medical Primatology, Part III. Basel: Karger, 1972;pp. 270–8.
59. Lieber CS, Rubin E. Alcoholic fatty liver in man on a high protein and low fat diet. Am J Med. 1968;44:200–6.
60. Baraona E, Julkunen R, Tannenbaum L, Lieber CS. Role of intestinal bacterial overgrowth in ethanol production and metabolism in rats. Gastroenterology. 1986;90:103–10.
61. Bjorkhem I. On the role of alcohol dehydrogenase in ω-oxidation of fatty acids. Eur J Biochem. 1972;30:441–51.
62. Bosron WF, Ehrig T, Li T-K. Genetic factors in alcohol metabolism and alcoholism. Semin Liver Dis. 1993;13:126–35.
63. Faller J, Fox IH. Evidence for increased urate production by activation of adenine nucleotide turnover. N Engl J Med. 1982;307:1598–602.
Lieber CS, Jones DP, DeCarli LM. Effects of prolonged ethanol intake: production of fatty liver despite adequate diets. J Clin Invest. 1965;44:1009–21.
64. Lieber CS, Schmid R. The effect of ethanol on fatty acid metabolism: Stimulation of hepatic fatty acid synthesis in vitro. J Clin Invest. 1961;40:394–9.
65. Lieber CS, DeCarli LM, Schmid R. Effects of ethanol on fatty acid metabolism in liver slices. Biochem Biophys Res Commun. 1959;1:302–6.
66. Galli A, Price D, Crabb D. High-level expression of rat class I alcohol dehydrogenase is sufficient for ethanol-induced fat accumulation in transduced HeLa cells. Hepatology. 1999;29:1164–70.
67. Videla L, Israel Y. Factors that modify the metabolism of ethanol in rat liver and adaptive changes produced by its chronic administration. Biochem J. 1970;118:275–81.
68. Jauhonen P, Baraona E, Miyakawa H, Lieber CS. Mechanism for selective perivenular hepatotoxicity of ethanol. Alcohol Clin Exp Res. 1982;6:350–7.
69. Jauhonen P, Baraona E, Lieber CS, Hassinen IE. Dependence of ethanol-induced redox shift on hepatic oxygen tensions prevailing in vivo. Alcohol. 1985;2:163–7.
70. Kato S, Kawase T, Alderman J, Lieber CS. Role of xanthine oxidase in ethanol-induced lipid peroxidation in rats. Gastroenterology. 1990;98:203–10.
71. Buhler R, Hess M, von Wartburg J-P. Immunohistochemical localization of human liver alcohol dehydrogenase in liver tissue, cultured fibroblasts and hela cells. Am J Pathol. 1982;108:89–99.

72. Day CP, Bashir R, James OF, Bassendine MF, Crabb DW, Thomasson HR et al. Investigation of the role of polymorphisms at the alcohol and aldehyde dehydrogenase loci in genetic predisposition to alcohol-related end-organ damage. Hepatology. 1991;14:798–801 (Erratum, Hepatology. 1991;15:750).
73. Poupon RE, Nalpas B, Coutelle C, Fleury B, Couzigou P, Higueret D and French Group for Research on Alcohol and Liver. Polymorphism of alcohol dehydrogenase, alcohol and aldehyde dehydrogenase activities; implications in alcoholic cirrhosis in white patients. Hepatology. 1992;15:1017–22.
74. Lieber CS. Cytochrome P4502E1: Its physiological and pathological role. Physiol Rev. 1997;77:517–44.
75. Lieber CS. Microsomal ethanol-oxidizing system (MEOS), the first 30 years (1968–1998) – a review. Alcohol Clin Exp Res. 1999;23:991–1007.
76. Meldolesi J. On the significance of the hypertrophy of the smooth endoplasmic reticulum in liver cells after administration of drugs. Biochem Pharmacol. 1967;16:125–31.
77. Conney AH. Pharmacological implications of microsomal enzyme induction. Pharmacol Rev. 1967;19:317–66.
78. Lane BP, Lieber CS. Effects of butylated hydroxytoluene on the ultrastructure of rat hepatocytes. Lab Invest. 1967;16:341–8.
79. Lieber CS, DeCarli LM. Ethanol oxidation by hepatic microsomes: Adaptive increase after ethanol feeding. Science. 1968;162:917–18.
80. Lieber CS, DeCarli LM. Hepatic microsomal ethanol oxidizing system: In vitro characteristics and adaptive properties in vivo. J Biol Chem. 1970;245:2505–12.
81. Teschke R, Hasumura Y, Joly JG, Ishii H, Lieber CS. Microsomal ethanol-oxidizing system (MEOS): Purification and properties of a rat liver system free of catalase and alcohol dehydrogenase. Biochem Biophys Res Commun. 1972;49:1187–93.
82. Teschke R, Hasumura Y, Lieber CS. Hepatic microsomal alcohol oxidizing system. Solubilization, isolation and characterization. Arch Biochem Biophys. 1974;163:404–15.
83. Ohnishi K, Lieber CS. Reconstitution of the microsomal ethanol-oxidizing system: qualitative and quantitative changes of cytochrome P-450 after chronic ethanol consumption. J Biol Chem. 1977;252:7124–31.
84. Koop DR, Morgan ET, Tarr GE, Coon MJ. Purification and characterization of a unique isozyme of cytochrome P-450 from liver microsomes of ethanol-treated rabbits. J Biol Chem. 1982;257:8472–80.
Miwa GT, Levin W, Thomas PE, Lu AYH. The direct oxidation of ethanol by catalase- and alcohol dehydrogenase-free reconstituted system containing cytochrome P-450. Arch Biochem Biophys. 1978;187:464–75.
85. Lasker JM, Raucy J, Kubota S, Bloswick BP, Black M, Lieber CS. Purification and characterization of human liver cytochrome P-450-ALC. Biochem Biophys Res Commun. 1987;148:232–8.
86. Tsutsumi M, Lasker JM, Shimizu M, Rosman AS, Lieber CS. The intralobular distribution of ethanol-inducible P450IIE1 in rat and human liver. Hepatology. 1989;10:437–46.
87. Takahashi T, Lasker JM, Rosman AS, Lieber CS. Induction of P450E1 in human liver by ethanol is due to a corresponding increase in encoding mRNA. Hepatology. 1993;17:236–45.
88. Salmela KS, Kessova IG, Tsyrlov IB, Lieber CS. Respective roles of human cytochrome P4502E1, 1A2, and 3A4 in the hepatic microsomal ethanol oxidizing system. Alcohol Clin Exp Res. 1998;22:2125–32.
89. Salaspuro MP, Lieber CS. Non-uniformity of blood ethanol elimination: its exaggeration after chronic consumption. Ann Clin Res. 1978;10:294–7.
90. Kater RMH, Tobon F, Iber FL. Increased rate of tolbutamide metabolism in alcoholic patients. JAMA. 1969;207:363–5.
91. Kater RMH, Roggin G, Tobon F, Zieve P, Iber FL. Increased rate of clearance of drugs from the circulation of alcoholics. Am J Med Sci. 1969;258:35–9.
92. Misra PS, Lefevre A, Ishii H, Rubin E, Lieber CS. Increase of ethanol meprobamate and pentobarbital metabolism after chronic ethanol administration in man and in rats. Am J Med. 1971;51:346–51.
93. Sotaniemi EA, Anttila M, Rautio A, Stengard J, Saukko P, Jarvensivu P. Propranolol and sotaiol metabolism after a drinking party. Clin Pharmacol Ther. 1981;29:705–10.
94. Hetu C, Joly J-G. Differences in the duration of the enhancement of liver mixed-function oxidase activities in ethanol-fed rats after withdrawal. Biochem Pharmacol. 1985;34:1211–16.

95. Vessell ES, Page JG, Passananti GT. Genetic environmental factors affecting ethanol metabolism in man. Clin Pharmacol Ther. 1971;12:192–201.
96. Carulli N, Manenti I, Gallo M, Salvioli GF. Alcohol-drugs interaction in man: Alcohol and tolbutamide. Eur J Clin Invest. 1971;1:421–4.
97. Pritchard JF, Schneck DW. Effects of ethanol and phenobarbital on the metabolism of propanolol by 9000 g rat liver supernatant. Biochem Pharmacol. 1977;26:2453–4.
98. Sellman R, Kanto J, Raijola E, Pekkarinen A. Human and animal study on elimination from plasma and metabolism of diazepam after chronic alcohol intake. Acta Pharmacol Toxicol. 1975;36:33–8.
99. Grassi GG, Grassi C. Ethanol-antibiotic interactions at hepatic level. J Clin Pharmacol Biopharmacol. 1975;11:216–25.
100. Teschke R, Moreno F, Petrides AS. Hepatic microsomal ethanol oxidizing system (MEOS) respective role of ethanol and carbohydrates for the enhanced activity after chronic alcohol consumption. Biochem Pharmacol. 1981;30:45–51.
101. Joly J-G, Hetu C. Effects of chronic ethanol administration in the rat: relative dependency on dietary lipids. Biochem Pharmacol. 1975;124:1475–80.
102. Mitchell JR, Mack C, Mezey E, Maddrey WC. The effects of variation in dietary protein and ethanol on hepatic microsomal drug metabolism in the rat. Hepatology. 1981;1:336–40.
103. Laethem RM, Balaxy M, Falck JR, Laethem CL, Koop DR. Formation of 19(S)-, 19(R)-, and 18(R)-hydroxyeicosatetraenoic acids by alcohol-inducible cytochrome P4502E1. J Biol Chem. 1993;268:12912–18.
104. Amet Y, Berthou F, Goasduff T, Salaun JP, Le Breton L, Menez JF. Evidence that cytochrome P450 2E1 is involved in the (ω-1)-hydroxylation of lauric acid in rat liver microsomes. Biochem Biophys Res Comm. 1994;203:1168–74.
105. Adas F, Betthou F, Picart D, Lozac'h P, Beauge F, Amet Y. Involvement of cytochrome P450 2E1 in the (omega-1)-hydroxylation of oleic acid in human and rat liver microsomes. J Lipid Res. 1998;39:1210–19.
106. Koop DR, Casazza JP. Identification of ethanol-inducible P-450 isozyme 3a as the acetone and acetol monooxygenase of rabbit microsomes. J Biol Chem. 1985;260:13607–12.
107. Koop DR, Crump BL, Nordblom GD, Coon MJ. Immunochemical evidence for induction of the alcohol oxidizing cytochrome P450 isozyme 3a (P-450IIE1) as a benzene and phenol hydroxylase. Toxicol Appl Pharmacol. 1989;98:278–88.
108. Yang CS, Yoo J-S, Ishizaki H, Hong J. Cytochrome P450IIE1: roles in nitrosamine metabolism and mechanisms of regulation. Drug Metab Rev. 1990;22:147–59.
109. Raucy JL, Lasker JM, Kramer JC, Salazer DE, Lieber CS, Corcoran GB. Induction of P450IIE1 in the obese rat. Mol Pharmacol. 1991;39:275–80.
110. Weltman MD, Farrell GC, Hall P, Ingelman-Sundberg M, Liddle C. Hepatic cytochrome P4502E1 is increased in patients with nonalcoholic steatohepatitis. Hepatology. 1998;27:128–33.
111. Tsutsumi M, Leo MA, Kim C, Tsutsumi M, Lasker J, Lowe N, Lieber CS. Interaction of ethanol with enflurane metabolism and toxicity: Role of P450IIE1. Alcohol Clin Exp Res. 1990;14:174–9.
112. Sato M, Matsuda Y, Lieber CS. Increased hepatotoxicity of acetaminophen after chronic ethanol consumption in the rat. Gastroenterology. 1981;80:149–8.
113. Whitecomb DC, Block GD. Association of acetaminophen hepatotoxicity with fasting and ethanol use. JAMA. 1994;272:1845–50.
114. Morton S, Mitchell MC. Effects of chronic ethanol feeding on glutathione turnover in the rat. Biochem Pharmacol. 1985;34:1559–63.
115. Speisky H, MacDonald A, Giles G, Orrego H, Israel Y. Increased loss of decreased synthesis of hepatic glutathione after acute ethanol administration. Biochem J. 1985;225:565–72.
117. Leo MA, Rosman A, Lieber CS. Differential depletion of carotenoids and tocopherol in liver diseases. Hepatology. 1993;17:977–86.
118. Lieber CS, Casini A, DeCarli LM, Kim C, Lowe N, Sasaki R, Leo MA. S-adenosyl-L-methionine attenuates alcohol-induced liver injury in the baboon. Hepatology. 1990;11:165–72.
119. Lieber CS. Role of S-adenosyl-L-methionine in the treatment of liver diseases. J Hepatol. 1999;30:1155–9.
120. Aleynik MK, Leo MA, Aleynik SI, Lieber CS. Polyenylphosphatidylcholine opposes the increase of cytochrome P4502E1 by ethanol and corrects its iron-induced decrease. Alcohol Clin Exp Res. 1999;23:96–100.

121. Patek AJ, Toth EG, Saunders ME, Castro GAM, Engel JJ. Alcohol and dietary factors in cirrhosis. Arch Intern Med. 1975;135:1053–7.
122. Iber FL. In alcoholism, the liver sets the pace. Nutr Today. 1971;6:2–9.
123. Mendenhall C, Bongiovanni G, Goldberg S, Miller B, Moore MJ, Rouster S et al. VA co-operative Study on Alcoholic Hepatitis III: Changes in protein-calorie malnutrition associated with 30 days of hospitalization with and without enteral nutritional therapy. J Parent Ent Nutr. 1985;9:590–6.
124. Morgan MY. Enteral nutrition in chronic liver disease. Acta Chir Scand. 1981;507:81–90.
125. Simko V, Connell AM, Banks B. Nutritional status in alcoholic with and without liver disease. Am J Clin Nutr. 1982;35:197–203.
126. World MJ, Ryle PR, Jones D, Shaw GK, Thomson AD. Differential effect of chronic alcohol intake and poor nutrition on body weight and fat stores. Alcohol Alcohol. 1984;19:281–90.
127. Liu S, Serdula MK, Williamson DF, Mokdad AH, Byers T. A prospective study of alcohol intake and change in body weight among US adults. Am J Epidemiol. 1994;140:912–20.
World MJ, Ryle PR, Pratt OE, Thompson AD. Alcohol and body weight. Alcohol Alcohol. 1984:19:1–6.
128. Armellini F, Zamboni M, Frigo L, Mandragona R, Robbi R, Micciolo R, Bosello O. Alcohol consumption, smoking habits and body fat distribution in Italian men and women aged 20–60 years. Eur J Clin Nutr. 1993;47:52–60.
129. Tremblay A, Buemann B, Theriault G, Bouchard C. Body fatness in active individuals reporting low lipid and alcohol intake. Eur J Clin Nutr. 1995;49:824–31.
130. Bebb HT, Houser HB, Witschi JC, Littell AS, Fuller RK. Calorie and nutrient contribution of alcoholic beverages to the usual diets of 155 adults. Am J Clin Nutr. 1971;24:1042–52.
131. Neville JN, Eagles JA, Samson G, Olson RE. Nutritional status of alcoholics. Am J Clin Nutr. 1968;21:1329–40.
132. Gruchow HW, Sobociaski KA, Barboriak JJ. Alcohol, nutrient intake, and hypertension in US adults. JAMA. 1985;253:1567–70.
133. Lieber CS. Perspectives: Do alcohol calories count? Am J Clin Nutr. 1991;54:976–82.
134. Hillers VN, Massey LK. Interrelationships of moderate and high alcohol consumption with diet and health status. Am J Clin Nutr. 1985;41:356–62.
135. Westerfeld WW, Schulman MP. Metabolism and caloric value of alcohol. JAMA. 1959;170:197–203.
136. Bonjour JP. Vitamins and alcoholism. I. Ascorbic acid. Int J Vitamin Nutr. 1979;49:434–41.
137. Gruchow HW, Sobocinski KA, Barboriak JJ, Scheller JG. Alcohol consumption, nutrient intake and relative body weight among US adults. Am J Clin Nutr. 1985;42:289–95.
138. Saville PD. Changes in bone mass with age and alcoholism. J Bone Joint Surg (Am). 1965;47:492–9.
139. Gascon-Barre M. Influence of chronic ethanol consumption on the metabolism and action of vitamin D. J Am Coll Nutr. 1985;4:565–74.
140. Nilsson BE. Conditions contributing to fracture of the femoral neck. Acta Chir Scand. 1970;136:383–4.
141. Solomon L. Arthropathy and necrosis of the femoral head. J Bone Joint Surg (Br). 1973;55:246–61.
142. Reisenauer AM, Buffington CAT, Villanueva JA, Halsted CH. Folate absorption in alcoholic pigs: in vivo intestinal perfusion studies. Am J Clin Nutr. 1989;50:1429–35.
143. Naughton CA, Chandler CJ, Duplantier RB, Halsted CH. Folate absorption in alcoholic pigs: in vitro hydrolysis and transport at the intestinal brush border membrane. Am J Clin Nutr. 1989;50:1436–41.
144. Said HM, Strum WB. Effect of ethanol and other aliphatic alcohols on the intestinal transport of folates. Digestion. 1986;35:129–35.
145. Halsted CH, Robles EZ, Mezey E. Decreased jejunal uptake of labeled folic acid (^{3}H-PGA) in alcoholic patients: Roles of alcohol and nutrition. N Engl J Med. 1971;285:701–6.
146. Racusen LC, Krawitt EL. Effect of folate deficiency and ethanol ingestion on intestinal folate absorption. Am J Dig Dis. 1977;22:915–20.
147. Lindenbaum J, Lieber CS. Alcohol and the hematologic system. In: Lieber CS, ed. Medical Disorders of Alcoholism. Pathogenesis and Treatment. Vol. 22. Philadelphia: WB Saunders, 1982:pp. 313–62.
148. Sullivan LW, Herbert V. Suppression of hematopoiesis by ethanol. J Clin Invest. 1964;43:2048–62.

149. Russell RM, Rosenberg IH, Wilson PD, Iber FL, Oaks EB, Giovetti AC et al. Increased urinary excretion and prolonged turnover time of folic acid during ethanol ingestion. Am J Clin Nutr. 1983;38:64–70.
150. Tamura T, Romero JJ, Watson JE, Gong EJ, Halsted CH. Hepatic folate metabolism in the chronic alcoholic monkey. J Lab Clin Med. 1981;97:654–61.
151. Tamura T, Halsted CH. Folate turnover in chronically alcoholic monkeys. J Lab Clin Med. 1983;101:623–8.
152. Herbert V. Vitamin B_{12}: An overview. In: Herbert V, ed. Vitamin B_{12} Deficiency. Round Table Series 66. London: Royal Society of Medicine Press, 1999; pp. 1–8.
153. Herbert V, Zalusky R, Davidson C. Correlation of folate deficiency with alcoholism and associated macrocytosis, anemia, and liver disease. Ann Intern Med. 1963;58:977–88.
154. Klipstein FA, Lindenbaum J. Studies of serum folate levels and folic acid clearances in patients with liver disease. Blood. 1965;25:443–56.
155. Herzlich B, Herbert V. Rapid collection of human intrinsic factor uncontaminated with cobalophilin (R binder). Am J Gastroenterol. 1986;81:678–80.
156. Lindenbaum J, Lieber CS. Effects of chronic ethanol administration on intestinal absorption in man in the absence of nutritional deficiency. Ann NY Acad Sci. 1975;252:228–34.
157. Lindenbaum J, Saha JR, Shea N, Lieber CS. Mechanisms of alcohol-induced malabsorption of vitamin B_{12}. Gastroenterology. 1973;64:762.
158. Findlay J, Sellers E, Forstner G. Lack of effect of alcohol on small intestinal binding of the vitamin B12 – intrinsic factor complex. Can J Physiol Pharmacol. 1976;54:469–76.
159. van der Beek EJ, Lowik MR, Hulshof KF, Kistemaker C. Combinations of low thiamine, riboflavin, vitamin B6 and vitamin C intake among Dutch adults. (Dutch Nutrition Surveillance System). J Am Coll Nutr. 1994;13:383–91.
160. Rosenthal WS, Adham NF, Lopez R, Cooperman JM. Riboflavin deficiency in complicated chronic alcoholism. Am J Clin Nutr. 1973;26:858–60.
161. Kim C-I, Roe DA. Development of fiboflavin deficiency in alcohol-fed hamsters drug-nutrient interactions. Drug-Nutr Interact. 1985;3:99–107.
162. Marotta F, Labadarios D, Frazer L, Girdwood A, Marks IN. Fat-soluble vitamin concentration in chronic alcohol-induced pancreatitis. Dig Dis Sci. 1994;39:993–8.
163. Bjorneboe GE, Bjorneboe A, Hagen BF, Mørland J, Drevon C. Reduced hepatic alphatocopherol content after long-term administration of ethanol to rats. Biochim Biophys Acta. 1987; 918:236–41.
164. Kawase T, Kato S, Lieber CS. Lipid peroxidation and antioxidant defense systems in rat liver after chronic ethanol feeding. Hepatology. 1989;10:815–21.
165. McColister R, Prasad AS, Doe RP. Normal renal magnesium clearance and the effect of water loading, chlorothiazide and ethanol on magnesium excretion. J Lab Clin Med. 1958;52:928–32.
166. Flink EB. Magnesium deficiency in alcoholism. Alcohol Clin Exp Res. 1986;10:590–4.
167. Abbott L, Nadler J, Rude RK. Magnesium deficiency in alcoholism: possible contribution to osteoporosis and cardiovascular disease in alcoholics. Alcohol Clin Exp Res. 1994;18:1076–82.
168. Wu C, Kenny MA. Circulating total and ionized magnesium after ethanol ingestion. Clin Chem. 1996;42:625–9.
169. Volini F, de la Huerga J, Kent G et al. Trace metal studies in liver disease using atomic absorption spectroscopy. In: Sunderman FW, Sunderman FW Jr, eds. Laboratory Diagnosis of Liver Disease. St. Louis: WH Green, 1968: pp. 199–206.
170. Chapman RW, Morgan MY, Bell R, Sherlock S. Hepatic iron uptake in alcoholic liver disease. Gastroenterology. 1983;84:143–7.
171. Chapman RW, Morgan MY, Boss AM, Sherlock S. Acute and chronic effects of alcohol on iron absorption. Dig Dis Sci. 1983;28:321–7.
172. Olynk J, Hall P, Sallie R, Reed W, Shilkin K, Mackinnon M. Computerized measurement of iron in liver biopsies: A comparison with biochemical iron measurement. Hepatology. 1990;12:26–30.
173. Bacon BR, Britton S. The pathology of hepatic iron overload: a free radical-mediated process? Hepatology. 1990;11:127–37.
174. Chojkier M, Houglum K, Solis-Herruzo J, Brenner DA. Stimulation of collagen gene expression by ascorbic acid in cultured human fibroblasts. A role for lipid peroxidation? J Biol Chem. 1989;264:16957–62.

175. Vallee BL, Wacker WEC, Bartholomay AF, Robin ED. Zinc metabolism in hepatic dysfunction. I. Serum zinc concentrations Laemne cirrhosis and their validation by sequential analysis. N Engl J Med. 1956;255:403–8.
176. Vallee BL, Wacker EC, Bartholomay AF, Hock F. Zinc metabolism in hepatic dysfunction. Correlations of metabolic patterns with biochemical findings. N Engl J Med. 1957;257:1055–65.
177. Sullivan JF. The relation of zincuria to water and electrolyte excretion in patients with hepatic cirrhosis. Gastroenterology. 1962;42:439–42.
178. Sullivan JF. Effect of alcohol on urinary zinc excretion. Q J Stud Alcohol. 1962;23:216–20.
179. Sandstead HH. Zinc nutrition in the United States. Am J Clin Nutr. 1973;26:1251–60.
180. Valberg LS, Flanagan PR, Ghent CN, Chamberlain MJ. Zinc absorption and leukocyte zinc in alcoholic and nonalcoholic cirrhosis. Dig Dis Sci. 1985;30:329–39.
181. Poo JL, Rosas-Romero R, Rodriguez F, Silencio JL, Muñoz R, Bourges H, Uribe M. Serum zinc concentrations in two cohorts of 153 healthy subjects and 100 cirrhotic patients from Mexico City. Dig Dis. 1995;13:136–42.
182. Hartoma TR, Sontaniemi RA, Pelkonen O, Ahlqvist J. Serum zinc and serum copper and indices of drug metabolism in alcoholics. Eur J Clin Pharmacol. 1977;12:147–51.
183. Sullivan JF, Williams RV, Burch RE. The metabolism of zinc and selenium in cirrhotic patients during six weeks of zinc ingestion. Alcohol Clin Exp Res. 1979;3:235–9.
184. Szutowski MM, Lipsaka M, Bandolet JP. Effect of ethanol on subcellular metal distribution in rat liver. Polish J Pharmacol Pharm. 1976;28:397–401.
185. Versieck J, Hoste J, Vanballenberghe L, Barbier F, Cornelis R, Wallput I. Serum molibdenium in diseases of the liver and biliary system. J Lab Clin Med. 1981;97:535–44.
186. Perlow W, Baraona E, Lieber CS. Symptomatic intestinal disaccharidase deficiency in alcoholics. Gastroenterology. 1977;72:680–4.
187. Marin GA, Ward NL, Fischer R. Effect of ethanol on pancreatic and biliary secretions in humans. Dig Dis. 1973;18:825–33.
188. Lefevre A, DeCarli LM, Lieber CS. Effect of ethanol on cholesterol and bile acid metabolism. J Lipid Res. 1972;13:48–55.
189. Knodell RG, Kinsey D, Boedeker EC, Collin D. Deoxycholate metabolism in alcoholic cirrhosis. Gastroenterology. 1976;71:196–201.
190. Thomson AD, Majumdar SK. The influence of ethanol on intestinal absorption and utilization of nutrients. Clin Gastroenterol. 1981;10:263–93.
191. Breen KJ, Buttigieg R, Iossifidis S, Lourensz C, Wood B. Jejunal uptake of thiamine hydrochloride in man: influence of alcoholism and alcohol. Am J Clin Nutr. 1985;42:121–6.
192. Katz D, Metz J, van der Westhuyzen J. Intestinal absorption of thiamine from yeast-containing sorghum beer. Am J Clin Nutr. 1985;42:666–70.
193. Lumeng L, Li T-K. Vitamin B_6 metabolism in chronic alcohol abuse. J Clin Invest. 1974;53:693–704.
194. Fonda ML, Brown SG, Pendleton MW. Concentration of vitamin B6 and activities of enzymes of B6 metabolism in the blood of alcoholic and nonalcoholic men. Alcohol Clin Exp Res. 1989;3:804–9.
195. Lumeng LJ. The role of acetaldehyde in mediating the deleterious effect of ethanol on pyridoxal 5′-phosphate metabolism. J Clin Invest. 1978;62:286–93.
196. Lumeng L, Schenker S, Li T-K, Brashear RE, Compton MC. Clearance and metabolisms of plasma pyridoxial 5′ phosphate in the dog. J Lab Clin Med. 1984;103:59–64.
197. Parker TH, Marshall JP, Roberts RK, Wang S, Schiff ER, Wilkinson GR, Schenker, S. Effect of acute alcohol ingestion on plasma pyridoxal 5′-phosphate. Am J Clin Nutr. 1979;32:1246–52.
198. Vech RL, Lumeng L, Li TK. Vitamin B6 metabolism in chronic alcohol abuse. The effect of ethanol oxidation on hepatic pyridoxal 5′-phosphate metabolism. J Clin Invest. 1975;55:1026–32.
199. Finkelstein JD, Martin JJ. Methionine metabolism in mammals. Adaptation to methionine excess. J Biol Chem. 1986;261:1582–7.
200. Hardwick DF, Applegarth DA, Cockcroft DM, Ross PM, Cder RJ. Pathogenesis of methionine-induced toxicity. Metabolism. 1970;19:381–91.
201. Iob V, Coon WW, Sloan W. Free amino acids in liver, plasma and muscle of patients with cirrhosis of the liver. J Surg Res. 1967;7:41–3.

202. Iber FL, Rosen H, Stanley MA, Levenson SM, Chalmers TC. The plasma amino acids in patients with liver failure. J Lab Clin Med. 1957;50:417–25.
203. Fischer JE, Yoshimura N, Aguirre A, James JH, Cummings MG, Abel RM, Deindoerfer F. Plasma amino acids in patients with hepatic encephalopathy. Am J Surg. 1974;127:40–7.
204. Montanari A, Simoni I, Vallisa D, Trifiro A, Colla R, Abbiati R et al. Free amino acids in plasma and skeletal muscle of patients with liver cirrhosis. Hepatology. 1988;8:1034–9.
205. Kinsell L, Harper HA, Barton HC, Michaels GD, Weiss HA. Rate of disappearance from plasma of intravenously administered methionine in patients with liver damage. Science. 1947;106:589–94.
206. Horowitz JH, Rypins EB, Henderson JM, Heymsfield SB, Moffitt SD, Bain RP et al. Evidence for impairment of transsulfuration pathway in cirrhosis. Gastroenterology. 1981;81:668–75.
207. Duce AM, Ortiz P, Cabrero C, Mato JM. S-adenosyl-L-methionine synthetase and phospholipid methyltransferase are inhibited in human cirrhosis. Hepatology. 1988;8:65–8.
208. Lu SC. Methionine adenosyltransferase and liver disease: It's all about SAM. Gastroenterology. 1998;114:403–7.
209. Avila MA, Carretero V, Rodriguez N, Mato J. Regulation by hypoxia of methionine adenosyltransferase activity and gene expression in rat hepatocytes. Gastroenterology. 1998;114:364–71.
210. Finkelstein JD, Cello FP, Kyle WE. Ethanol-induced changes in methionine metabolism in rat liver. Biochem Biophys Res Commun. 1974;61:475–81.
211. Hirata F, Axelrod J. Phospholipid methylation and biological signal transmission. Science. 1980;209:1082–90.
212. Hirata F, Viveros OH, Diliberto EJ Jr, Axelrod J. Identification and properties of two methyltransferases in conversion of phosphatidylethanolamine to phosphatidylcholine. Proc Natl Acad Sci USA. 1978;75:1718–21.
213. Yamada S, Mak KM, Lieber CS. Chronic ethanol consumption alters rat liver plasma membranes and potentiates release of alkaline phosphatase. Gastroenterology. 1985;88:1799–806.
214. Stramentinoli G, Gualano M, Galli-Kienle G. Intestinal absorption of S-adenosyl-L-methionine. J Pharmacol Exp Ther. 1979;209:323–6.
215. Bornbardieri G, Pappalardo G, Bernardi L, Barra D, Di Palma A, Castrini G. Intestinal absorption of S-adenosyl-L-methionine in humans. Int J Clin Pharmacol Ther Toxicol. 1983;21:186–8.
216. Hoffinan DR, Marion DW, Cornatzer WE, Duerra JA. S-adenosylmethionine and S-adenosylhomocysteine metabolism in isolated rat liver. J Biol Chem. 1980;255:10822–7.
217. Travers J, Varela I, Mato JM. Effect of exogenous S-adenosyl-L-methionine on phosphatidylcholine synthesis by isolated rat hepatocytes. Biochem Pharmacol. 1984;33:1562–4.
218. Pezzoli C, Stramentinoli G, Galli-Kienele M, Plaff E. Uptake and metabolism of S-adenosyl-L-methionine by isolated rat hepatocytes. Biochem Biophys Res Commun. 1978;85:1031–8.
219. Engstrom MA, Benevenga NJ. Rates of oxidation of the methionine and S-adenosylmethionine methyl carbons in isolated rat hepatocytes. J Nutr. 1987;117:1820–6.
220. Giulidori P, Stramentinoli G. A radioenzymatic method for S-adenosyl-L-methionine determination in biological fluids. Anal Biochem. 1984;137:217–20.
221. Giudici GA, Le Grazie C, Di Padova C. The use of ademethionine (SAMe) in the treatment of cholestatic liver disorders: meta-analysis of clinical trials. In: Mato JM, Lieber C, Kaplowitz N, Caballero A, eds. Methionine Metabolism: Molecular Mechanism and Clinical Implications. Madrid: CSIC Press, 1992;67–79.
222. Frezza M, Pozzato G, Chiesa L, Stramentinoli G, Di Padova C. Reversal of intrahepatic cholestasis of pregnancy in women after high dose S-adenosyl-L-methionine administration. Hepatology. 1984;4:274–8.
223. Frezza M, Surrenti C, Manzillo G, Fiaccadori F, Bortolini M, Di Padova C. Oral S-adenosylmethionine in the symptomatic treatment of intrahepatic cholestasis: a double-blind placebo controlled study. Gastroenterology. 1990;99:211–15.
224. Vendemiale G, Altomare E, Trizio T, Le Grazie C, Di Padova C, Salerno MT et al. Effect of oral S-adenosyl-L-methionine on hepatic glutathione in patients with liver disease. Scand J Gastroenterol. 1989;24:407–15.
225. Mato JM, Cámara J, Fernández de Paz J, Caballería L, Coll S, Caballero A et al. S-Adenosylmethionine in alcoholic liver cirrhosis: A randomized, placebo-controlled, double-blind, multicentre clinical trial. J Hepatol. 1999;30:1081–9.

226. Lieber CS, Robins SJ, Li J, DeCarli, Mak KM, Fasulo JM, Leo MA. Phosphatidylcholine protects against fibrosis and cirrhosis in the baboon. Gastroenterology. 1994;106:152–9.
227. Lieber CS, Leo MA, Mak KM, DeCarli LM, Sato S. Choline fails to prevent liver fibrosis in ethanol-fed baboons but causes toxicity. Hepatology. 1985;5:561–72.
228. Zeisel S, Busztajn JK. Choline and human nutrition. Annu Rev Nutr. 1994;14:269–96.
229. Nanji AA, French SW. Dietary linoleic acid is required for development of experimentally induced alcoholic liver injury. Life Sci. 1989;44:223–7.
230. Lekim D, Graf E. Tierexperimentelle Studien zur Pharmakokinetik der 'essentiellen' Phospholipide (EPL). Drug Res Arznèimittel-Forsch. 1976;26:1772–82.
231. Zern MA, Leo MA, Giambrone MA, Lieber CS. Increased type I procollagen mRNA levels and in vitro protein synthesis in the baboon model of chronic alcoholic liver disease. Gastroenterology. 1985;89:1123–31.
232. Poniachik J, Baraona E, Lieber CS. Dilinoleoylphosphatidylcholine (DLPC) prevents hepatic stellate cell activation. Hepatology. 1996;24:462A.
233. Arai M, Leo MA, Nakano M, Gordon ER, Lieber CS. Biochemical and morphological alterations of baboon hepatic mitochondria after chronic ethanol consumption. Hepatology. 1984;4:165–74.
234. Arai M, Gordon ER, Lieber CS. Decreased cytochrome oxidase activity in hepatic mitochondria after chronic ethanol consumption and the possible role of decreased cytochrome aa_3 content and changes in phospholipids. Biochim Biophys Acta. 1984;797:320–7.
235. Navder KP, Baraona E, Lieber CS. Polyenylphosphatidylcholine attenuates alcohol-induced fatty liver and hyperlipemia in rats. J Nutr. 1997;127:1800–6.
236. Hoek JB, Thomas AP, Rooney TA, Higashi K, Rubin E. Ethanol and signal transduction in the liver. Fed Am Soc Exp Biol J. 1992;6:2386–96.
237. Ma X, Zhao J, Lieber CS. Polyenylphosphatidylcholine attenuates non-alcoholic hepatic fibrosis and accelerates its regression. J Hepatol. 1996;24:604–13.
238. Li J-J, Kim C-I, Leo MA, Mak KM, Rojkind M, Lieber CS. Polyunsaturated lecithin prevents acetaldehyde-mediated hepatic collagen accumulation by stimulating collagenase activity in cultured stellate cells. Hepatology. 1992;15:373–81.
239. Lieber CS, Leo MA, Aleynik SI, Aleynik MK, DeCarli LM. Polyenylphosphatidylcholine decreases alcohol-induced oxidative stress in the baboon. Alcohol Clin Exp Res. 1997;21:375–9.
240. Niederau C, Strohmeyer G, Heinges T, Peter K, Gopfert E, Leich Study Group. Polyunsaturated phosphatidyl-choline and interferon alpha for treatment of chronic hepatitis B and C: a multi-center, randomized, double blind, placebo-controlled trial. Hepato Gastroenterol. 1998;45:797–804.
241. Leo MA, Lieber CS. Alcohol, vitamin A, and beta-carotene: Adverse interactions, including hepatotoxicity and carcinogenicity. Am J Clin Nutr. 1999;69:1071–85.
242. Vahlquist A, Sjolund K, Norden A, Pererson PA, Stigmar G, Johansson B. Plasma vitamin A transport and visual dark adaptation in diseases of the intestine and liver. Scand J Clin Lab Invest. 1978;38:301–8.
243. Leo MA, Lieber CS. Hepatic vitamin A depletion in alcoholic liver injury. N Engl J Med. 1982;307:597–601.
244. Sato M, Lieber CS. Changes in vitamin A status after acute ethanol administration in the rat. J Nutr. 1982;112:1188–96.
245. Sato M, Lieber CS. Increased metabolism of retinoic acid after chronic ethanol consumption in rat liver microsomes. Arch Biochem Biophys. 1982;213:557–64.
246. Duester G. Involvement of alcohol dehydrogenase, short-chain dehydrogenase/reductase, acetaldehyde dehydrogenase, and cytochrome P450 in the control of retinoid signaling by activation of retinoic acid synthesis. Biochemistry. 1996;35:12221–7.
247. Leo MA, Lowe N, Lieber CS. Decreased hepatic vitamin A after drug administration in men and in rats. Am J Clin Nutr. 1984;40:1131–6.
248. Reddy TV, Weisburger EK. Hepatic vitamin A status of rats during feeding of hepatocarcinogen 2-aminoanthrequinone. Cancer Lett. 1980;10:39–44.
249. Leo MA, Lowe N, Lieber CS. Potentiation of ethanol-induced hepatic vitamin A depletion by phenobarbital and butylated hydroxytoluene. J Nutr. 1987;117:70–6.
250. Roberts AB, Lamb LC, Spron MB. Metabolism of all-*trans*-retinoic acid in hamster liver microsomes: Oxidation of 4-hydroxy- to 4-keto retinoic acid. Arch Biochem Biophys. 1980;234:374–83.

251. Leo MA, Iida S, Lieber CS. Retinoic acid metabolism by a system reconstituted with cytochrome P-450. Arch Biochem Biophys. 1984;234:305–12.
252. Leo MA, Lieber CS. New pathway for retinol metabolism in liver microsomes. J Biol Chem. 1985;260:5228–31.
253. Tomita S, Okuyama E, Ohnishi T, Ichikawa Y. Characteristic properties of a retinoic acid synthetic cytochrome P-450 purified from liver microsomes of 3-methylcholanthrene-induced rats. Biochimica Biophys Acta. 1996;1290:273–81.
254a. Leo MA, Kim C, Lieber CS. NAD+-dependent retinol dehydrogenase in liver microsomes. Arch Biochem Biophys. 1987;259:241–9.
254b. Leo MA, Kim CI, Lowe N, Lieber CS. Increased hepatic retinal dehydrogenase activity after phenobarbital and ethanol administration. Biochem Pharmacol. 1989;38:97–103.
255. Zachman RD, Olson JA. A comparison of retinene reductase and alcohol dehydrogenase of rat liver. J Biochem Chem. 1961;236:2309–13.
256. Mezey E, Holt PR. The inhibitory effect of ethanol on retinol oxidation by human liver and cattle retina. Exp Mol Pathol. 1971;15:148–56.
257. Leo MA, Lieber CS. Normal testicular structure and reproductive function in deermice lacking retinol and alcohol dehydrogenase activity. J Clin Invest. 1984;73:593–6.
258. Leo MA, Lasker JM, Raucy JL, Kim C, Black M, Lieber CS. Metabolism of retinol and retinoic acid by human liver cytochrome P450IIC8. Arch Biochem Biophys. 1989;269:305–12.
259. Leo MA, Sato M, Lieber CS. Effect of hepatic vitamin A depletion on the liver in humans and rats. Gastroenterology. 1983;84:562–72.
260. Leo MA, Arai M, Sato M, Lieber CS. Exacerbation by ethanol of liver injury due to vitamin A deficiency and excess. In: CS Lieber, ed. Biological Approach to Alcoholism: Update. Research Monograph-11, DHHS Publication No. (ADM) 83–1261, Superintendent of Documents. Washington, DC: US Government Printing Office; 1983: pp. 195–233.
261. Davis BH, Vucic A. The effect of retinol on Ito cell proliferation in vitro. Hepatology. 1988;8:788–93.
262. Davis BH, Kramer RJ, Davidson NO. Retinoic acid modulates rat Ito cell proliferation, collagen, and transforming growth factor β production. J Clin Invest. 1990;86:2062–70.
Anonymous. Vitamin A, retinol, carotene, and cancer prevention (editorial). Br Med J. 1980;281:957–8.
263. Friedman SL, Wei S, Blaner W. Retinol release by activated rat hepatic lipocytes: regulation by Kupffer cell-conditioned medium and PDGF. Am J Physiol. 1993;264:G947–52.
Sporn MB. Prevention of epithelial cancer by vitamin A and its synthetic analogs. In: Hiatt HH, Watson JD, Winsten JA, eds. Origins of Human Cancer. New York: Cold Spring Harbor, 1977.
264. Atukorala S, Basu TK, Dickerson WT, Donaldson D, Sakula A. Vitamin A, zinc and lung cancer. Br J Cancer. 1979;40:927–31.
265. Basu TK, Donaldson D, Jenner M, Williams DG, Sakula A. Plasma, vitamin A in patients with carcinoma. Br J Cancer. 1976;33:119–21.
266. Wald N, Idle M, Boreham J, Bailey A. Low serum vitamin A and subsequent risk of cancer. Lancet. 1980;2:813–15.
267. Kark JS, Smith AH, Switzer BR, Hames CG. Serum vitamin A (retinol) and cancer incidence in Evans County, Georgia. J Natl Cancer Inst. 1981;66:7–16.
268. Auerbach O, Stout AP, Hammond EC, Garfinkel L. Changes in bronchial epithelium in relation to cigarette smoking and in relation to lung cancer. N Engl J Med. 1961;265:253–67.
269. Becci PJ, McDowell EM, Trump BF. The respiratory epithelium. IV. Histogenesis of epidermoid nietaplasia and carcinoma *in situ* in the hamster. J Natl Cancer Inst. 1978;61:577–86.
270. Harris CC, Kaufman DG, Sporn MB, Saffiotti U. Histogenesis of squamous metaplasia and squamous cell carcinoma of the respiratory epithelium in an animal model. Cancer Chemother Rep. 1973;4:43–54.
271. Saffiotti U, Montesano R, Sellakumar AR, Borg SA. Experimental cancer of the lung. Inhibition by vitamin A of the induction of tracheobronchial squamous metaplasia and squamous cell tumor. Cancer. 1967;20:857–64.
272. Schreiber H, Saccomanno G, Martin DH, Brennan L. Sequential cytological changes during development of respiratory tract tumor induced in hamsters by benzo(a)pyrene fenric oxide. Cancer Res. 1974;34:689–98.

273. Stenback F, Sellakumar. A. Squamous metaplasia and respiratory tumors induced by intratracheal instillations of 7, 12-dimethylbenz(a)anthracene in Syrian golden hamsters. Eur J Cancer. 1974;10:483–6.
274. Trump BF, McDowell EM, Glavin F, Barett LA, Becci PJ, Schorch W, Kaiser HE. The respiratory epithelium. III. Histogenesis of epidermoid metaplasia and carcinoma in situ in the human. J Natl Cancer Inst. 1978;61:563–75.
275. Umiker W, Storey C. Bronchogenic carcinoma in situ. Report of a case with positive biopsy, cytological examination, and lobectomy. Cancer. 1952;5:369–74.
276. Weller RW. Metaplasia of bronchial epithelium: a postmortem study. Am J Clin Pathol. 1953;23:768–74.
277. Williams MJ. Extensive carcinoma in situ or the bronchial mucosa associated with two invasive bronchogenic carcinomas. Report of a case. Cancer. 1952;5:740–7.
278. Valentine. EH. Squamous metaplasia of the bronchus. A study of metaplastic change occurring in the epithelium of the major bronchus in cancerous and noncancerous cases. Cancer. 1957;10:272–9.
279. Mak KM, Leo MA, Lieber CS. Potentiation by ethanol consumption of tracheal squamous metaplasia caused by vitamin A deficiency in rats. J Natl Cancer Inst. 1987;79:1001–10.
280. Kvale G, Bielke F, Gart JJ. Dietary habits and lung cancer risk. Int J Cancer. 1983;31:397–405.
281. Pollack ES, Nomura AMY, Heilbrum L, Steimmermann GN, Green SB. Prospective study of alcohol consumption and cancer. N Engl J Med. 1984;310:617–21.
282. Leo MA, Lowe N, Lieber CS. Interaction of drugs and retinol. Biochem Pharmacol. 1986;35:3949–53.
283. Wang X, Liu C, Chung J, Stickel F, Seitz HK, Russell RM. Chronic alcohol intake reduces retinoic acid concentration and enhances AP-1 (c-Jun and c-Fos) expression in rat liver. Hepatology. 1998;28:744–50.
284. Duester G. Alcohol dehydrogenase as a critical mediator of retinoic acid synthesis from vitamin A in the mouse embryo. J Nutr. 1998;128:459S–62S.
285. Haselbeck RJ, Duester G. Regional restriction of alcohol/retinol dehydrogenases along the mouse gastrointestinal epithelium. Alcohol Clin Exp Res. 1997;21:1484–90.
286. Duester G. A hypothetical mechanism for fetal alcohol syndrome involving ethanol inhibition of retinoic acid synthesis at the alcohol dehydrogenase step. Alcohol Clin Exp Res. 1991;15:565–72.
287. Pullarkat RK. Hypothesis. Prenatal ethanol-induced birth defects and retinoic acid. Alcohol Clin Exp Res. 1991;15:565–7.
288. Deltour L, Ang HL, Duester G. Ethanol inhibition of retinoic acid synthesis as a potential mechanism for fetal alcohol syndrome. FASEB J. 1996;10:1050–7.
289. Chen H, Namkung J, Juchau MR. Effects of ethanol on biotransformation of all-trans-retinol and all-trans-retinal to all-trans-retinoic acid in rat conceptal cytosol. Alcohol Clin Exp Res. 1996;20:942–7.
290. Kedishvili NY, Gough WH, Chernoff EAG, Hurley TD, Stone CL, Bowman KD et al. cDNA sequence and catalytic properties of a chick embryo alcohol dehydrogenase that oxidizes retinol and $3\beta,5''$-hydroxysteroids. J Biol Chem. 1997;272:7494–500.
291. Tuyns AJ, Riboli E, Doornbos G, Pequignot G. Diet and esophageal cancer in Calvados (France). Nutr Cancer. 1987;9:81–92.
292. DeCarli A, Liati P, Negri E, Franceschi S, La Vecchia C. Vitamin A and other dietary factors in the etiology of esoghageal cancer. Nutr Cancer. 1987;10:29–37.
293. Graham S, Marshall J, Haughey B, Brasure J, Fredenheim J, Zielezny M et al. Nutritional epidemiology of cancer of the esophagus. Am J Epidemiol. 1990;131:454–67.
294. Soprano DR, Soprano KJ. Retinoids as teratogens. Annu Rev Nutr. 1995;111–32.
295. Lammer EJ, Chen DT, Hoar RM, Agnish ND, Benke PJ, Braun JT et al. Retinoic acid embryopathy. N Engl J Med. 1985;313:837–41.
296. Rothman KJ, Moore LL, Singer MR, Nguyen U, Mannino S, Milunsky A. Teratogenicity of high vitamin A intake. N Engl J Med. 1995:333:1369–73.
297. Oakley GP, Erickson JD. Vitamin A and birth defects. N Eng J Med. 1995;333:1414–15.
298. Karl PI, Gordon BH, Lieber CS, Fisher SE. Acetaldehyde production and transfer by the perfused human placental cotyledon. Science. 1988;242:273–5.
299. Abel EL, Sokol RJ. A revised conservative estimate of the incidence of FAS and its economic impact. Alcohol Clin Exp Res. 1991;15:514–24.

300. Whitby KE, Collins TFX, Welsh JJ, Black TN, Llynn T, Sharckelford M et al. Developmental effects of combined exposure to ethanol and vitamin A. Food Chem Toxicol. 1994;32:305–20.
301. Russell RM, Boyer JL, Bagheri SA, Hruban Z. Hepatic injury from chronic hypervitaminosis A resulting in portal hypertension and ascites. N Engl J Med. 1974;291:435–40.
302. Farrell GC, Bathal PS, Powell LW. Abnormal liver function in chronic hypervitaminosis A. Dig Dis Sci. 1977;22:724–8.
303. Geubel AP, DeGalocsy C, Alves N, Rahier J, Dive C. Liver damage caused by therapeutic vitamin A administration: estimate of dose related toxicity in 41 cases. Gastroenterology. 1991;100:1701–9.
304. Leo MA, Arai M, Sato M, Lieber CS. Hepatotoxicity of vitamin A and ethanol in the rat. Gastroenterology. 1982;82:194–205.
305. Worner TM, Gordon G, Leo MA, Lieber CS. Treatment with vitamin A of sexual dysfunction in male alcoholics. Am J Clin Nutr. 1988;48:1431–5.
306. Minuk GY, Kelly JK, Hwang WS. Vitamin A hepatoxicity in multiple family members. Hepatology. 1988;8:272–5.
307. Leo MA, Lieber CS. Hypervitaminosis A: A liver lover's lament. Hepatology. 1988;8:412–17.
308. Leo MA, Lieber CS. Hepatic fibrosis after long term administration of ethanol and moderate vitamin A supplementation in the rat. Hepatology. 1983;3:1–11.
309. Olson JA. Recommended dietary intakes (RDI) of vitamin A in humans. Am J Clin Nutr. 1987;45:704–16.
310. Heywood R, Palmer AK, Gregson RL, Hummler H. The toxicity of beta-carotene. Toxicity. 1985;36:91–100.
311. Ahmed S, Leo MA, Lieber CS. Interactions between alcohol and beta-carotene in patients with alcoholic liver disease. Am J Clin Nutr. 1994;60:430–6.
312. Ward RJ, Peters TJ. The antioxidant status of patients with either alcohol-induced liver damage or myopathy. Alcohol Alcohol. 1992;27:359–65.
313. Forman MR, Beecher GR, Lanza E, Reichman ME, Graubard BI, Campbell WS et al. Effect of alcohol consumption on plasma carotenoid concentrations in premenopausal women: A controlled dietary study. Am J Clin Nutr. 1995;62:131–5.
314. Leo MA, Kim CI, Lowe N, Lieber CS. Interaction of ethanol with β-carotene: Delayed blood clearance and enhanced hepatotoxicity. Hepatology. 1992;15:883–91.
315. Leo MA, Aleynik S, Aleynik M, Lieber CS. β-Carotene beadlets potentiate hepatotoxicity of alcohol. Am J Clin Nutr. 1997;66:1461–9.
316. Greenberg ER, Baron JA, Karagas MR, Stukel TA, Nierenberg DW, Stevens MM et al. Mortality associated with low plasma concentration of beta carotene and the effect of oral supplementation. JAMA. 1996;275:699–703.
317. Hennekens CH, Buring JE, Manson JE, Stamfer M, Rosner B, Cook NR et al. Lack of effect of long-term supplementation with beta carotene on the incidence of malignant neoplasms and cardiovascular disease. N Engl J Med. 1996;334:1145–9.
318. Bowan HT, Omaye ST. Oxidative changes associated with beta-carotene and alpha-tocopherol enrichment of human low-density lipoproteins. J Am Coll Nutr. 1998;17:171–9.
319. α-Tocopherol, β-carotene and Cancer Prevention Study Group. The effect of vitamin E and β-carotene on the incidence of lung cancer and other cancers in male smokers. N Engl J Med. 1994;330:1029–35.
320. Omenn GS, Goodman GE, Thornquist MD, Balmes J, Cullen MR, Glass A et al. Effects of a combination of beta carotene and vitamin A on lung cancer and cardiovascular disease. N Engl J Med. 1996;334:1150–5.
321. Leo MA, Lieber CS. Beta carotene, vitamin E, and lung cancer. N Engl J Med. 1994;331:612.
322. Garro AJ, Gordon BHJ, Lieber CS. Alcohol Abuse: Carcinogenic effects and fetal alcohol-syndrome. In: Lieber CS, ed. Medical and Nutritional Complications of Alcoholism: Mechanisms and Management. New York: Plenum Press, 1992; p. 459.
323. Paolini M, Forti GC, Perocco P, Pedulli GF, Abdel-Rahmans SZ, Legators MS. Co-carcinogenic effect of β-carotene. Nature. 1999;398:760–1.
324. Jewell C, O'Brien N. Effect of dietary supplementation with carotenoids on xenobiotic metabolizing enzymes in the liver, lung, kidney and small intestine of the rat. Br J Nutr. 1999;81:235–42.
325. Burton GW, Ingold KU. β-Carotene: An unusual type of lipid antioxidant. Science. 1984;224:569–73.

326. Lowe GM, Booth LA, Young AJ, Biton RF. Lycopene and β-carotene protect against oxidative damage in HT29 cells at low concentrations but rapidly lose this capacity at higher doses. Free Rad Res. 1999;30:141–51.
327. Woods JA, Bilton RF, Young AJ. β-Carotene enhances hydrogen peroxide-induced DNA damage in human hepatocellular Hep G2 cells. FEBS Lett. 1999;449:255–8.
328. Albanes D, Heinonen OP, Taylor PR, Virtamo J, Edwards BK, Rautalahti M et al. α-Tocopherol and β-carotene supplements and lung cancer incidence in the Alpha-Tocopherol, Beta-Carotene Cancer Prevention Study: Effects of base-line characteristics and study compliance. J Natl Cancer Inst. 1996;88:1560–71.
329. Omenn GS, Goodman GE, Thornquist MD, Balmes J, Cullen MR, Glass A et al. Risk factors for lung cancer and for intervention effects in CARET, the beta-carotene and retinol efficacy trial. J Natl Cancer Inst. 1996;88:1550–9.
330. Albanes D, Virtamo J, Taylor PR, Rautalahti M, Pietinen P, Heinonen OP. Effects of supplemental β-carotene, cigarette smoking, and alcohol consumption on serum carotenoids in the alpha tocopherol, beta-carotene cancer prevention study. Am J Clin Nutr. 1997;66:366–72.
331. Leo MA, Seitz HK, Maier H, Lieber CS. Carotenoid, retinoid and vitamin E status of the orpharyngeal mucosa in the alcoholic. Alcohol Alcohol. 1995;30:163–70.
332. Bishayee A, Sarkar A, Chatterjee M. Further evidence for chemopreventive potential of beta-carotene against experimental carcinogenesis: diethylnitrosamine-initiated and phenobarbital-promoted hepatocarcinogenesis is prevented more effectively by beta-carotene than by retinoic acid. Nutr Cancer. 2000;37:89–98.
333. Kune GA, Bannerman S, Field B, Watson LF, Cleland H, Merenstein D, Vitetta L. Diet, alcohol, smoking, serum β-carotene, and vitamin A in male nonmelanocytic skin cancer patients and controls. Nutr Cancer. 1992;18:237–44.
334. Menkes MS, Comstock GW, Vuilleumier JP, Helsing KJ, Rider AA, Brookmeyer R. Serum beta-carotene, vitamins A and E, selenium, and the risk of lung cancer. N Engl J Med. 1986;315:1250–4.
335. Bode JL, Goebell H, Stahler M. Changes in alcohol dehydrogenase activity in rat liver following protein deficiency and ethanol. Z Gesamte Exp Med. 1970;152:111–24.
336. Bode CH, Buchwald B, Goebell H. Inhibition of ethanol breakdown due to protein deficiency in man. German Med. 1971;1:149–51.
337. Meijer AJ, Van Woebkon GM, Williamson JR, Tager JM. Rate-limiting factors in the oxidation of ethanol by isolated rat liver cells. Biochem J. 1975;150:205–9.
338. Korsten MA, Matsuzaki S, Feinman L, Lieber CS. High blood acetaldehyde levels after ethanol administration: Differences between alcoholic and non-alcoholic subjects. N Engl J Med. 1975;292:386–9.
339. Lieber CS, Lasker JM, DeCarli LM, Saeli J, Wojtowicz T. Role of acetone, dietary fat and total energy intake in induction of hepatic microsomal ethanol oxidizing system. J Pharmacol Exp Ther. 1988;1247:791–5.
340. Israel Y, Kalant H, Orrego H, Khanna JM, Videla L, Phillips JM. Experimental alcohol-induced hepatic necrosis: Suppression by propylthiouracil. Proc Natl Acad Sci USA. 1975;72:1137–41.
341. Kessler BJ, Lieber JB, Bronfin GJ, Sass M. The hepatic blood flow and splanchnic oxygen consumption in alcohol fatty liver. J Clin Invest. 1954;33:1338–45.
342. Sato N, Kamada T, Kawano S, Hayashi N, Kishida Y, Meren H et al. Effect of acute and chronic ethanol consumption on hepatic tissue oxygen tension in rats. Pharmacology. 1983;18:443–7.
343. Shaw S, Heller E, Friedman H, Baraona E, Lieber CS. Increased hepatic oxygenation following ethanol administration in the baboon. Proc Soc Exp Biol Med. 1977;56:509–13.
344. Stein SW, Lieber CS, Leevy CM, Cherrick GR, Abelmann WH. The effect of ethanol upon systemic hepatic blood flow in man. Am J Clin Nutr. 1963;13:68–74.
345. Carmichael FJ, Saldivia V, Israel Y, McKaigney JP, Orrego H. Ethanol-induced increase in portal hepatic blood flow: interference by anesthetic agents. Hepatology. 1987;7:89–94.
346. Lieber CS, Baraona E, Hernández-Muñoz R, Kubota S, Sato N, Kawano S et al. Impaired oxygen utilization: A new mechanism for the hepatotoxicity of ethanol in sub-human primates. J Clin Invest. 1989;83:1682–90.

347. Casini A, Cunningham M, Rojkind M, Lieber CS. Acetaldehyde increases procollagen type I and fibronectin gene transcription in cultured rat fat-storing cells through a protein synthesis-dependent mechanism. Hepatology. 1991;13:758–65.
348. Lieber CS, DeCarli LM. Reduced nicotinamide-adenine dinucleotide phosphate oxidase: Activity enhanced by ethanol consumption. Science. 1970;170:78–80.
349. Dai Y, Rashba-Step J, Cederbaum AI. Stable expression of human cytochrome P4502E1 in HepG2 cells: characterization of catalytic activities and production of reactive oxygen intermediates. Biochemistry. 1993;32:6928–37.
350. Ekstrom G, Ingelman-Sundberg M. Rat liver microsomal NADPH-supported oxidase activity and lipid peroxidation dependent on ethanol-inducible cytochrome P-450 (P-450IIE1). Biochem Pharmacol. 1989;38:1313–19.
351. Castillo T, Koop DR, Kamimura S, Triadafilopoulos G, Tsukamoto. Role of cytochrome P-450 2E1 in ethanol-, carbon tetrachloride- and iron-dependent microsomal lipid peroxidation. Hepatology. 1992;16:992–6.
352. Albano E, Tomasi A, Goria-Gatti L, Poli G, Vannini B, Dianzani MU. Free radical metabolism of alcohols in rat liver microsomes. Free Rad Res Commun. 1987;3:243.
353. Reinke L, Lai EK, DuBose CM, McCay PB, Janzen EG. Reactive free radical generation in vivo in heart and liver of ethanol-fed rats: Correlation with radical formation in vitro. Proc Natl Acad Sci USA. 1987;84:8223–7.
354. Reinke LA, Kotake Y, McCay PB, Janzen EG. Spin trapping studies of hepatic free radicals formed following the acute administration of ethanol to rats: in vivo detection of l-hydroxyethyl radicals with PBN. Free Rad Biol Med. 1991;11:31–9.
355. Koivisto T, Mishin VM, Mak KM, Cohen PA, Lieber, CS. Induction of cytochrome P-4502E1 by ethanol in rat Kupffer cells. Alcohol Clin Exp Res. 1996;20:207–12.
356. Müller A, Sies H. Role of alcohol dehydrogenase activity and of acetaldehyde in ethanol-induced ethane and pentane production by isolated perfused rat liver. Biochem J. 1982;206:153–6.
357. Müller A, Sies H. Inhibition of ethanol- and aldehyde-induced release of ethane from isolated perfused rat liver by Pargyline and Disulfiram. Pharmacol Biochem Behav. 1983;18:429–32.
358. Shaw S, Rubin KP, Lieber CS. Depressed hepatic glutathione and increased diene conjugates in alcoholic liver disease: Evidence of lipid peroxidation. Dig Dis Sci. 1983;28:585–9.
359. Hirano T, Kaplowitz N, Tsukamoto H, Kamimura S, Fernandez-Checa JC. Hepatic mitochondrial glutathione depletion and progression of experimental alcoholic liver disease in rats. Hepatology. 1992;6:1423–7.
360. Gebhardt AC, Lucas D, Ménez JF, Seitz HK. Chlormethiazole inhibition of cytochrome P450 2E1 as assessed by chlorzoxazone hydroxylation in humans. Hepatology. 1997;26:957–61.
361. Fang C, Lindros KO, Badger TM, Ronis MJJ, Ingelman-Sundberg M. Zonated expression of cytokines in rat liver: effect of chronic ethanol and the cytochrome P450 2E1 inhibitor, chlormethiazole. Hepatology. 1998;27:1304–10.
362. Eap CB, Schnyder C, Besson J, Savary L, Buclin T. Inhibition of CYP2E1 by chlormethiazole as measured by chlorzoxazone pharmacokinetics in patients with alcoholism and in healthy volunteers. Clin Pharmacol Ther. 1998;64:52–7.
363. French S, Morimoto M, Reitz R, Koop D, Klopfenstein B, Estes K et al. Lipid peroxidation, CYP2E1 and arachidonic acid metabolism in alcoholic liver disease in rats. J Nutr. 1997;127:907S–11S.
364. Kim ND, Kwak MK, Kim SG. Inhibition of cytochrome P450 2E1 expression by 2-(allylthio) pyrazine, a potential chemoprotective agent: hepatoprotective effects. Biochem Pharmacol. 1997;53:261–9.
365. Morimoto M, Hagbjork AL, Nanji AA, Ingelman-Sundberg M, Lindros KO, Fu PC et al. Role of cytochrome P450 2E1 in alcoholic liver disease pathogenesis. Alcohol. 1993;10:459–64.
366. Morimoto M, Hagbjork AL, Wan YJY, Fu PC, Clot P, Albano E et al. Modulation of experimental alcohol-induced liver disease by cytochrome P450 2E1 inhibitors. Hepatology. 1995;21:1610–17.
367. Mathews, JM, Etheridge AS, Raymer JH, Black SR, Pulliam DW, Bucher JR. Selective inhibition of cytochrome P450 2E1 in vivo and in vitro with trans-1,2-dichloroethylene. Chem Res Toxicol. 1998;11:778–85.
368. Aleynik SI, Leo MA, Aleynik MK, Lieber CS. Polyenylphosphatidylcholine prevents carbon tetrachloride induced lipid peroxidation while it attenuates liver injury and fibrosis. J Hepatol. 1997;26:554–61.

369. Aleynik SI, Leo MA, Takeshige U, Aleynik M, Lieber CS. Dilinoleoylphosphatidylcholine (DLPC) is the active antioxidant of polyenylphosphatidylcholine (PPC). Gastroenterology. 1997;112:1209.
370. Navder KP, Baraona E, Lieber CS. Polyenylphosphatidylcholine decreases alcoholic hyperlipemia without affecting the alcohol-induced rise of HDL-cholesterol. Life Sci. 1997;61:1907–14.
371. Vendemiale G, Jayatilleke E, Shaw S, Lieber CS. Depression of biliary glutathione excretion by chronic ethanol feeding in the rat. Life Sci. 1984;34:1065–73.
372. Vendemiale G, Grattagliano I, Signorile A, Altomare E. Ethanol-induced changes of intracellular thiol compartmentation and protein redox status in the rat liver: effect of tauro-ursodeoxycholate. J Hepatol. 1998;28:46–53.
373. Plevris JN, Hayes PC, Bouchier IAD. Ursodeoxychoic acid in the treatment of alcoholic liver disease. Eur J Gastroenterol Hepatol. 1991;3:653–6.
374. Kerai MD, Waterfield CJ, Kenyon SH, Asker DS, Timbrell JA. Taurine: protective properties against ethanol-induced hepatic steatosis and lipid peroxidation during chronic ethanol consumption in rats. Amino Acids. 1998;15:53–76.
375. Tabouy L, Zamora AJ, Oliva L, Montet AM, Beauge F, Montet JC. Ursodeoxycholate protects against ethanol-induced liver mitochondrial injury. Life Sci. 1998;63:2259–70.
376. Oliva L, Beauge F, Choquart D, Montet AM, Guitaoui M, Montet JC. Ursodeoxycholate alleviates alcoholic fatty liver damage in rats. Alcohol Clin Exp Res. 1998;22:1538–43.
377. Neuman MG, Cameron RG, Shear NH, Bellentani S, Tiribelli C. Effects of tauroursodeoxycholic and ursodeoxycholic acid on ethanol-induced cell injuries in the human hep G2 cell line. Gastroenterology. 1995;109:555–63.
378. von Herbay A, de Groot H, Hegi U, Stremmel W, Strohmeyer G, Sies H. Low vitamin E content in plasma of patients with alcoholic liver disease, hemochromatosis and Wilson's disease. J Hepatol. 1994;20:41–6.
379. Ferenci P, Dragosics B, Dittrich H, Frank H, Benda L, Loch H et al. Randomized controlled trial of silymarin treatment in patients with cirrhosis of the liver. J Hepatol. 1989;9:105–13.
380. Trinchet JC, Coste T, Levy VG, Vivet F, Duchatelle V, Legendre C et al. Treatment of alcoholic hepatitis with silymarin: A double-blind comparitive study in 116 patients. Gastroenterol Clin Biol. 1989;13:120–4.
381. Zhang H, Loney LA, Potter BJ. Effect of chronic alcohol feeding on hepatic iron status and ferritin uptake by rat hepatocytes. Alcohol Clin Exp Res. 1993;17:394–400.
382. Valenzuela A, Fernandez V, Videla LA. Hepatic and biliary levels of glutathione and lipid peroxides following iron overload in the rat: Effect of simultaneous ethanol administration. Toxicol Appl Pharmacol. 1983;70:87–95.
383. Lieber CS, Spritz N, DeCarli LM. Role of dietary, adipose and endogenously synthesized fatty acids in the pathogenesis of the alcoholic fatty liver. J Clin Invest. 1966;45:51–62.
384. Lieber CS, Spritz N. Effects of prolonged ethanol intake in man: Role of dietary, adipose, and endogenously synthesized fatty acids in the pathogenesis of the alcoholic fatty liver. J Clin Invest. 1966;45:1400–11.
385. Lieber CS, DeCarli LM. Quantitative relationship between the amount of dietary fat and the severity of the alcoholic fatty liver. Am J Clin Nutr. 1970;23:474–8.
386. Lieber CS, DeCarli LM. Study of agents for the prevention of the fatty liver produced by prolonged alcohol intake. Gastroenterology. 1966;50:316–22.
387. Lieber CS, Lefevre A, Spritz N, Feinman L, DeCarli LM. Difference in hepatic metabolism of long and medium-chain fatty acids: The role of fatty acid chain length in the production of the alcoholic fatty liver. J Clin Invest. 1967;46:1451–60.
388. Nanji AA, Yang EK, Fogt F, Sadrzadeh SMH, Dannenberg AJ. Medium chain triglycerides and vitamin E reduce the severity of established experimental alcoholic liver disease. J Pharmacol Exp Ther. 1996;277:1694–700.
389. Nolan JP. Intestinal endotoxins as mediators of hepatic injury – an idea whose time has come again. Hepatology. 1989;10:887–91.
390. Nolan JP, Camara DS. Intestinal endotoxins as co-factors in liver injury. Immunol Invest. 1989;18:325–37.
391. Adachi Y, Moore LE, Bradford BU, Gao W, Thurman RG. Antibiotics prevent liver injury in rats following long term exposure to ethanol. Gastroenterology. 1995;108:218–24.

392. Decker K. Biologically active products of stimulated liver macrophages (Kupffer Cells). J Biochem. 1990;192:245–61.
393. Matsuoka M, Tsukamoto H. Stimulation of hepatic lipocyte collagen production by Kupffer cell-derived transforming growth factor beta: implication for a pathogenetic role in alcoholic liver fibrogenesis. Hepatology. 1990;11:599–605.
394. Kamimura S, Tsukamoto H. Cytokine gene expression by Kupffer cells in experimental alcoholic liver disease. Hepatology. 1995;22:1304–9.
395. Bautista AP. The role of Kupffer cells and reactive oxygen species in hepatic injury during acute and chronic alcohol intoxication. Alcohol Clin Exp Res. 1998;22:255S–9S.
396. Batey R, Cao Q, Madsen G, Pang G, Russell A, Clancy R. Decreased tumor necrosis factor-α and interleukin-1α production from intrahepatic mononuclear cells in chronic ethanol consumption and up regulation by endotoxin. Alcohol Clin Exp Res. 1998;22:150–6.
397. Tsukamoto H. Molecular mechanism of induced hepatic macrophage cytokine gene expression in experimental alcoholic liver injury. Alcohol Clin Exp Res. 1998;22:253S–4S.
398. Shibayama Y, Asaka S, Nakata K. Endotoxin hepatotoxicity augmented by ethanol. Exp Mol Pathol. 1991;55:196–301.
399. Khoruts A, Stahnke L, McClain CJ, Logan G, Allen JI. Circulating tumor necrosis factor, interleukin-1 and interleukin-6 concentrations in chronic alcoholic patients. Hepatology. 1991;13:267–76.
400. Sheron N, Bird G, Goka J, Alexander G, Williams R. Elevated plasma interleukin-6 and increased severity and mortality in alcoholic hepatitis. Clin Exp Immunol. 1991;84:449–53.
401. Iimuro Y, Gallucci RM, Luster MI, Kono H, Thurman RG. Antibodies to tumor necrosis factor alfa attenuate hepatic necrosis and inflammation caused by chronic exposure to ethanol in the rat. Hepatology. 1997;26:1530–7.
402. Czaja MJ, Xu J, Ah E. Prevention of carbon tetrachloride-induced rat liver injury by soluble tumor necrosis factor. Gastroenterology. 1995;108:1849–54.
403. Tu G-C, Cao W-N, Zhou F, Israel Y. Tetranucleotide GGGA mofit in primary RNA transcripts. J Biol Chem. 1998;273:25125–31.
404. Maddrey WC, Roftnott JK, Bedine MS, Weber FL Jr, Mezey E, White RI Jr. Corticosteroid therapy of alcoholic hepatitis. Gastroenterology. 1978;75:193–9.
405. Carithers RL Jr, Henong F, Dienl AM et al. Methylprednisolone therapy in patients with severe alcoholic hepatitis: A randomized multicenter trial. Ann Intern Med. 1989;110:685–90.
406. Lieber CS, Lefevre A, Luffman F. The effect of prednisolone on the increased blood ammonia level in Eck fistula dogs. Rev Belg Pathol. 1958;26:414–25.
407. Imperiale TF, McCullough AJ. Do corticosteroids reduce mortality from alcoholic hepatitis? A meta-analysis of the randomized trials. Ann Intern Med. 1990;113:299–307.
408. Ramond M-J, Poynard T, Rueff S et al. A randomized trial of prednisolone in patients with severe alcoholic hepatitis. N Engl J Med. 1992;326:507–12.
409. Trinchet JC, Balkau S, Poupon RE, Heintzmann F, Callard P, Gotheil C et al. Treatment of severe alcoholic hepatitis by infusion of insulin and glucagon: A multicenter sequential trial. Hepatology. 1992;15:76–81.
410. Oneta CM, Mak KM, Lieber CS. Dilinoleoylphosphatidylcholine selectively modulates lipopolysaccharide-induced Kupffer cell activation. Hepatology. 1998;28:634A.
411. Oneta CM, Mak KM, Lieber CS. Dilinoleoylphosphatidylcholine selectively modulates lipopolysaccharide-induced Kupffer cell activation. J Lab Clin Med. 1999;134:466–70.
412. Paronetto F. Immunologic reactions in alcoholic liver disease. In: Lieber CS, ed. Medical and Nutritional Complications of Alcoholism: Mechanisms and Management. New York: Plenum Press, 1992: pp. 283–305.
413. Falchuk KR, Fiske S, Federman C, Trey C. Pericentral hepatic fibrosis and intracellular hyaline in diabetes mellitus. Gastroenterology. 1980;78:535–41.
414. Feinman L, Lieber CS. Hepatic collagen metabolism: effect of alcohol consumption in rats and baboons. Science. 1972;176:795.
415. Patrick RS. Alcohol as a stimulus to hepatic fibrogenesis. J Alcohol. 1973;8:13–27.
416. Mezey E, Potter JJ, Iber FL, Maddrey WC. Hepatic collagen proline hydroxylase activity in alcoholic hepatitis: effect of d-penicillamine. J Lab Clin Med. 1979;93:92–100.
417. Mak KM, Lieber CS. Alterations in endothelial fenestrations in liver sinusoids of baboons fed alcohol: a scanning electron microscopic study. Hepatology. 1984;4:386–91.

418. Ma X, Svegliati-Baroni G, Poniachik J, Baraona E, Lieber CS. Collagen synthesis by liver stellate cells is released from its normal feedback regulation by acetaldehyde-induced modification of the carboxyl-terminal propeptide of procollagen. Alcohol Clin Exp Res. 1997;21:1204–11.
419. Poniachik J, Baraona E, Zhao J, Lieber CS. Dilinoleoylphosphatidylcholine decreases hepatic stellate cell activation. J Lab Clin Med. 1999 (in press).
420. Geesin JC, Hendricks LJ, Falkenstein PA, Gordon JS, Berg RA. Regulation of collagen synthesis by ascorbic acid: Characterization of the role of ascorbate stimulated lipid peroxidation. Arch Biochem Biophys. 1991;290:127–32.
421. Tsukamoto H. Oxidative stress, antioxidants, and alcoholic liver fibrogenesis. Alcohol. 1993;10:465–7.
422. Kershenobich D, Vargas F, Garcia-Tsao G, Perez Tamayo R, Gent M, Rojkind M. Colchicine in the treatment of cirrhosis of the liver. N Engl J Med. 1988;318:1709–13.
423. Boyer LJ, Ransohoff FD. Is colchicine effective therapy for cirrhosis? N Engl J Med. 1988;318:1751–2.
424. Rosman AS, Waraich A, Galvin K, Casiano J, Paronetto F, Lieber CS. Alcoholism is associated with hepatitis C but not hepatitis B in an urban population. Am J Gastroenterol. 1996;91:498–505.
425. Consensus Conference: Liver transplantation. JAMA. 1983;250:2961–4.
426. Bird GLA, O'Grady JG, Harvey FAH et al. Liver transplantation in patients with alcoholic cirrhosis: Selection criteria and rates of survival and relapse. Br Med J. 1990;301:15–17.
427. Osorio RW, Ascher NL, Avery M, Baccetti P, Roberts JP, Lake JR. Predicting recidivism after orthotopic liver transplantation for alcoholic liver disease. Hepatology. 1994;20:105–10.
428. Lucey MR, Merion RM, Henley KS et al. Selection for and outcome of liver transplantation in alcoholic liver disease. Gastroenterology. 1992;102:1736–41.
429. Bonet H, Manez R, Kramer D et al. Liver transplantation for alcoholic liver disease: Survival of patients transplanted with alcoholic hepatitis plus cirrhosis as compared with those with cirrhosis alone. Alcohol Clin Exp Res. 1993;17:1102–6.
430. Schiff ER. Hepatitis and alcohol. Hepatology. 1997;26:39S–42S.
431. Tsutsumi M, Ishizaki M, Takada A. Relative risk for the development of hepatocellular carcinoma in alcoholic patients with cirrhosis: A multiple logistic-regression coefficient analysis. Alcohol Clin Exp Res. 1996;20:758–62.
432. Wiley TE, McCarthy M, Breidi L, McCarthy M, Layden TJ. Impact of alcohol on the histological and clinical progression of hepatitis C infection. Hepatology. 1998;28:805–9.
433. Lieber CS. Pathogenesis and natural course of alcoholic liver disease. In: Schmid R, Bianchi L, Blum HE, Gerok W, Maier KP, Stalder GA, eds. Acute and Chronic Liver Disease: Molecular Biology and Clinics. Symposium No. 87. Section III: Toxic Liver Diseases, Lancaster, UK: Kluwer Academic Publishers, 1996: pp. 109–25.
434. Lieber CS. Hepatic, metabolic and toxic effects of ethanol: 1991 update. Alcohol: Clin Exp Res. 1991;15:573–92.
435. Lieber CS. Hepatic and other medical disorders of alcoholism: from pathogenesis to treatment. J Stud Alcohol. 1998;59:9–25.

16
The effect of ursodeoxycholic acid on fibrosis markers in alcoholic liver disease

J. M. C. STENNER, R. P. JAZRAWI, H. A. AHMED, A. VERMA and T. C. NORTHFIELD

INTRODUCTION

It is estimated that only 10–20% of chronic alcohol abusers ever progress to have significant liver disease[1,2], but this is not to say the remainder are also immune to the social and economic effects of this chemical. Significant alcoholic liver disease is the occurrence of alcoholic hepatitis or fibrosis, indeed, even mild degrees of fibrosis may predict those patients who may progress to cirrhosis[3]. Prognosis in alcoholic liver disease is dependent on many factors but the presence of alcoholic hepatitis and cirrhosis is associated with an almost 50% 5 year mortality[4,5]. Thus the aim of treatment is to treat both the inflammatory alcoholic hepatitis and to prevent fibrosis. Abstinence is undoubtedly the best therapy, but many patients present with established fibrosis or find it impossible to stop drinking completely. More active treatments have been tried. Corticosteroids are recommended in patients with hepatic encephalopathy, jaundice and alcoholic hepatitis where there is no intercurrent infection and show a short term survival benefit, if used appropriately[6]. Other treatments such as, colchicine[7,8], anabolic steroids[9–11] and propylthiouracil[12,13] have been advocated but are not commonly used in clinical practice. There is therefore a need for a pharmaceutical intervention that could improve liver function in patients with alcoholic liver disease that is safe, well tolerated and effective.

UDCA AND FIBROTIC LIVER DISEASE

Ursodeoxycholic acid (UDCA), a hydrophilic bile acid, has been shown to be beneficial in cholestatic liver diseases. It is well tolerated and has a very low toxicity. In primary biliary cirrhosis, UDCA improves survival[14], delays the time to transplant[15] and improves liver histology[16,17]. UDCA has also been used in viral hepatitis, cholestatic liver disease of pregnancy and primary sclerosis cholangitis. Although the exact mechanism of action has not been fully determined it is notable that in this wide range of conditions, taking UDCA usually improves liver function tests particularly alkaline phosphatase (ALP), γ glutamyl transpeptidase (γGT), alanine aminotransferase (ALT) and bilirubin. These enzymes should be better termed as liver damage tests as they correlate poorly with function but reflect ongoing damage to the liver parenchyma or bile ducts. It is difficult to see why a reduction in the markers should be anything other than beneficial, except at the point of end stage liver failure, but it is widely accepted that they are poor markers of long-term outcome and disease progression.

The best proof of the efficacy of a drug treatment is to show a survival benefit in the treatment group. However, in diseases that have a long and incompletely understood natural history such data are difficult to obtain. Therefore there is considerable interest in interim measures that determine whether a drug could have a long-term benefit. While it is possible to measure aspects of liver function using the clearance of a variety of substances (e.g. galactose, bromosulphthalen, aminopyrine), the most widely practised measurement is of hepatic fibrosis. This is logical as the development of fibrosis denotes progressive disease. Whatever the aetiology, the risk of the complications of liver disease, e.g. portal hypertension, ascites, variceal haemorrhage and hepatocellular carcinoma, rises with the degree of fibrosis and this has an impact on both morbidity and mortality. The current gold standard for the assessment of hepatic fibrosis is by liver biopsy. However this procedure is not well suited for studying the effect of potential therapeutic drugs. It is painful and disliked by patients. It has significant morbidity and mortality and is subject to sampling error[18–20]. Furthermore, hepatic fibrosis is dynamic, it can progress (fibrogenesis) or regress (fibrolysis) and the balance between these two processes cannot be determined from a liver biopsy. As a result there are ethical, theoretical and practical difficulties to obtaining repeated same-patient liver biopsies that are currently required for researching liver disease – particularly alcoholic liver disease!

An alternative to biopsy for the assessment of fibrosis is to use serum markers of fibrosis.

SERUM MARKERS OF FIBROSIS

A serum marker of fibrosis is the generic term for an ever-expanding range of macromolecules whose serum levels have been shown to correlate with hepatic fibrosis[21–23]. In contrast to a liver biopsy, fibrosis markers are safe and easy to perform, can be measured repeatedly and there is the potential to measure markers that reflect either fibrogenesis or fibrolysis. It is for these reasons serum markers of fibrosis have been attractive as a research tool in progressive liver disorders.

FIBROSIS MARKERS AND ALCOHOLIC LIVER DISEASE

Fibrosis markers have been measured in alcoholic liver disease. As with most studies involving fibrosis markers these have primarily been about correlating serum levels with the degree of histological fibrosis. The consensus of this work has been that whilst there is an excellent statistical correlation with histological fibrosis scores, fibrosis markers lack the sensitivity to distinguish between early stages of fibrosis and normal[24,25]. The very highest levels are always recorded in patients with ongoing alcoholic hepatitis which may be of clinical relevance. The potential of measuring serial levels of fibrosis markers in an individual patient was shown by Niemala et al.[26]. They showed a significant fall in both procollagen III N terminal peptide (PIIIP) and laminin, but not collagen IV, in patients with alcoholic liver disease who significantly reduced their alcohol intake against a group of similar patients who continued drinking, in whom there was no such fall. Those patients in the reduced alcohol group showed an improvement in their clinical condition. This work supports the contention that changes in the levels of fibrosis markers over a period of time represent a corresponding change in hepatitic fibrosis. This has been convincingly demonstrated in work looking at the effect of interferon in viral hepatitis. There have been a number of studies that have shown that levels of fibrosis markers return towards normal in patients who attain complete remission following therapy[27–29]. These patients also show improvement in histology thus linking the biopsy proven change in fibrosis with serum markers of fibrosis.

FIBROSIS MARKERS AND UDCA IN PBC

Fibrosis markers have been used in the assessment of PBC and the effect of UDCA in this condition. Much of the work has been on the value of the markers in predicting those patients who will progress[30–33]. In addition there are data showing that fibrosis markers change with changes in disease-related fibrosis[34]. However, Beukers et al.[35] showed no relationship between fibrosis markers and histological disease progression, but it is difficult to interpret the data without the absolute values. Equally in the apparently negative report of the value of serial measurements by Poupon[30] there was no convincing change in clinical condition and hence the lack of change in fibrosis markers may have represented the true situation. In another similar study there is certainly a strong trend to a reduction in PIIIP levels in the group treated with UDCA (16% decrease vs. 6% increase)[41]. By contrast Oesterling et al.[36] showed a slight fall in PIIIP levels, as an indication of decreased fibrogenesis, but also a rise in collagen VI, an indication of fibrolysis, the clinically desirable pattern, in those patients on UDCA.

UDCA AND ALCOHOLIC LIVER DISEASE

Alcoholic liver disease can present with cholestatic features, namely jaundice and raised alkaline phosphatase and therefore UDCA may have the beneficial effect shown in other cholestatic liver diseases. UDCA has been shown to reduce the cytotoxicity of ethanol in a cell culture model of alcoholic liver disease[37] and to reduce the degree of fibrosis in the bile duct ligated rat model of cholestatic liver disease[38].

In 1991 Plevris et al.[39] showed a significant improvement in ALT, γGT and bilirubin in 11 patients with cirrhosis given UDCA in a 4-week cross-over study. Cicognani et al. reported at the DDW 1999 in abstract form, data of a 6 month, double-blind randomized placebo controlled study in 30 patients suspected of having alcoholic steatosis (not biopsy confirmed). They also showed a significant improvement in ALT and γGT. It is important to note that no assessment of fibrosis was made in either of these studies and as previously discussed evidence that therapy is having an effect on fibrosis is of major importance.

We have completed a study using fibrosis markers as a measure of the effect of UDCA in patients with alcoholic liver disease. The fibrosis markers used in this study were PIIIP and hyaluronic acid as markers of fibrogenesis, and undulin and collagen VI as markers of fibrolysis.

Fifty patients with biopsy confirmed alcoholic liver disease (48 cirrhosis, two steatosis) were randomized to 6 months of UDCA 10–15 mg/kg/day or to placebo. Patients were excluded if they had evidence of decompensated liver disease, or an entry PIIIP below 0.5 μg/ml. The patients were seen monthly for clinical assessment and serum sampling. Alcohol intake was assessed by history and carbohydrate deficient transferrin (%CDT) levels in serum. Compliance was assessed by tablet count and serum UDCA levels. The fibrosis markers PIIIP and hyaluronic acid were measured using commercial assays, collagen VI and undulin were measured in Professor Schuppan's laboratory.

Forty-seven patients completed 3 months' treatment (23 UDCA, 24 placebo) and 39 patients completed the 6-month study period (20 UDCA, 19 placebo). Two patients were withdrawn from analysis after enrolment, as they had no fibrosis on liver biopsy. There was a significant improvement in γGT and ALT ($p < 0.05$) but not ALP, INR or total bilirubin in the treatment group. There was a significant fall in PIIIP levels in both groups, which was more pronounced in the treatment group; the difference between the treatment group and the placebo group was significant at 6 months ($p < 0.02$). There were no significant differences between the treatment and placebo groups with respect to hyaluronic acid, collagen VI or undulin (Table 1).

During the period of the trial the mean %CDT levels in the placebo and UDCA groups did not alter, although higher in the placebo group (Fig. 1). This

Table 1 Data expressed as percentage change from entry value

	UDCA		*Placebo*	
	3 months	*6 months*	*3 months*	*6 months*
PIIIP	−16.3*	−28*+	−4.2	−10.4*
Hyaluronic acid	12.5	−8.8	4.2	−10.1
Collagen VI	−6	−10	−2	−1
Undulin	−4	0	−2	−2
ALP	6.4	−3.5	−5.3	−10.9
χGT	−47*+	−47.8*+	−10.3	7.2
ALT	−20.1*+	−11.8*+	7.7	16.7

* Significant within treatment group (compared to baseline)
+ Significant between treatment groups

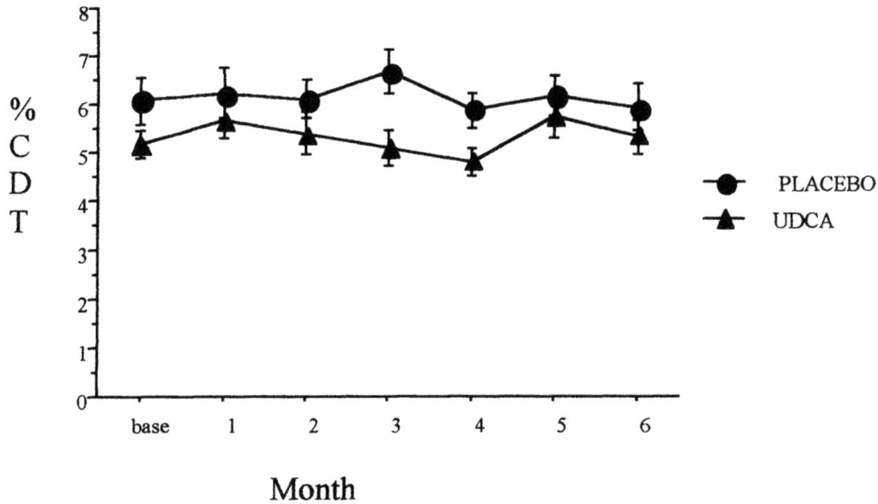

Figure 1 Mean %CDT over time in UDCA and placebo groups.

suggests that the significant change and differences in the PIIIP levels, in this study, was not due to different alcohol intake, which was effectively a constant, but rather to the UDCA treatment.

The lack of change in undulin and collagen VI, markers of the breakdown of fibrosis tissue, may be due to the fact that the study patients were well-compensated cirrhotics with very little potential for fibrolysis. The studies that have shown a change in these markers have been in patients with fibrosis[36,40].

Hyaluronic acid levels would have been expected to mirror changes in PIIIP. That this did not occur may suggest that UDCA, in alcoholic liver disease, affects liver production/ clearance of these markers in different ways, or that the trial period was insufficient. A further consideration must be that patients were selected for having a raised PIIIP level and therefore if UDCA were having a beneficial effect on fibrosis, changes in this marker would be more readily detectable.

SUMMARY

UDCA has been consistently shown to improve liver enzyme levels in alcoholic liver disease. UDCA may also have a beneficial effect in alcoholic liver disease by reducing the amount of ongoing fibrogenesis on the evidence of significantly reduced levels of the serum marker of fibrosis PIIIP. Further work on the effect of UDCA in alcoholic liver disease is now indicated. A longer trial with both clinical and histological outcome measures can be justified now that there is evidence that UDCA may have antifibrotic effect.

ACKNOWLEDGEMENTS

To the Falk Foundation for supporting the UDCA in alcoholic liver disease trial; Professor Schuppan for the undulin and collagen VI measurements; Cortecs for supervising the trial; Medicomp for data support.

REFERENCES

1. Lelbach WK. Epidemiology of alcoholic liver disease. Prog Liver Dis. 1976;5:494–515.
2. Leevy CM. Cirrhosis in alcoholics. Med Clin North Am. 1968;52:1445–55.
3. Marbet UA, Bianchi L, Meury U, Stalder GA. Long-term histological evaluation of the natural history and prognostic factors of alcoholic liver disease. J Hepatol. 1987;4:364–72.
4. Powell WJ Jr, Klatskin G. Duration of survival in patients with Laennec's cirrhosis. Influence of alcohol withdrawal, and possible effects of recent changes in general management of the disease. Am J Med. 1968;44:406–20.
5. D'Amico G, Morabito A, Pagliaro L, Marubini E. Survival and prognostic indicators in compensated and decompensated cirrhosis. Dig Dis Sci. 1986;31:468–75.
6. Ramond MJ, Poynard T, Rueff B, Mathurin P, Theodore C, Chaput JC et al. A randomized trial of prednisolone in patients with severe alcoholic hepatitis. N Engl J Med. 1992;326:507–12.
7. Trinchet JC, Beaugrand M, Callard P, Hartmann DJ, Gotheil C, Nusgens BV et al. Treatment of alcoholic hepatitis with colchicine. Results of a randomized double blind trial. Gastroenterol Clin Biol. 1989;13:551–5.
8. Akriviadis EA, Steindel H, Pinto PC, Fong TL, Kanel G, Reynolds TB et al. Failure of colchicine to improve short-term survival in patients with alcoholic hepatitis. Gastroenterology. 1990;99:811–18.
9. Bonkovsky HL, Fiellin DA, Smith GS, Slaker DP, Simon D, Galambos JT. A randomized, controlled trial of treatment of alcoholic hepatitis with parenteral nutrition and oxandrolone. I. Short-term effects on liver function. Am J Gastroenterol. 1991;86:1200–8.
10. Mendenhall CL, Anderson S, Garcia-Pont P, Goldberg S, Kiernan T, Seeff LB et al. Short-term and long-term survival in patients with alcoholic hepatitis treated with oxandrolone and prednisolone. N Engl J Med. 1984;311:1464–70.
11. Mendenhall CL, Moritz TE, Roselle GA, Morgan TR, Nemchausky BA, Tamburro CH et al. A study of oral nutritional support with oxandrolone in malnourished patients with alcoholic hepatitis: results of a Department of Veterans Affairs cooperative study. Hepatology. 1993;17:564–76.
12. Orrego H, Kalant H, Israel Y, Blake J, Medline A, Rankin JG et al. Effect of short-term therapy with propylthiouracil in patients with alcoholic liver disease. Gastroenterology. 1979;76:105–15.
13. Orrego H, Blake JE, Blendis LM, Compton KV, Israel Y. Long-term treatment of alcoholic liver disease with propylthiouracil. N Engl J Med. 1987;317:1421–7.
14. Poupon RE, Bonnand AM, Chretien Y, Poupon R. Ten-year survival in ursodeoxycholic acid-treated patients with primary biliary cirrhosis. The UDCA-PBC Study Group. Hepatology. 1999;29:1668–71.
15. Heathcote EJ, Stone J, Cauch-Dudek K, Poupon R, Chazouilleres O, Lindor KD et al. Effect of pretransplantation ursodeoxycholic acid therapy on the outcome of liver transplantation in patients with primary biliary cirrhosis (see comments). Liver Transpl Surg. 1999;5:269–74.
16. Angulo P, Batts KP, Therneau TM, Jorgensen RA, Dickson ER, Lindor KD. Long-term ursodeoxycholic acid delays histological progression in primary biliary cirrhosis. Hepatology. 1999;29:644–7.
17. Degott C, Zafrani ES, Callard P, Balkau B, Poupon RE, Poupon R. Histopathological study of primary biliary cirrhosis and the effect of ursodeoxycholic acid treatment on histology progression. Hepatology. 1999;29:1007–12.
18. Maharaj B, Maharaj RJ, Leary WP, Cooppan RM, Naran AD, Pirie D et al. Sampling variability and its influence on the diagnostic yield of percutaneous needle biopsy of the liver. Lancet. 1986;1:523–5.
19. Bedossa P, Poynard T, Naveau S, Martin ED, Agostini H, Chaput JC. Observer variation in assessment of liver biopsies of alcoholic patients. Alcohol Clin Exp Res. 1988;12:173–8.

20. Piccinino F, Sagnelli E, Pasquale G, Giusti G. Complications following percutaneous liver biopsy. A multicentre retrospective study on 68 276 biopsies. J Hepatol. 1986;2:165–73.
21. Schuppan D, Stolzel U, Oesterling C, Somasundaram R. Serum assays for liver fibrosis. J Hepatol. 1995;22(2 Suppl):82–8.
22. Ruwart MJ, Wilkinson KF, Rush BD, Vidmar TJ, Peters KM, Henley KS et al. The integrated value of serum procollagen III peptide over time predicts hepatic hydroxyproline content and stainable collagen in a model of dietary cirrhosis in the rat (see comments). Hepatology. 1989;10:801–6.
23. Oberti F, Valsesia E, Pilette C, Rousselet MC, Bedossa P, Aube C et al. Noninvasive diagnosis of hepatic fibrosis or cirrhosis. Gastroenterology. 1997;113:1609–16.
24. Sato S, Nouchi T, Worner TM, Lieber CS. Liver fibrosis in alcoholics. Detection by Fab radioimmunoassay of serum procollagen III peptides. JAMA. 1986;256:1471–3.
25. Bell H, Raknerud N, Orjasaeter H, Haug E. Serum procollagen III peptide in alcoholic and other chronic liver diseases. Scand J Gastroenterol. 1989;24:1217–22.
26. Niemela O, Risteli J, Blake JE, Risteli L, Compton KV, Orrego H. Markers of fibrogenesis and basement membrane formation in alcoholic liver disease. Relation to severity, presence of hepatitis, and alcohol intake (see comments). Gastroenterology. 1990;98:1612–19.
27. Suou T, Hosho K, Kishimoto Y, Horie Y, Kawasaki H. Long-term decrease in serum N-terminal propeptide of type III procollagen in patients with chronic hepatitis C treated with interferon alfa. Hepatology. 1995;22:426–31.
28. Fabris P, Marranconi F, Bozzola L, Biasin MR, De Lazzari F, Plebani M et al. Fibrogenesis serum markers in patients with chronic hepatitis C treated with alpha-IFN (see comments). J Gastroenterol. 1999;34:345–50.
29. Gallorini A, Plebani M, Pontisso P, Chemello L, Masiero M, Mantovani G et al. Serum markers of hepatic fibrogenesis in chronic hepatitis type C treated with alfa-2A interferon. Liver. 1994;14:257–64.
30. Poupon RE, Balkau B, Guechot J, Heintzmann F. Predictive factors in ursodeoxycholic acid-treated patients with primary biliary cirrhosis: role of serum markers of connective tissue. Hepatology. 1994;19:635–40.
31. Nyberg A, Lindqvist U, Engstrom-Laurent A. Serum hyaluronan and aminoterminal propeptide of type III procollagen in primary biliary cirrhosis: relation to clinical symptoms, liver histopathology and outcome. J Intern Med. 1992;231:485–91.
32. Eriksson S, Zettervall O. The N-terminal propeptide of collagen type III in serum as a prognostic indicator in primary biliary cirrhosis. J Hepatol. 1986;2:370–8.
33. Babbs C, Smith A, Hunt LP, Rowan BP, Haboubi NY, Warnes TW. Type III procollagen peptide: a marker of disease activity and prognosis in primary biliary cirrhosis. Lancet. 1988;1:1021–4.
34. Nyberg A, Engstrom-Laurent A, Loof L. Serum hyaluronate in primary biliary cirrhosis – a biochemical marker for progressive liver damage. Hepatology. 1988;8:142–6.
35. Beukers R, van Zanten RA, Schalm SW. Serial determination of type III procollagen amino propeptide serum levels in patients with histologically progressive and non-progressive primary biliary cirrhosis. J Hepatol. 1992;14:22–9.
36. Oesterling C, Aksu T, Somasundaram R. Serum markers of collagen synthesis and breakdown suggest an antifibrotic effect of ursodeoxycholic acid in patients with PBC stage I–IV. Gut. 1995;37(Suppl 2):A121 (abstract).
37. Neuman MG, Cameron RG, Shear NH, Bellentani S, Tiribelli C. Effect of tauroursodeoxycholic and ursodeoxycholic acid on ethanol-induced cell injuries in the human Hep G2 cell line. Gastroenterology. 1995;109:555–63.
38. Poo JL, Feldmann G, Erlinger S, Braillon A, Gaudin C, Dumont M et al. Ursodeoxycholic acid limits liver histologic alterations and portal hypertension induced by bile duct ligation in the rat. Gastroenterology. 1992;102:1752–9.
39. Plevris J, Hayes P, Bouchier I. Ursodeoxycholic acid in the treatment of alcoholic liver disease. Eur J Gastroenterol Hepatol. 1991;3:653–6.
40. Shahin M, Schuppan D, Waldherr R, Risteli J, Risteli L, Savolainen ER et al. Serum procollagen peptides and collagen type VI for the assessment of activity and degree of hepatic fibrosis in schistosomiasis and alcoholic liver disease. Hepatology. 1992;15:637–44.
41. Vuoristo M, Farkkila M, Karvonen AL et al. A placebo-controlled trial of primary biliary cirrhosis treatment with colchicine and ursodeoxycholic acid. Gastroenterology. 1995;108:1470–8.

17
Drugs and toxins – drug handling

U. A. MEYER

BASIC CONCEPTS OF DRUG AND XENOBIOTIC METABOLISM IN THE LIVER

Most pharmacologically or toxologically active molecules are lipophilic and remain unionized or only partially ionized at physiological pH. After glomerular filtration in the kidney they would be reabsorbed and remain in the organism. Biotransformation means that a lipid-soluble xenobiotic or endobiotic compound is enzymatically transformed by so-called functionalization reactions (phase I) and/or conjugation (phase II) reactions, into polar, watersoluble and excretable metabolites (Table 1). The major organ for drug biotransformation is the liver. The metabolic products are often less active than the parent drug or may even be inactive. However, some biotransformation products (metabolites) may have enhanced activity or toxic effects, including mutagenesis, teratogenesis and carcinogenesis. Thus biotransformation may include both detoxification and toxification processes.

Although every tissue has some ability to metabolize xenobiotics, the liver is the principal organ of biotransformation. At the subcellular level, the major enzymes of biotransformation are either anchored in the membranes of the endoplasmatic reticulum (cytochrome P450-monooxygenases (CYPs), epoxide

Table 1 Drug metabolizing enzymes

Phase I *Conversion of functional groups*	*Phase II* *Derivatization, Conjugation*
Dehydrogenases	Acetyltransferases
Esterases	Glucuronosyltransferases
Monooxygenases	GSH-transferases
Oxidases	Glycine/taurine conjugation
Reductases	Methyltransferases Sulfotransferases

hydrolase, glucuronyl-transferases) or are cytosolic enzymes (acetyltransferases, sulfotransferases, xanthine oxidase).

One of the major enzyme systems that determines the organism's capability of dealing with drugs and chemicals is the cytochrome P450 monooxygenases. The enzyme system consists of two protein components: a haemoprotein called cytochrome P-450 of 45–55 kDa molecular weight and a flavoprotein called NADPH-cytochrome P-450 reductase. Cytochrome P-450 is the substrate- and oxygen-binding site of the enzyme system, while the reductase serves as an electron carrier, shuttling electrons from NADPH to the cytochrome P-450-substrate complex.

The multiplicity and complexity of drug-metabolizing enzyme systems is indeed astonishing. The cytochrome P450 system by last count comprises close to 1000 genes in all species tested of which at least 50–100 are expressed in each human, and this is only one system[1]. The families of UDPG-glucuronosyl transferases and glutathione-transferases also comprise considerable numbers of genes, other enzyme systems appear less complex (e.g. N-acetyltransferase) and others have not been sufficiently studied (e.g. esterases, sulfotransferases) to evaluate their complexity.

For clinical medicine an important practical concept also emerges from this information. If drugs in common clinical use are considered, only six of the numerous cytochromes P450 play a major role in their metabolism, prominent among them in regard to a number of substrate drugs are CYP3A4 and CYP2D6, CYP2C9, CYP2C19, CYP1A2, CYP2E1. For purposes such as predicting interactions or polymorphic metabolism, knowledge of the major features of these 6 P450 enzymes appears sufficient. Clinically important continuously updated information on these enzymes is available on several internet sites, e.g. http://www.dml.georgetown.edu/depts/pharmacology/ davetab. html; http://www. afp.org/afp/980101ap/cupp.html;http://drnelson.utmem.edu/ P450lect.html

GENETIC, ENVIRONMENTAL AND DISEASE FACTORS REGULATING DRUG-METABOLISM

Numerous factors influence the concentration and activity of drug-metabolizing enzymes including age, nutrition, liver disease, environmental chemicals (e.g. cigarette smoking) and drugs themselves. A major source of interindividual differences in drug metabolism are common genetic polymorphisms, i.e. inherited deficiencies of single drug-metabolizing enzymes, such as CYP2C19, CYP2D6 and N-acetyltransferase 2 (NAT2, see http://www.imm.se/CYPalleles/). Recent studies also indicate that there are major interethnic differences in drug metabolism, particularly in the expression of cytochromes P450 and glucuronosyltransferases, including different frequencies of genetic polymorphisms.

Induction

A large number of CYPs (and also other drug metabolizing enzymes such as glucuronosyltransferases, epoxide hydrolase, etc.) are selectively induced by drugs such as phenobarbital, rifampicin, dexamethasone, or by cigarette smoke and exposure to other chemicals. The induction response is dose dependent and reversible. There has been major progress in understanding the molecular mechanism of induction. Induction most often occurs at the level of transcription and prototypical inducers include polycyclic aromatic hydrocarbons (e.g. TCDD), phenobarbital (PB), peroxisome proliferators (e.g. clofibrate) and steroids (e.g. dexamethasone). Each of these classes of compounds induces a different but overlapping pattern of enzymes. Recent advances in our understanding of the induction response suggest the following general mechanism of transcriptional activation. The xenobiotics of the four major groups of inducers interact with intracellular proteins either of the basic helix-loop-helix class (polycyclic aromatic hydrocarbons, AhR system) or with so-called orphan nuclear receptors such as PPAR (peroxisome proliferators), CAR (phenobarbital) or PXR (CYP3A4 inducers such as rifampicin, dexamethasone). Each of these intracellular proteins then forms heterodimers with other proteins (Arnt for AhR, RXR for PPAR, CAR and PXR) and the heterodimer binds to DNA recognition motifs, becoming a genuine transcription factor. Although many of the details of these mechanisms remain to be elucidated, the new findings provide new approaches to understand how small lipid-soluble molecules change the cellular phenotype and affect the metabolism of drugs and other xenobiotics to inactive, active or toxic metabolites[1–6].

Inhibition

Since one P450 enzyme may bind many different substrates, competition at the site of drug binding by cosubstrates or other chemicals may cause inhibition. Known potent inhibitors of P450 enzymes are quinidine (CYP2D6), cimetidine (numerous P450s), furafylline, fluvoxamine (CYP1A2), gestodene (CYP3A subfamily).

Disease

Severe liver disease (hepatitis, cirrhosis, liver cancer), diabetes and starvation may affect drug metabolism by multiple mechanisms. Of particular importance are drugs whose metabolism is limited by liver blood flow (e.g. propropolol, lidocaine, nifedipine, verapamil, etc.). In cirrhosis with portal-systemic shunts these drugs can reach very high (toxic) plasma concentrations. The effects of severe liver disease on different cytochrome P450 enzymes have recently been evaluated[7].

ROLE OF DRUG METABOLISM IN HEPATOTOXICITY

Numerous drugs and other xenobiotics are toxic to the liver. In fact, recent reviews list between 500 and 1000 drugs as potential hepatotoxins[8,9]. The specific toxicity of drugs in the liver is predominantly accounted for by the fact that the liver is the major site of biotransformation of drugs and that this process may lead to the production of reactive metabolites. These metabolites then mediate toxicity close to or within the tissue where they are generated (Fig. 1). There are three types of toxic products generated through oxidative drug metabolism: electrophiles, free radicals and reactive oxygen molecules.

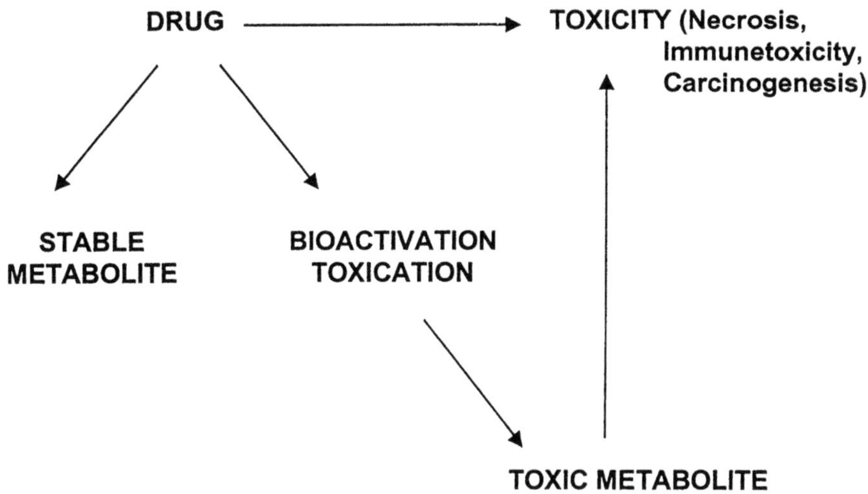

Figure 1 Relationship between drug metabolism and drug toxicity.

Electrophiles are substances which seek electrons (positive charge density) and will form electron sharing covalent bonds with substances which can donate electrons (negative charge density nucleophiles). Electrophilic metabolites vary in their inherent reactivity so that some may preferentially attack thiol groups (acetaminophen metabolite, bromobenzene) or amino groups (halothane metabolite) on proteins including thiol-containing proteins that regulate calcium homeostasis.

Free radicals are atoms, ions or molecules which have an unpaired electron and will remove an electron from other substances leading to a new free radical. Drug free radicals tend preferentially to attack unsaturated fatty acids in membrane phospholipids leading to lipid peroxidation. Examples are carbon tetrachloride and again halothane. A chain reaction of free radical exchange ensues with the ultimate breakdown of fatty acids.

Reactive oxygen species (ROS) undergo a series of reactions. O_2^- (superoxide anion), the initial form produced, is rapidly converted to H_2O_2 by the action of superoxide dismutase. H_2O_2 can be converted to $\cdot OH$ (hydroxyl radical) which is a potent oxidizing agent. This process of so-called redox cycling occurs when a reduced substrate such as doxorubicin reoxidizes in the presence of oxygen. The effects of $\cdot OH$ include lipid peroxidation, protein thiol oxidation or attack on other cellular constituents.

CELLULAR DEFENCE MECHANISMS

The effects of reactive metabolites on cellular constituents, such as proteins and membrane phospholipids, may be counteracted by cellular defence. Important factors are glutathione (GSH) and D-α-toxopherol (vitamin E). Some electrophilic drug metabolites, such as N-acetyl-benzoquinoneimine (NABQI), are so-called soft electrophiles. These chemicals will react preferentially with a soft nucleophile such as the thiol group. The thiol of GSH is preferentially attacked rather than protein thiols. Although the abundance of GSH may account partially for this preference, the high degree of preference for GSH suggests that the reaction is catalysed by a GSH S-transferase. Defence against free radicals is mediated by scavengers which can interrupt the free radical chain reaction of lipid peroxidation. Many endogenous substances may be important in this regard, such as ascorbic acid or vitamin A. However, the key free radical scavenger which protects against lipid peroxidation is α-tocopherol. This is present in membranes and can interrupt the free radical chain reaction. Numerous enzyme systems, including superoxide dismutase, catalase, epoxide hydrolases and GSH-peroxidases, GSH-reductases and GSH-S-transferases also are involved in the protection against oxidizing effects of electrophiles, radicals and ROS.

REACTIVE METABOLITES AND HEPATOCELLULAR DAMAGE

The biochemical consequences of reactive metabolites, namely covalent binding, lipid peroxidation and protein-thiol oxidation, are probably important in mediating toxicity. However, the extent of these chemical phenomena do not always correlate with injury. Therefore, uncertainty exists as to their strict relevance to the pathogenesis of toxicity in many instances. Reactive metabolites may lead to covalent binding, lipid peroxidation, protein thiol oxidation of both a large excess of non-critical targets and a small number of critical targets. Much controversy exists as to the identification of these critical targets which mediate the final pathway to cell death. Most likely, a combination of factors act in concert and with varying targets. Covalent binding may alternatively play a key role in the pathogenesis of hepatotoxicity by initiating an immune response rather than directly causing necrosis. A drug metabolite may thus serve as a hapten leading to sensitization.

Recent studies have shown that a sustained rise in cytosolic calcium can lead to cell death or contribute to toxicity, along with other factors. Covalent binding or oxidation of the thiol groups of calcium, pumps (ATPases) can lead to increased cytosolic calcium. Lipid peroxidation, by changing the physicochemical properties of the membranes, can increase calcium permeability or impair pumping. A sustained rise in calcium activates a variety of degradative enzymes, such as proteases, phospholipases and endonucleases. Increased cytosolic calcium can lead to recycling of calcium in and out of the mitochondria which can impair mitochondrial function.

CONCLUSIONS

The enzymatic reactions of drug biotransformation in the liver can lead to inactive, active or toxic metabolites. The balance between toxification and detoxification of the parent drug and its metabolites determines the generation of toxicity or the resistance to toxicity. Genetic and environmental factors influence this balance and determine the individual risk to toxicity. The knowledge of these individual factors increasingly allows identification of patients at risk.

REFERENCES

1. Nelson DR, Koymans L, Kamataki T, Stegeman JJ, Feyereisen R, Waxman DJ et al. P450 superfamily: update on new sequences, gene mapping, accession numbers and nomenclature. Pharmacogenetics. 1996;6:1–42.
2. Kliewer AS, Lehmann JM ,Willson TM. Orphan nuclear receptors: shifting endocrinology into reverse. Science. 1999;284:757–60.
3. Waxman DJ. P450 gene induction by strcturally diverse xenochemicals: central role of nuclear receptors CAR, PXR, and PPAR[1]. Arch Biochem Biophys. 1999;369:11–23.
4. Savas U, Griffin KJ, Johnson EF. Molecular mechanisms of cytochrome P-450 induction by xenobiotics: an expanded role for nuclear hormone receptors. Mol Pharmacol. 1999;56:851–7.
5. Früh FW, Zanger UM, Meyer UA. Extent and character of phenobarbital-mediated changes in gene expression in liver. Mol Pharmacol. 1997;51:363–9.
6. Handschin C, Meyer UA. A conserved nuclear receptor consensus sequence (DR-4) mediates transcriptional activation of the chicken CYP2H1 gene by phenobarbital in a hepatoma cell line. J Biol Chem. 2000;(in press).
7. George J, Murray M, Byth K, Farrell GC. Differential alterations of cytochrome P450 proteins in livers from patients with severe chronic liver disease. Hepatology. 1995;21:120–8.
8. Farrell GC. Drug-induced Liver Disease. London: Churchill Livingstone, 1994.
9. Sturgill MG, Lambert GH. Xenobiotic-induced hepatotoxicity: mechanisms of liver injury and methods of monitoring hepatic function. Clin Chem. 1997;43:1512–26.

18
Drug- and toxin-induced liver injury: diagnosis, natural course and therapy

P. J. MEIER-ABT

The liver is the major detoxification organ of the body: as a consequence, it represents the major target organ for numerous drugs, environmental toxins and other xenobiotic substances. New drugs continue to appear on the market that during phase IV monitoring turn out to be hepatotoxic in a proportion of susceptible patients and must eventually be recalled from the market because of their liver toxicity. Recent reports of fatal liver injury from drugs of abuse and environmental toxins further illustrate that continuous efforts are required to early detect potential hepatotoxins, to study the mechanisms of their hepatotoxicity and to develop more effective strategies to prevent and treat drug- and toxin-induced liver injury. This short summary concentrates on some general principles of diagnosis and therapy of drug-induced liver injury, points to some specific new information related to paracetamol induced hepatocellular necrosis, drug- and toxin-induced microvesicular steatosis and drug-induced cholestasis and includes a few recent examples of liver disasters caused by food- and water-borne environmental toxins. For more detailed information the reader is referred to the literature including comprehensive state of the art reviews, book chapters and monographs[1–5].

DRUG-INDUCED LIVER INJURY

Drug-induced liver injury is a major challenge for both the pharmaceutical industry (drug development) and the physician (diagnosis and therapy). The frequency of clinical drug hepatotoxicity often remains unrecognized. Its prevalence among various causes of liver disease is estimated to range from 2 to 5% of cases with jaundice, to ~10% of cases with hepatitis and to 10–15% (up to 50% in England due to the popularity of paracetamol) of cases with fulminant hepatic failure[1].

Diagnosis

Diagnosis of drug-induced liver disease is sometimes obvious, but more frequently difficult. It should be suspected in almost any kind of liver disease. The initial diagnostic steps include: (1) establishing a list of medications and comparing the chronology of each treatment with that of the liver disease; newly marketed drugs should be carefully monitored, since their potential hepatotoxicity is frequently recognized only during phase IV pharmacovigilance (e.g. nimesulide[6,7]); (2) gathering information about individual risk factors for adverse drug reactions (e.g. previous adverse drug reactions, biotransformation polymorphisms, immunoallergic manifestations); (3) comparing the type of liver disease with that produced by the ingested and potentially hepatotoxic drugs, and (4) excluding other causes of liver disease by specific investigations (e.g. viral serology); specific serological markers are available with only a few drugs such as halothane hepatitis (antitrifluoracetylated proteins), iproniazid hepatitis (anti-M6 autoantibody), tienilic acid hepatitis (anti-LKM2 autoantibody) and dihydralazine hepatitis (anti-liver microsome autoantibody). In severe, acute and in suspected chronic cases liver biopsy helps to establish a definite diagnosis. The last step in the diagnosis is essentially based on the improvement of the liver disease within weeks following the cessation of the treatment.

Drugs can induce a wide spectrum of liver pathology, including acute hepatocellular necrosis (e.g. paracetamol), acute cytolytic hepatitis (e.g. halothane), pure hepatocellular cholestasis (e.g. oestrogens, anabolic steroids, cyclosporine), microvesicular steatosis (e.g. aspirine, nucleoside analogs, tetracyclines, valproic acid), steatohepatitis (e.g. amiodarone), vanishing bile duct syndrome (e.g. ajmaline), perisinusoidal fibrosis (e.g. methotrexate, vitamin A), vascular lesions (e.g. chemotherapeutic agents) and adenomas (e.g. oral contraceptives). Although liver biopsy is the gold standard for definite classification of drug-induced liver disorders, in numerous cases liver biopsy is not necessary for the diagnosis, and therefore is rarely performed. In these cases the term liver injury should be used and classified according to an international consensus report into hepatocellular, cholestatic and mixed, based on serum enzyme (ALT, AST, AP) and bilirubin elevations, and into fulminant, acute and chronic based on the time of appearance and duration of liver abnormalities[8].

Natural course

The natural course of drug-induced liver injury greatly varies with the type of drug involved and the underlying liver pathology. If not already decreased (or transplanted) because of fulminant hepatitis, most cases of drug-induced hepatocellular injuries resolve with the cessation of the treatment.

Paracetamol overdose

Acute paracetamol (acetaminophen) overdose is characterized by three phases consisting of initial acute gastrointestinal symptoms ($\leq$24 h), an asymptomatic period (~2 days) and clinically apparent hepatic injury 3–5 days after ingestion. The critical acute hepatotoxic dose of paracetamol is around 7.5 g (children

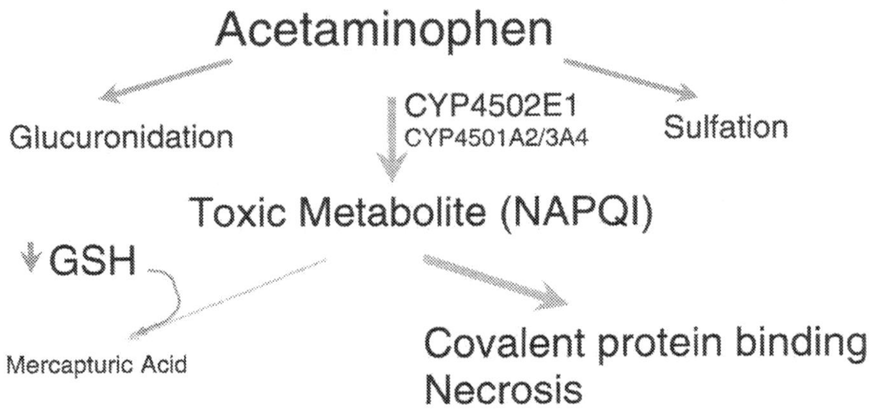

Figure 1 Mechanisms of paracetamol (acetaminophen) induced hepatocellular necrosis.

150 mg/kg) in normal adults. In patients with risk factors such as chronic alcohol abuse, however, the acute hepatotoxic dose can be as low as 3 g due to the induction of CYP2E1/1A2 and a decrease of hepatocellular glutathione (GSH) levels. Both these mechanisms lead to an increased formation and accumulation of the toxic metabolite N-acetyl-p-benzoquinoneimine (NAPQI) in centrilobular hepatocytes (Fig. 1) and thus increase the sensitivity of perivenous hepatocytes towards paracetamol. Because the ingested dose may be wrongly estimated and because vomiting may have decreased the amount of paracetamol actually absorbed, it is useful to measure paracetamol plasma levels, starting 4 h after the ingestion. Those patients whose plasma paracetamol concentrations are above a line joining points of 1.0 mmol/l (150 mg/l) at 4 h and 0.19 mmol/l (30 mg/l) at 12 h after ingestion (on a semilogarithmic plot) are at risk of developing severe liver damage and must be treated with N-acetylcysteine[9]. In alcoholic patients a lower treatment line joining plots of 0.66 mmol/l (100 mg/l) at 4 h to 0.10 mmol/l (15 mg/l) at 15 h is recommended. Patients presenting more than 15 h after paracetamol ingestion should be commenced on N-acetylcysteine immediately and the treatment should be discontinued only when the investigations reveal no evidence of liver damage[10].

In contrast to acute poisoning, induction of autoprotection against hepatocellular necrosis has been reported in chronic paracetamol overdose. For example, daily abuse of increasing paracetamol doses of up to 65 g/day for 2 years was tolerated in a 32-year-old white male without any evidence of liver injury[11]. This surprising clinical observation was experimentally reproduced in mice, which developed a minimal hepatotoxicity and a 400% increase in LD_{50} to a normally supralethal paracetamol dose after pretreatment with increasing subtoxic paracetamol doses for 8 days[11]. Mechanistically the authors provide evidence that selective down-regulation of CYP2E1/1A2 and GSH rebound through hepatocyte proliferation are essential features for the development of autoprotection against chronic paracetamol overdose.

Drug-induced microvesicular steatosis and steatohepatitis

Severe, acute or even fatal liver injury with initially relatively low levels of serum transaminases can occur with drug-induced mitochondrial dysfunction leading to microvesicular steatosis and steatohepatitis[12]. Mitochondrial *β*-oxidation of fatty acids is particularly sensitive to inhibition by aspirin, valproic acid, tetracyclines and some non-steroidal anti-inflammatory drugs (e.g. 2-acylpropionate derivatives). Patients at risk are very young children (valproic acid), children with viral infections (aspirin; Reye's syndrome), patients treated concomitantly with cytochrome P450 inducers (e.g. phenytoin, carbamazepine) and patients with inherited disorders of mitochondrial *β*-oxidation and/or urea cycle enzymes. While the incidence of Reye's syndrome decreased following the avoidance of aspirin in febrile children, valproic acid induced severe fatty liver injury continues to be observed at an incidence of ~1/40 000. Valproic acid is a branched chain fatty acid that forms acyl-coenzyme A thereby (Fig. 2) depleting the intramitochondrial pool of coenzyme A. Furthermore, it is desaturated by cytochrome P450 to Δ_4-valproate, which is oxidized in mitochondria to the electrophilic Δ_4,Δ_2-valproyl-coenzyme A, a metabolite that can inactivate *β*-oxidation enzymes (Fig. 2). Clinically, valproate-induced overt hepatotoxicity is characterized by prodromes including lethargy, nausea and vomiting followed by jaundice, elevated serum ammonia levels and other signs of metabolic liver failure. Increased serum transaminases occur only at a relatively late stage of liver injury when the mitochondrial energy crisis can no longer support the survival of hepatocytes. Valproate should be stopped if any prodromal symptoms and/or signs of hepatic insufficiency (e.g. abnormalities of serum bilirubin, albumin, coagulation factors) develop. The monthly control of serum transaminases during the first 6 months of valproate therapy is controversial, since silent increases of serum transaminases occur in 16–67% of patients treated with valproate, and increased serum transaminases are a late sign of potentially fatal microvesicular steatosis (see above). To prevent severe hepatotoxicity valproate should not be given to children under 3 years of age or in combination with

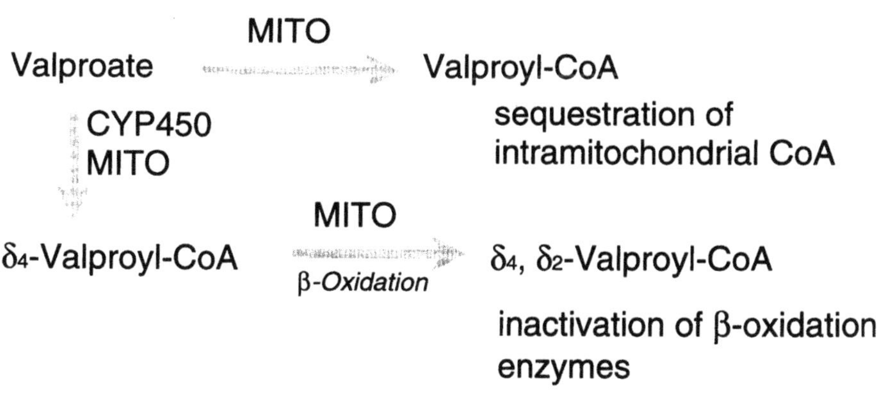

Figure 2 Mechanisms of valproate induced hepatotoxicity.

cytochrome P450 inducers or with other mitochondrial damaging drugs. The latter also include the dideoxynucleotide antiviral drugs (e.g. zidovudine, zalcibaine, didanosine), which can be incorporated by DNA polymerase γ into mitochondrial DNA (mtDNA) leading to termination of mtDNA replication and, thus, to an acquired equivalent of a mitochondrial cytopathy[12].

Drug-induced cholestasis

Drug-induced cholestasis can occur without (pure hepatocellular cholestasis) (Table 1) or with (mixed liver injury) hepatitis. In addition, chronic cholestasis can be caused by some drugs due to the induction of the vanishing bile duct syndrome (e.g. chlorpromazine, ajmaline derivatives, flucloxacillin, amoxacillin/clavulonic acid). Recent progress in the identification of the canalicular transport systems involved in hepatic bile formation[13] has shown that the inherited failure to express the phosphatidylcholine flippase MDR3 or the bile salt export pump BSEP at the canalicular membrane forms the basis of progressive familiar intrahepatic cholestasis type 3 (PFIC3) and type 2 (PFIC2), respectively[14]. Based on

Table 1 Drug-induced cholestasis

Cholestasis without hepatitis
Oestrogens, 17a-alkylated androgenic steroids, cyclosporin A, rifamycin/rifampicin, others
Cholestasis with hepatitis
Chlorpromazine and other phenothiazines, tricyclic antidepressants, macrolide antibiotics, others
Chronic Cholestasis (vanishing bile duct syndrome)
Chlorpromazine, flucloxacillin, others

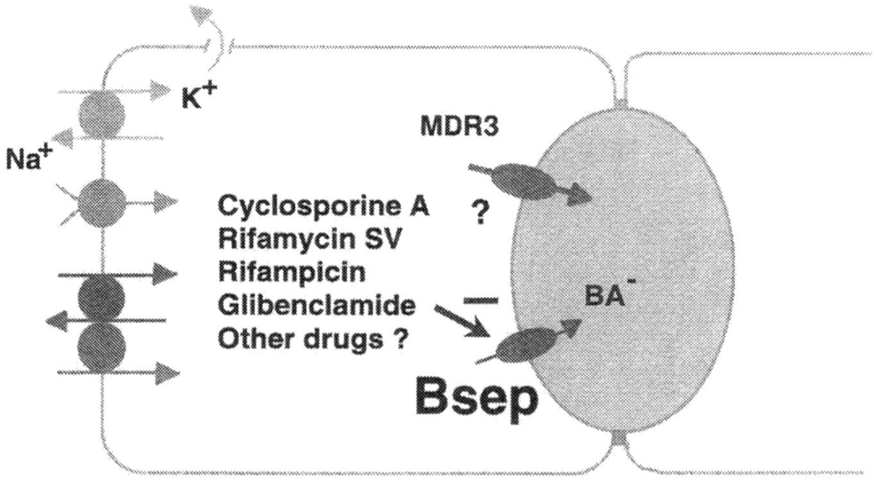

Figure 3 Drug-induced cholestasis caused by inhibition of the canalicular bile salt export pump. For details see text and Ref. 15.

these inherited forms of cholestatic liver diseases it must be assumed that some acquired forms of drug-induced cholestasis might also be caused by inhibition of the canalicular excretory systems. In fact, recent investigations indicate that a variety of potentially cholestatic drugs including cyclosporine A, rifamycin, rifampicin and glibenclamide are potent inhibitors of the canalicular bile salt export pump BSEP (Fig. 3)[15]. Hence, their administration in combination and/or their administration to patients with a preexisting decrease of BSEP function (e.g. disease related; genetic polymorphisms) could induce a clinically relevant failure of canalicular bile salt secretion. As a consequence cytotoxic bile salts will accumulate within hepatocytes and serum and induce hepatocellular apoptosis and necrosis leading to increased serum transaminases and the full picture of severe clinical cholestasis. It is probable that similar acquired forms of cholestasis can also be caused by drug- and toxin-induced inhibition of the canalicular phosphatidylcholine flippase MDR3 although this assumption remains to be investigated. As in PFIC3, inhibition of MDR3 would decrease the canalicular secretion of phospholipids and thus impair the formation of mixed micelles in bile. As a consequence the intrabiliary concentration of free bile salts will be increased and could include toxic bile duct damage leading eventually to the vanishing bile duct syndrome. Although further details of the pathogenesis of drug-induced cholestasis remain to be elucidated in future studies, the recent progress in the understanding of the molecular hepatobiliary transport processes have paved the way for the development of better prevention and treatment strategies for drug- and toxin-induced cholestatic liver disease.

Therapy

Therapy of drug-induced liver injury requires in the first place the rapid identification of the offending drug and the cessation of its administration. Cases with fulminant liver injury must be prepared for potential liver transplantation. Any case with suspected or proven paracetamol overdose must be treated with N-acetylcysteine as early as possible[9] to prevent impending hepatocellular necrosis. Whether N-acetylcysteine and/or other antioxidative agents (e.g. S-adenosylmethionine) protect against toxic liver injury induced by other drugs has not been established. The same is true for the suggested hepatoprotective effects of corticosteroids in autoimmune drug-induced hepatitis. In prolonged cholestasis ursodeoxycholate may be of benefit and supplementation of fat-soluble vitamins or medium chain triglycerides must be provided. Further, cholestyramine or colestipol may help reduce pruritis.

TOXIN-INDUCED LIVER INJURY

Toxic liver injury by nonpharmaceutical agents encompasses, in principle, the same mechanisms and types of liver pathology as drug-induced liver injury.

Diagnosis of toxic liver injury is obvious in acute poisoning with well known hepatotoxic agents including *Amanita* mushrooms and chlorinated hydrocarbons (e.g. carbon tetrachloride, trichloroethylene). More difficult is the identification of drugs of abuse, e.g. cocaine, ecstasy (3,4-methylenedioxymethamphetamine)[16]; herbal medicines[17] and bacterial toxins[18–20] as causes of fulminant and acute liver failure. The same is true for toxin-induced chronic liver disease as exemplified by pyrrolizidine alkaloids induced veno-occlusive disease[17]. The medicinal plant *Germander* has produced instances of chronic hepatitis and cirrhosis[21]. In such cases the identification of the causative hepatotoxic agent often requires, besides careful gathering of information from the patient and relatives, complex analytical chemistry and other specific laboratory investigations.

The natural course of toxic liver injury can be fulminant, acute or chronic, depending on the type and dose of the ingested toxin. *Amanita* mushroom poisoning is characterized by an initial 6–12 h asymptomatic phase and a 1–4 day gastroenteritis phase (severe vomiting and diarrhoea) during which increasing signs of toxic liver injury develop. In severe cases terminal liver failure with hepatic encephalopathy usually develops 4–8 days after mushroom ingestion. Fulminant, acute and chronic forms of liver diseases have been reported for a variety of hepatotoxins including drugs of abuse and herbal medicines (see above).

Two recent reports of fatal liver injury induced by food- and water-borne environmental toxins deserve special attention. First, a 17-year-old boy died because of emetic toxin-induced fulminant liver failure[18]. The boy consumed spaghetti with homemade pesto that was heavily contaminated with *Bacillus cereus*, a widely recognized food-borne pathogen. *Bacillus cereus* produces emetic toxin, a cyclic peptide that is unusually resistant to heat and proteolysis. Histological examination of the boy's liver showed diffuse microvesicular steatosis, a finding indicative of decreased mitochondrial β-oxidation[22]. In fact, emetic toxin has been shown to impair mitochondrial fatty acid metabolism and to uncouple oxidative phosphorylation in isolated mitochondria[18]. Hence, the mechanism of emetic toxin induced hepatotoxicity is similar to the mitochondrial energy crisis induced by aspirin in Reye's syndrome and in valproate-induced hepatotoxicity (see above). Second, fatal liver failure and death due to microcystin intoxication recently occurred in a haemodialysis unit in Brazil[19,20]: 60 patients died. The water used for haemodialysis was taken from a lake with massive overgrowth of cyanobacteria (blue-green algae). The primary target organs of microcystins are the liver and brain. Microcystins inhibit protein phosphatases 1 and 2A, disrupt the cytoskeleton and lead to massive hepatocellular necrosis and hepatic haemorrhage[23]. Recent personal observations indicate that uptake of microcystins into hepatocytes and across the blood–brain barrier is mediated by the human organic anion transporting polypeptide OATP and can be inhibited by other high affinity OATP substrates such as BSP and dehydroepiandrosteronesulfate (DHEAS).

Therapy of toxic liver injury includes interruption of the toxic exposure, early decontamination in acute poisoning (e.g. oral activated charcoal) and adequate supportive measures. With the exception of N-acetylcysteine in paracetamol poisoning (see above), specific antidotal therapy with antioxidative agents has not been established for any forms of toxic liver injury. In *Amanita* mushroom poisoning silibinin and high doses of penicillin G are generally recommended, although their efficacy has also not been definitely demonstrated in controlled clinical trials. In most cases of fulminant toxic hepatitis liver transplantation remains the only therapeutic option.

REFERENCES

1. Pessayre D, Larrey D, Biour M. Drug-induced liver injury. In: Bircher J, Benhamou JP, McIntyre N, Rizzetto M, Rodés J, eds. Oxford Textbook of Clinical Hepatology, 2nd edn, Vol 2. Oxford: Oxford Medical Publications, 1999: pp. 1261–1315.
2. Kahl R. Toxic liver injury. In: Bircher J, Benhamou JP, McIntyre N, Rizzetto M, Rodés J, eds. Oxford Textbook of Clinical Hepatology, Vol 2. Oxford: Oxford Medical Publications, 1999: pp. 1319–34.
3. Zimmerman HJ. Hepatotoxicity. The Adverse Effects of Drugs and Other Chemicals on the Liver, 2nd edn. Philadelphia: Lippincott Williams & Wilkins, 1999.
4. Farrell GC. Drug-induced Liver Disease. London: Churchill Livingstone, 1994.
5. Stricker BHCH. Drug-induced Hepatic Injury, 2nd edition. Amsterdam: Elsevier, 1992.
6. Steenbergen WV, Peeters P, De Bondt J, Staessen D, Büscher H, Laporta T et al. Nimesulide-induced acute hepatitis: evidence from six cases. J Hepatol. 1998;29:135–41.
7. McCormick PA, Kennedy F, Curry M, Traynor O. COX 2 inhibitor and fulminant hepatic failure. Lancet. 1999;353:40–1.
8. Benichou C. Criteria for drug-induced hepatitis. Report of an international consensus meeting. J Hepatol. 1990;11:272–6.
9. Vale JA, Proudfoot AT. Paracetamol (acetaminophen) poisoning. Lancet. 1995;346:547–52.
10. O'Grady JG. Paracetamol-induced acute liver failure: prevention and management. J Hepatol. 1997;26(Suppl.1):41–6.
11. Shayiq RM, Roberts DW, Rothstein K, Snawder JE, Benson W, Ma X, Black M. Repeat exposure to incremental doses of acetaminophen provides protection against acetaminophen-induced lethality in mice: an explanation for high acetaminophen dosage in humans without hepatic injury. Hepatology. 1999;29:451–63.
12. Fromenty B, Berson A, Pessayre D. Microvesicular steatosis and steatohepatitis: role of mitochondrial dysfunction and lipid peroxidation. J Hepatol. 1997;26(Suppl. 1):13–22.
13. Trauner M, Meier PJ, Boyer JL. Molecular pathogenesis of cholestasis. N Engl J Med. 1998;339:1217–27.
14. Trauner M, Meier PJ, Boyer JL. Molecular regulation of hepatocellular transport systems in cholestasis. J Hepatol. 1999;31:165–78.
15. Stieger B, Fattinger K, Madon J, Kullak-Ublick GA, Meier PJ. Drug and estrogen induced cholestasis through inhibition of the hepatocellular bile salt export pump. Gastroenterology. 2000;118:422–30.
16. Selim K, Kaplowitz N. Hepatotoxicity of psychotropic drugs. Hepatology. 1999;29:1347–51.
17. Larrey D. Hepatotoxicity of herbal medicine. J Hepatol. 1997;26 (Suppl. 1):47–51.
18. Mahler H, Pasi A, Kramer JM, Schulte P, Scoging AC, Bar W, Kraehenbuhl S. Fulminant liver failure in association with the emetic toxin of *Bacillus cereus*. N Engl J Med. 1997;336:1142–8.
19. Pouria S, de Andrade A, Barbosa J, Cavalcanti RL, Barreto VT, Ward CJ et al. Fatal microcystin intoxication in haemodialysis unit in Caruaru, Brazil. Lancet. 1998;352:21–6.
20. Jochimsen EM, Carmichael WW, An JS, Cardo DM, Cookson ST, Holmes CEM et al. Liver failure and death after exposure to microcysteins at a hemodialysis center in Brazil. N Engl J Med. 1998;338:873–8.
21. Ben Yahia M, Mavier P, Metreau JM, Zafrani ES, Fabre M, Gatineau-Saillant G et al. Hépatite chronique active et cirrhose induites par la germandrée petit-chêne à propos de trois cas. Gatroenterol Clin Biol. 1993;17:959–62.
22. Fromenty B, Pessayre D. Inhibition of mitochondrial beta-oxidation as a mechanism of hepatotoxicity. Pharmacol Ther. 1995;67:101–54.
23. Dawson RM. The toxicology of microcysteins. Toxicon. 1998;36:953–62.

Section IV
Metabolic liver diseases

19
Liver-directed gene therapy: 2000 and beyond

S. J. LEE, M. TAKAHASHI, Y. KAWASHITA, A. KADAKOL, S. S. GHOSH, B. PARASHAR, N. ROY CHOWDHURY and J. ROY CHOWDHURY

The discovery of molecular genetic mechanisms of many liver diseases and advances in the methods of gene transfer in vivo have brought successful liver-directed gene therapy close to clinical application. Various options available for liver-directed gene therapy have been reviewed recently[1]. In the present article, we discuss in brief the current goals, methods and challenges of gene therapy for liver diseases at the turn of the century.

Gene therapy strategies are being developed for the treatment of inherited, as well as acquired, disorders of the liver. A partial list of inherited liver diseases that are current targets of gene therapy is shown in Table 1. Gene therapy is also being explored in the treatment of acquired liver diseases, such as viral infections, cirrhosis and primary and metastatic liver tumours. Several diseases, such as haemophilia and diabetes, for which liver is not the primary pathophysiological site are also targets of liver-directed gene therapy. In addition, gene transfer to the liver is being investigated as means of abrogation of immune rejection of allogeneic or xenogeneic organ or cell transplants.

Table 1 A partial list of inherited metabolic disorders that are current targets of liver-directed gene therapy

Crigler-Najjar syndrome type 1
Ornithine transcarbamylase deficiency
Haemophilia A and B (deficiency of coagulation factor VIII and IX, respectively)
Familial hypercholesterolaemia
Mucopolysaccharidosis VII
Maple syrup urine disease
Hereditary tyrosinaemia-1
Wilson's disease

Strategies for liver-directed gene therapy can be classified into several broad groups. Gene transfer to the liver may replace missing functional gene products. Metabolic diseases, listed in Table 1, are examples of such conditions. The liver could be used to generate proteins, such as the coagulation factors, insulin or growth hormone. In some circumstances genes may be transferred to the liver to express proteins that are normally not produced in the liver. For example, the catalytic subunit of the apolipoprotein B mRNA editing enzyme (APOBEC-1)[2], which is normally expressed in the intestine but not in the liver of many mammals, including humans, could be expressed ectopically in the liver to reduce the plasma concentration of low density lipoproteins. The liver can be used also to generate non-physiological (pharmacological) proteins, such as vaccines, single-chain antibodies, dominant-negative proteins, immunomodulatory substances and agents that induce or inhibit apoptosis. Another approach is to down-regulate the expression of a specific gene by transferring synthetic antisense RNAs or ribozymes or genes that express antisense RNAs, ribozymes or dominant-negative proteins for the treatment of viral diseases, hypercholesterolaemia, primary or secondary liver tumours, and mutant α_1-antitrypsin deposition in the liver. Recently, site-directed gene repair in vivo has been performed successfully in mammalian liver, using synthetic oligomers designed to hybridize to specific genomic sequences, thereby triggering the mismatch repair enzyme system of the cell to correct mutations or single-base deletions[3].

Gene transfer into the liver may be accomplished by transplantation of normal or transduced isolated hepatocytes, via in situ injection or perfusion, or through systemic administration of vectors. Both viral and non-viral gene transfer methods have been used for these purposes.

GENE TRANSFER TO THE LIVER USING NON-VIRAL VEHICLES

Transient expression of a transgene may be obtained by direct injection of DNA into the liver parenchyma or gene introduction using ballistics. In experimental animals, rapid injection of a plasmid in a volume large enough to cause temporary congestive cardiac failure results in transient expression in the liver.

Liposomes offer a more practical method of gene delivery. Nucleic acids incorporated into amphiphilic lipids with net positive or negative charge, with or without endosome-destabilizing properties have been used to transfer genes to the liver[4]. Incorporation of molecules with specific affinity for hepatocytes could enhance liver-specific delivery of liposomes[5]. The asialoglycoprotein receptor (AsGPr), which is preferentially expressed in hepatocytes, has been utilized successfully for liver-targeted gene transfer[6]. Galactose-terminated peptides, such as asialoorosomucoid or asialofetuin, or other densely galactosylated substances, e.g. lactosylated polyethyleneimine[3,7] or galactocerebroside-containing liposomes[3] have been used to transfer genes to hepatocytes via receptor-mediated endocytosis. Similarly, the mannose receptor has been used to target nucleic acids to non-parenchymal liver cells[8,9].

Delivery of DNA into the liver by physical or endocytotic methods results in short-term transgene expression. Endocytosed molecules are mostly translocated to lysosomes for degradation, limiting their translocation to the nucleus. Partial hepatectomy[10] or administration of colchicine[11] after endocytotic gene delivery extended the persistence of the transgene in cytoplasmic vesicles for several months, probably by interfering with the transport to lysosomes by transient disruption of the microtubular network. Agents that destabilize the endosomal vesicles e.g. polyetheleneimine, or viral or bacterial fusogenic proteins, could release the endocytosed genes into the cytoplasm, thereby enhancing translocation into the nucleus[12,13]. Components of the haemagglutinating virus of Japan have been incorporated into liposomes to enhance gene transfer[14] or to target genes to hepatocytes via the asialoglycoprotein receptor[15]. As recombinant viruses have a natural ability to express transgenes for a longer duration, virus-based vectors are being used by a large number of investigators for liver-directed gene therapy.

RECOMBINANT VIRUSES AS GENE DELIVERY VEHICLES

Many viruses have specific mechanisms to enter mammalian cells via physiological receptors, exit from endosomal vesicles to translocate into the nucleus and express viral genes with or without integration into the chromosomes. Genetically engineered viruses that express desired transgenes, but not the viral proteins, have been used extensively for gene transfer. Factors that need to be considered in determining the desirability of a recombinant virus for a specific application include available infectious titre, ability to infect non-dividing cells, efficiency of integration into the host genome, repeatability of administration and safety of the vector system. Some viral vectors that are commonly used in liver-directed gene therapy are described in brief.

Retrovirus-based vectors

Retroviruses stably insert a complementary DNA copy of their RNA genome into the host chromosome as a requirement of their life cycle. Their ability to be faithfully transmitted to the progeny cells and to accommodate relatively large genes make them attractive in gene therapy applications[16,17]. However, Moloney's murine leukaemia virus (MoMuLV)-based retroviruses require cell division for integration[17], making them inefficient for gene delivery to hepatocytes, which are normally quiescent. To circumvent this limitation, new vectors, based on other classes of retroviruses that can infect non-dividing cells, such as lentiviruses, are being developed. The RNA genome of retroviruses encodes three major viral proteins, gag, pol and env. The coding region is flanked on either side by the long terminal repeats (LTRs) that contain a promoter, enhancers and polyadenylation signals, that are needed for viral transcription. The ψ sequence allows packaging of the viral RNA into viral particles. Following entry of the virus into a mammalian cell via surface receptors, the RNA genome is reverse-transcribed into double stranded DNA provirus, which forms a part of a nucleoprotein complex, termed the pre-integration complex (PIC). In the case of murine leukaemia retroviruses, the pre-integration complexes do not pass through intact nuclear membranes. Therefore, integration into the host genome requires mitosis-associated dissolution of nuclear envelope[18].

The U3 region within the 3′ LTR carries promoters and enhancers necessary for the transcription of the integrated provirus. Deletions introduced into this region are transmitted to the 5′ region of the viral DNA during reverse transcription. The resulting viral DNA lacks both 5′ and 3′ U3 regions, preventing the initiation of transcription from the viral LTRs. Absence of the 3′ promoter in these self-inactivating vectors eliminates the possibility of undesirable activation of an oncogene by the integrated proviral genome, thereby increasing their biosafety[19]. Replication-defective retroviruses are generated by replacing most or all viral genes by target transgenes. The recombinant viral particles are produced by transfecting the recombinant DNA into packaging cell lines that provide the viral proteins in *trans*.

Interaction of viral envelope glycoproteins with specific receptors on the host cell surface is required for internalization of the virus and is the major determinant of the host range of the recombinant vector. Exchanging the *env* gene of one virus with that of another results in the generation of pseudotyped viruses that exhibit the host range properties of the virus from which the envelope is derived[20]. For example, replacement of retroviral envelopes with vesicular stomatitis virus G glycoprotein (VSV-G) generates psuedotyped virus particles, that have a wider host range, are not inactivated by human plasma and can be concentrated by centrifugation.

To facilitate transgene expression in non-dividing cells, vectors based on lentiviruses, such as human immunodeficiency virus (HIV-1), are being developed[21]. The basic mode of replication of lentiviruses is similar to that of murine retroviruses, but in contrast to the situation in MoMuLV, the lentiviral pre-integration complexes are actively transported through intact nuclear membranes, permitting integration into the genome of quiescent cells[21]. Recombinant lentiviruses show promise in liver-directed gene therapy. However gene transfer efficiency that would be sufficient for clinical benefit has not been demonstrated with these vectors, and it is uncertain whether lentiviruses can integrate into totally quiescent hepatocytes (G-0) in vivo.

Recombinant adeno-associated virus

Adeno-associated virus-2 (AAV-2) is a small (4.7 kb) single stranded DNA virus of the parvovirus family. The wildtype virus integrates on the q13.4-ter arm of human chromosome 19[22]. In the presence of a helper virus, such as adenovirus[23] or herpes simplex virus[24], AAV sequences are rescued from the integration site, resulting in productive infection. In the absence of a helper virus, the viral genome remains integrated in the host chromosome for long periods. The AAV genome contains three promoters (p5, p19, and p40), a polyadenylation signal, a gene each for a non-structural protein, Rep, and a structural protein, Cap. On both ends of these genes, there are 145 bp inverted terminal repeats (ITR) that form hairpin structures and are required for integration of the virus into the host genome[24]. The 3′-OH end of the ITR hairpin primes second-strand synthesis, generating a double-stranded AAV genome. Rep catalyses nicking at the terminal resolution site, producing a linear duplex which is the substrate for a new round of replication. Synthesis of the second strand is needed for gene expression and, probably, also for integration.

The site-specificity of recombinant AAV is lost in vectors in which the AAV coding sequences are deleted. Latent AAV as well as AAV vectors can persist in host cells as an episome or as an integrated viral genome. High-titre recombinant AAV, used in recent studies, has produced levels of gene expression in the liver[25], that could be potentially useful in disorders, such as coagulation factor IX deficiency.

Simian virus 40-based vectors

Recombinant simian virus 40 (SV40) is capable of infecting both dividing and non-dividing cells[26]. SV40 is a non-enveloped DNA virus of the papova virus family with a circular double stranded genome of about 5.2 kb without terminal repeats. The large (Tag) and small (tag) T antigens, that are expressed by differential splicing of a common RNA transcript are required for transcription of the viral structural proteins, VP1, VP2 and VP3[27]. The recombinant viral genome is generated by replacing the Tag gene by the target gene. Viral particles are generated by transfecting the recircularized recombionant viral genome into COS-7 cells, that provide Tag in *trans*. As the recombinant SV40 lacks the Tag gene, it does not replicate and express viral structural proteins. The absence of Tag also abrogates the immunogenicity of the recombinant SV40[26]. The recombinant SV40 system can accommodate up to 4.7 kb of exogenous DNA. The virus has been purified and concentrated to a titre of up to 10^{12} pfu/ml by sucrose gradient centrifugation. The ability of SV40 to infect non-dividing cells makes it attractive for liver-directed gene therapy[26]. Preliminary studies suggest that the recombinant SV40 integrates into the host chromosomal DNA rapidly and efficiently, without detectable cytotoxicity.

Recombinant adenovirus

Vectors derived from human adenovirus type 5 and type 2, have been investigated extensively. These vectors can be generated at high titres, express transgenes in both dividing and non-dividing cells[27] and can transfer genes to a wide variety of cells in culture. After systemic administration in rodents, the virus localizes preferentially and efficiently into the liver[28]. Nearly 100% transduction has been achieved in hepatocytes in vitro and in vivo, using these vectors. Adenoviral vectors are produced by disrupting the E1 gene which encodes transcription factors required for the expression of other adenoviral genes by cloning the transgene of interest into this region of an adenovirus shuttle vector. The recombinant virus is generated in a helper cell line that provides the viral proteins in *trans*.

Although adenoviral vectors are highly efficient in transferring genes to the liver in vivo, the episomal nature of these vectors limits its persistence within host cells[29]. The duration of transgene expression is further reduced by host anti-virus immune response, which precludes gene expression following subsequent administration of the vector[27]. Strategies to abrogate the host immune response by modification of the vector or the host are being investigated. Sequences encoding viral structural genes have been deleted progressively to produce gutless vectors[27]. However, despite the lack of de novo expression in cells the recombinant adenoviruses remain immunogenic because of the presence of viral proteins provided in *trans* by the packaging cells. Other approaches utilize the expression of immunomodulatory genes, such as adenoviral E3, by the recombinant vector[30]. The E3 genes may inhibit multiple pathways of the antiviral immune response, including the down-regulation of MHC class I expression in the host cell, and inhibition of action of TNFα[31].

An alternative approach aims at inducing host tolerance specifically to antigens present in the recombinant virus. Injection of recombinant adenovirus into newborn rats[28], intrathymic inoculation of adenoviral proteins in young adult rats[32], and oral administration of small doses of adenoviral proteins in adult rats[33] have all resulted in abrogation of both humoral and cell-mediated arms of host immune response against adenoviral antigens. Oral tolerization is mediated by suppressor cells, which reside in peripheral lymphatic tissues, and can prevent both primary and booster responses to adenoviral vectors[33,34]. Immune ignorance, but not tolerance to adenoviral vectors, can also be achieved by short-term immunosuppression with tacrolimus around the time of virus administration[35]. Because long-term tolerance is not induced by this method, immunosuppression must be used around the time of administration of each dose of the vector. Inhibition of co-stimulation between antigen presenting cells and cytotoxic lymphocytes by the administration of CTLA4-Ig and CD-40 antibodies to the host has resulted in some prolongation of expression of transgenes introduced via adenoviral vectors[36]. These methods now permit repeated administration of adenoviral vectors for long-term gene therapy, but safety concerns persist regarding tolerization of human hosts to adenoviruses, which are human pathogens.

Recombinant baculovirus

Vectors based on the recombinant baculovirus *Autographa californica* nuclear polyhedrosis (AcNPV) are commonly used for generating recombinant proteins in insect cells. Among mammalian cells, hepatocytes can be transduced by baculoviral vectors[37]. The endogenous polyhedrin promoter of the virus is inactive in mammalian cells, but transgene expression can be expressed from internal promoters that function in mammalian cells. Baculoviral vectors can accommodate a large amount of exogenous DNA. Although its in vivo gene transferring ability has not been demonstrated and its immunogenicity has not been well characterized, recombinant viruses consisting partly of baculoviral sequences and partly of sequences from other viruses are being explored for application in specific situations.

Recombinant herpes simplex virus-1 (HSV-1)

HSV-1 is a 150 kb double stranded DNA virus which can infect a broad range of dividing and non-dividing cell types[38]. However, long-term gene expression in the liver has not been achieved with the currently available HSV vectors.

SITE-DIRECTED GENE REPAIR

A strategy to correct single nucleotide mutations in genomic DNA, based on cellular gene repair mechanisms, has been reported[39]. Synthetic oligonucleotides that mediate this process consist of a chimaeric molecule of duplex structure. Single-stranded hairpin caps flank the double-stranded region of the molecule. The upper strand consists of five or more central DNA residues, flanked by 2′ orthomethyl RNA residues, and is complementary to the target genomic DNA sequence, except for a single mismatch at the middle of the central DNA residues. The RNA sequences are flanked by additional DNA sequences, which form T loops at each end of the double stranded secondary structure. The lower strand consists of DNA residues and is complementary to the sequence of the RNA/DNA chimaeric upper strand. The RNA residues may promote pairing with the complementary genomic sequence, increasing the efficiency and specificity of the gene repair. The mismatched nucleotide may trigger the cellular mismatch repair enzyme, providing the desired gene correction. The chimaeric oligonucleotides have been delivered to hepatocytes by receptor-mediated endocytosis, using lactosylated polyethyleneimine or galacto-cerebroside-containing liposomes, which are recognized by asialoglycoprotein receptors at the surface of hepatocytes. Using this technology, it has been possible to insert a missing guanosine residue into the bilirubin-UDP-glucuronosyl-transferase gene (*UGT1A1*) of mutant Gunn rats, an animal model for Crigler–Najjar syndrome type 1[3]. Correction of the genetic lesion resulted in the generation of normally active bilirubin-UGT in the Gunn rat liver, with consequent biliary excretion of bilirubin glucuronides and reduction of serum bilirubin concentrations. With further understanding of the mechanism of gene repair by this method, site-directed gene repair may become a viable alternative to gene replacement for the treatment of some inherited and acquired disorders.

EX VIVO GENE THERAPY

The first long-term gene therapy for a metabolic liver disease was performed by the ex vivo approach[40]. Primary hepatocytes isolated from a resected segment of the liver from a Watanabe heritable hyperlipidaemic rabbit (WHHL, a model for familial hypercholesterolaemia), were transduced with a retroviral vector expressing the gene for low-density lipoprotein receptor (LDLR). The phenotypically corrected hepatocytes were then transplanted back into the donor. This method requires integration of the therapeutic gene into the hepatocyte genome. As the hepatocyte donor was the same as the recipient, immunosuppression was not required. The procedure resulted in modest, but long-term reduction of serum LDL levels[40]. Subsequently, this approach was used in several patients with familial hypercholesterolaemia[41]. Although in vivo expression of the transgene was demonstrated, the clinical effect did not reach a therapeutically beneficial level. Efficiency of the ex vivo approach is restricted by the number of hepatocytes that can be harvested from a resected liver segment, inefficient transduction by MoMuLV-based vectors, and the number of phenotypically corrected hepatocytes that can be harvested and transplanted. Although the enthusiasm for ex vivo gene therapy is low at this time, research in various laboratories may provide partial solution to these problems. Improved cell culture methods[42,43], conditional and reversible immortalization of hepatocytes and improved titre of retroviral or adeno-associated viral vectors may improve the chances of successful application of this method in clinical situations.

Although none of the currently available methods of gene transfer to the liver is suitable for all types of applications, a wide choice of non-viral and viral vectors for gene transfer to the liver is now available for specific applications. Newer vectors that are continuously being developed are expected to replace the current generation of vectors in the coming decades. Both gene replacement and gene repair are expected to become important therapeutic modalities during the first quarter of the new century.

ACKNOWLEDGEMENTS

This work was supported in part by the following grants from the National Institute of Health: ROI-DK 46 057 (to JRC) and ROI-DK 39 137 (to NRC).

REFERENCES

1. Ghosh SS, Takahashi M, Thummala NR, Parashar B, Roy Chowdhury N, Roy Chowdhury J. Liver-directed gene therapy: promises, problems and prospects at the turn of the century. J Hepatol. 2000, in press.
2. Greeve J, Jona VK, Roy-Chowdhury N et al. Hepatic gene transfer of the catalytic subunit of the apolypoprotein B mRNA editing enzyme, APOBEC-1, leads to reduction of LDL in normal and Watanabe heritable hyperlipidemic rabbits. J Lipid Res. 1996;37:2001–17.
3. Kren B, Parashar B, Bandopadhyay P, Roy Chowdhury N, Roy Chowdhury J, Steer CJ. Correction of the UDP-glucuronosyltransferase gene defect in the Gunn rat model of Crigler-Najjar syndrome type I. Proc Natl Acad Sci USA. 1999;96:10349–54.
4. Litzinger DC, Brown JM, Wala I et al. Fate of cationic liposomes and their complex with oligonucleotide in vivo. Biochim Biophys Acta. 1996;1281:139–49.
5. Hara T, Aramaki Y, Takada S, Koike K, Tsuchiya S. Receptor-mediated transfer of pSV2CAT DNA to mouse liver cells using asialofetuin-labeled liposomes. Gene Ther. 1995;2:784–8.
6. Smith RM, Wu GY. Hepatocyte-directed gene delivery by receptor-mediated endocytosis. Semin Liver Dis. 1999;19:83–92.
7. Zanta MA, Boussif O, Adib A, Behr JP. In vitro gene delivery to hepatocytes with galactosylated polyethylenimine. Bioconjug Chem. 1997;8:839–44.
8. Franssen EJ, Jansen RW, Vaalburg M, Meijer DK. Hepatic and intrahepatic targeting of an anti-inflammatory agent with human serum albumin and neoglycoproteins as carrier molecules. Biochem Pharmacol. 1993;45:1215–26.
9. Nishikawa M, Kamijo A, Fujita T, Takakura Y, Sezaki H, Hashida M. Synthesis and pharmacokinetics of a new liver-specific carrier, glycosylated carboxymethyl-dextran, and its application to drug targeting. Pharm Res. 1993;10:1253–61.
10. Bommineni VR, Chowdhury NR, Wu GY et al. Depolymerization of hepatocellular microtubules after partial hepatectomy. J Biol Chem. 1994;269:25200–5.
11. Roy Chowdhury N, Hays RM, Bommineni VR et al. Microtubular disruption prolongs the expression of human bilirubin-uridinediphosphoglucuronate-glucuronosyltransferase-1 gene transferred into Gunn rat livers. J Biol Chem. 1996;271:2341–6.
12. Hara T, Kuwasawa H, Aramaki Y et al. Effects of fusogenic and DNA-binding amphiphilic compounds on the receptor-mediated gene transfer into hepatic cells by asialofetuin-labeled liposomes. Biochim Biophys Acta. 1996;1278:51–8.
13. Wu G, Zhan P, Sze LL, Rosenberg AR, Wu CH. Incorporation of adenovirus into a ligand-based DNA carrier system results in retention of original receptor specificity and enhances targeted gene expression. J Biol Chem. 1994;269:11542–6.
14. Hirano T, Fujimoto J, Veki T, Yamamoto H, Takeuchi M, Okamoto E et al. HVJ liposome-mediated gene transfer into hepatocytes in vivo. J Hepatol. 1998;29:910–14.

15. Ramani K, Hassan Q, Venkatiah B, Hasnain SE, Sarkar DP. Site-specific gene delivery in vivo through engineered Sendai viral envelopes. Proc Natl Acad Sci USA. 1998;95:11886–90.
16. Verma IM, Somia N. Gene therapy – promises, problems and prospects. Nature. 1997;389:239–42.
17. Kalpana GV. Retroviral vectors for liver-directed gene therapy. Semin Liver Dis. 1999;19:27–37.
18. Roe T, Reynolds TC, Yu G et al. Integration of murine leukemia virus depends on mitosis. EMBO J. 1993;12:2099–108.
19. Coffin JM, Hughes SH, Vermus HE. Retroviruses 1. Cold Spring Harbor, NY: Cold Spring Harbor Press, 1997.
20. Miller AD. Development of applications of retroviral vectors. In: Coffin JM, Hughes SH, Vermus HE, eds. Retroviruses. Cold Spring Harbor, NY: Cold Spring Harbor Press, 1997: pp. 437–73.
21. Bukrynsky MI, Haffar OK. HIV-1 nuclear import; matrix protein is back on center stage, this time with Vpr. Mol Med. 1998;4:138–43.
22. Samulsky RJ, Zhu X, Xiao X, Brook JD, Housman DE, Epstein N, Hunter LA. Targeted integration of adenoassociated virus (AAV) into human chromosome 19. EMBO J. 1991;10:3941–50.
23. Atchison RW, Casto BC, Hammon W. Adenovirus helps adenoassociated virus replication. Science. 1965;149:754–6.
24. Buller RM, Janik JE, Sebring ED, Rose JA. Herpes simplex virus types 1 and 2 completely help adenoassociated virus replication. J Virol. 1981;40:241–7.
25. Snyder RO, Miao CH, Patijn GA et al. Persistent and therapeutic concentrations of human factor IX in mice after hepatic gene transfer of recombinant AAV vectors. Nature Genet. 1997;16:270–6.
26. Strayer DS, Zern MA. Gene delivery to the liver using simian virus 40-derived vectors. Semin Liver Dis. 1999;19:71–81.
27. Chiocca S, Cotton M. Characteristics of Adenovirus Vectors. In: Chiocca EA and Breakfield XO, eds. Gene Therapy for Neurological Disorders and Brain Tumors, 1st edn. Totowa, NJ: Humana Press, 1998: pp. 39–52.
28. Takahashi M, Ilan Y, Sengupta K, Roy Chowdhury N, Roy Chowdhury J. Induction of tolerance to recombinant adenoviruses by injection into newborn rats: Long term amelioration of hyperbilirubinemia in Gunn rats. J Biol Chem. 1996;271:26536–42.
29. Horwitz MS. Adenovirudae and their replication. In: Fields BN, Knipe DM, eds. Virology. New York: Raven Press, 1990: pp. 1679–721.
30. Ilan Y, Droguett G, Roy Chowdhury N, Li Y, Sengupta K, Thummala NR et al. Insertion of the adenoviral E3 region into a recombinant viral vector prevents antiviral humoral and cellular immune responses and permits long-term gene expression. Proc Natl Acad Sci USA. 1997;94:2587–92.
31. Horwitz MS, Tufariello J, Grunhaus A, Fejer G. Model systems for studying the effects of adenovirus E3 genes on virulence in vivo. Curr Topics Microbiol Immunol. 1995;199:195–211.
32. Ilan Y, Attavar P, Takahashi M, Davidson A, Horwitz, M, Guida J et al. Induction of central tolerance by intrathymic inoculation of adenoviral antigens into the host thymus permits long term gene therapy in Gunn rats. J Clin Invest. 1996;98:2640–7.
33. Ilan Y, Prakash R, Davidson A, Jona VK, Droguett G, Horwitz MS et al. Oral tolerization to adenoviral antigens permits long term gene expression using recombinant adenoviral vectors. J Clin Invest. 1997;99:1098–106.
34. Ilan Y, Sauter B, Roy Chowdhury N, Reddy B, Thummala NR, Groguett G et al. Oral tolerization to adenoviral proteins permits repeated adenovirus-mediated gene therapy in rats with preexisting immunity to adenovirus. Hepatology. 1998;27:1368–76.
35. Ilan Y, Jona VK, Sengupta K, Davidson A, Horwitz MS, Roy-Chowdhury N, Roy-Chowdhury J. Transient immunosuppression with fk506 permits long-term expression of therapeutic genes introduced into the liver using recombinant adenoviruses. Hepatology. 1997;26:949–56.
36. Wilson CB, Embree LJ, Schowalter D, Albert R, Aruffo A, Hollenbaugh D et al. Transient inhibition of CD28 and CD40 ligand interactions prolongs adenovirus-mediated transgene expression in the lung and facilitates expression after secondary vector administration. J Virol. 1998;72:7542–50.
37. Hoffmann C, Sandig V, Jennings G. Efficient gene transfer into human hepatocytes by baculovirus vectors. Proc Natl Acad Sci USA. 1995;92:10099–103.

38. Fung Y, Federoff HG, Brownlee M et al. Rapid and efficient gene transfer in human hepatocytes by herpes viral vectors. Hepatology. 1995;22:723–9.
39. Yoon K, Cole-Strauss A, Kmiec EB. Targeted gene correction of episomal DNA in mammalian cells mediated by a chimeric RNA·DNA oligonucleotide. Proc Natl Acad Sci USA. 1996;93:2071–6.
40. Roy Chowdhury J, Grossman M, Gupta S et al. Long term improvement of hypercholesterolemia after ex vivo gene therapy in LDL-receptor deficient rabbits. Science. 1991;254:1802–5.
41. Grossman M, Raper SE, Kozarsky K et al. Successful ex vivo gene therapy directed to the liver in a patient with familial hypercholesterolemia. Nature Genet. 1994;6:335–41.
42. Block GD, Locker J, Bowen WC, Petersen BE, Katyal S, Strom SC et al. Population expansion, clonal growth and specific differentiation patterns in primary cultures of hepatocytes induced by HGF/SF, EGF and TGF alpha in a chemically defined (HGM) medium. J Cell Biol. 1996;132:1133–49.
43. Block GD, Roy Chowdhury J. General principles of ex vivo gene transfer into hepatocytes. In Mito M, Sawa M, eds. Hepatocyte Transplantation, New York: Karger-Landes, 1997: pp. 219–33.

20 Haemochromatosis: pathogenesis and diagnosis

B. R. BACON, R. E. FLEMING and R. S. BRITTON

INTRODUCTION

Hereditary haemochromatosis (HH) is a common inherited disorder of iron overload characterized by an increased absorption of iron from the proximal gastrointestinal tract with deposition of iron predominantly in the parenchymal cells of the liver, the pancreas, and other endocrine organs, the heart, joints, and the skin[1,2]. If undiagnosed and untreated, cirrhosis of the liver and hepatocellular cancer can result. In addition, diabetes, heart failure, arthropathy, and an increase in skin pigmentation can occur[1,2]. Marcel Simon and colleagues[3] in Rennes, France provided definitive proof of the genetic nature of HH demonstrating the close linkage of the disease to the short arm of chromosome 6 in the region of HLA-A3. In 1996, using a positional cloning technique a research group at Mercator Genetics identified the gene responsible for HH[4]. The HH gene was shown to be a novel major histocompatibility complex (MHC) class 1-like gene and was initially named *HLA-H* with subsequent renaming to *HFE*. Numerous studies show that on average about 85–90% of patients with typical clinical features of HH are homozygous for a single missense mutation in *HFE* resulting in the substitution of tyrosine for cysteine at amino acid 282 (C282Y)[5]. A second mutation of *HFE* resulting in a substitution of aspartate for histidine at amino acid 63 (H63D) was also identified[4] but is not associated with the same degree of iron loading as is C282Y[5]. The cloning of *HFE* has established a foundation for a new era of molecular and cell biological studies in the pathophysiology of HH. This chapter will review the current understanding of the structure and cell biology of the HFE protein, and will present a working hypothesis to explain the effect of the HFE protein on iron absorption. In addition, current diagnostic strategies for HH will be described. Several recent reviews also have covered these areas[1,2,5–10].

HFE PROTEIN AND ITS ASSOCIATION WITH β2-MICROGLOBULIN

The *HFE* gene encodes a 343 amino acid protein, consisting of a 22 amino acid signal peptide, a large extracellular domain, a single transmembrane domain and a short cytoplasmic tail[4,5]. The structure of HFE protein characterizes it as a MHC class I-like protein. The extracellular domain consists of three loops ($\alpha1$, $\alpha2$, $\alpha3$) with disulphide bonds within the second and third loops. Crystallographic studies show that the $\alpha1$ and $\alpha2$ loops form a platform of antiparallel β strands topped by two antiparallel α helices[11]. The groove between the antiparallel α helices is analogous to the peptide-binding groove in antigen-presenting MHC class I proteins but is physically narrower, thus precluding peptide binding[11]. Therefore, HFE protein does not appear to function in antigen presentation.

The $\alpha3$ loop of HFE protein, like the homologous region of MHC class I molecules, is the site of binding with $\beta2$-microglobulin ($\beta2$M). Physical association between HFE protein and $\beta2$M has been demonstrated in human duodenum[12] and placenta[13], as well as in cultured cells[14–16]. Interestingly, the major mutation responsible for HH results in the conversion of cysteine 282 in the $\alpha3$ loop to a tyrosine (C282Y) and abolishes the disulphide bond in the $\alpha3$ domain[4]. As a result, the binding of the C282Y mutant protein to $\beta2$M is diminished and the intracellular trafficking and surface presentation of the mutant protein is impaired[14,15]. The importance of the HFE protein–$\beta2$M association for normal function of HFE protein is emphasized by the finding that $\beta2$M-knockout mice have iron overload with an HH-like phenotype[17,18].

CELL BIOLOGY OF HFE PROTEIN

Localization

HFE mRNA is found in many tissues, with the exception of brain and lymphoblasts[4]. Expression of HFE protein has been observed in intestine, oesophagus, stomach, colon, liver (sinusoidal lining cells, bile duct epithelial cells), placenta and leukocytes[12,13,19,20]. The duodenum is the primary site of iron absorption and shows a distinctive pattern of HFE protein immunostaining, with prominent expression in the crypt enterocytes and little expression in villal cells[12,19]. We have postulated that HFE protein in duodenal crypt cells may play a key role in regulating dietary iron absorption (see working hypothesis below).

Physical association with transferrin receptor

The first mechanistic link between HFE protein and cellular iron metabolism was made with the finding that HFE protein forms a stable complex with the transferrin receptor (TfR)[12,13,21–24]. HFE protein has been shown to physically associate with TfR in placental synctiotrophoblasts[13], the site of maternal–fetal iron transport, and in duodenal crypt enterocytes[12], the site of regulation of dietary iron absorption. The TfR plays a key role in the cellular uptake of transferrin-bound iron[5,25]. Studies in transfected cells suggest that the HFE protein–TfR complex forms shortly after the biosynthesis of each protein, and this complex may traffic to the cell surface[16]. After binding diferric transferrin, the TfR undergoes endocytosis and recycling. Within the cell, HFE protein has been found co-localized with TfR within acidic vesicles[16]. The association between HFE protein and TfR is pH dependent, with dissociation of the complex occurring when the pH is decreased from 7.4 to 6.0[11]. Taken together, these results suggest that the complex of HFE protein, TfR and diferric transferrin may undergo endocytosis, and that when the endocytotic vesicles become acidified, HFE protein dissociates from TfR. The fate of HFE protein after this dissociation occurs is not clear. The effect of HFE protein on TfR-mediated iron uptake by cells is discussed below.

Intracellular trafficking of normal and mutant HFE protein

Transfected cells over-expresssing HFE protein have been utilized to study the trafficking of the wild-type and mutant proteins. Feder et al.[14] demonstrated that wild-type HFE protein is bound to β2M in 293 cells, and that this interaction is abrogated by the C282Y mutation, but not the H63D mutation. Both wild-type and H63D HFE proteins are expressed on the cell surface, while the C282Y mutant protein is retained intracellularly. Waheed et al.[15] showed that both wild-type and H63D HFE proteins are associated with β2M and are expressed on the cell surface of COS-7 cells, but these capabilities are lost by the C282Y protein. The C282Y mutant protein is retained in the ER and middle Golgi compartment, fails to undergo late Golgi processing, and is subject to accelerated degradation. Thus, C282Y HFE protein binds inefficiently to β2M, disrupting its trafficking to the cell surface, and facilitating its intracellular degradation.

Effect on HFE protein on TfR-mediated iron uptake pathway in cultured cells

Given the physical association between HFE protein and TfR, a number of investigators have examined the effect of HFE protein on the TfR-mediated iron uptake pathway. These studies have used cultured cells in which normal HFE protein is overexpressed by transfection. Feder et al.[21] observed that wild-type HFE protein decreases the affinity of the TfR for diferric transferrin, and that H63D protein does not have this effect. In addition, they demonstrated that addition of soluble wild-type HFE/β2M heterodimers to cultured cells also decreases the apparent affinity of the TfR for its ligand. However, it should be noted that TfR has a very high affinity for diferrric transferrin, so that the observed HFE-induced decrease in affinity of TfR for transferrin is unlikely to have functional consequences under physiologic conditions, where diferric transferrin levels are supramaximal to saturate TfR.

Gross et al.[16] showed that normal HFE protein and TfR are capable of associating with each other within 30 min of their synthesis in cultured cells. HFE protein and TfR could be co-immunoprecipitated throughout the biosynthetic pathway, and excess HFE protein is rapidly degraded, whereas the HFE–TfR complex is stable. They also reported that at the cell surface, normal HFE protein is complexed with TfR, decreasing the affinity of TfR for transferrin. HFE protein does not remain at the cell surface, but trafficks with TfR to transferrin-positive internal compartments. Cells expressing normal HFE protein have decreased ferritin levels relative to control cells, suggesting decreased intracellular iron levels[16]. Roy et al.[26] extended these studies to show that expression of normal HFE protein reduces cellular iron accumulation from transferrin by 33% but does not affect the endocytic or exocytic rates of TfR cycling. They proposed that normal HFE protein may reduce cellular acquisition of iron from transferrin within endocytic compartments. Somewhat different results on TfR dynamics were observed by Salter-Cid et al.[27], who reported that expression of normal HFE protein reduces the number of functional transferrin binding sites and impairs TfR internalization, thus reducing the uptake of transferrin-bound iron. Two other groups have recently reported that overexpression of wild-type HFE protein in HeLa cells induces an iron-deficient phenotype, with decreased ferritin levels and increased iron regulatory protein activity[28,29]. In both studies, expression of HFE protein resulted in a decrease in cellular iron accumulation from diferric transferrin.

Therefore, the results from five studies suggest that over-expression of normal HFE protein results in an iron-deficient phenotype, probably due to a decrease in iron acquisition from transferrin[16,26–29]. However, it is difficult to explain the HH characteristics of increased dietary iron absorption and iron-spared Kupffer cells if normal HFE protein results in an iron-deficient cellular phenotype: these HH characteristics would be better explained if mutant HFE protein caused an iron-deficient phenotype in intestinal crypt cells and Kupffer cells. It should be noted that these studies using cultured cells did not examine the effect of mutant HFE protein on cellular iron status, and did not co-express β2M, which plays an important role in normal trafficking of HFE protein. More experimental investigation is needed to address these issues in cell types that normally express HFE protein. In addition, the recent reports that HFE protein may interfere with the binding of diferric transferrin to TfR[23,24] will trigger additional studies to see if this interaction occurs in cells and in vivo.

TRANSGENIC MOUSE MODELS TO STUDY THE FUNCTION OF HFE PROTEIN

Transgenic technology has provided important information about the functional consequences of *HFE* gene disruption in the whole animal. Three groups[30–32] have created HFE knockout mice (*HFE –/–*): these mice have increased hepatic iron levels[30–32], elevated transferrin saturation[30] and increased intestinal iron absorption[31]. Interestingly, mice that are homozygous for the C282Y mutation have less severe iron loading than *HFE –/–* mice, indicating that the C282Y mutation is not a null allele[32]. These results indicate that lack of functional HFE protein results in iron overload, and that normal HFE protein acts directly or indirectly to suppress iron absorption. Transgenic mice over-expressing normal HFE protein are anaemic, supporting the concept that HFE protein acts to restrict iron absorption (Sly, Fleming et al., unpublished observation). We have postulated that this effect of HFE protein may occur at the level of the duodenal crypt cell, through facilitation of TfR-mediated iron uptake[33].

WORKING HYPOTHESIS TO EXPLAIN EFFECT OF HFE PROTEIN ON IRON ABSORPTION

A key feature of HH that is shared by *HFE –/–* mice is an increase in intestinal iron absorption[1,2]. Enterocytes in the duodenal crypts are thought to play an important role in sensing body iron status, and then maturing into villus cells that are programmed to absorb an appropriate amount of dietary iron. An iron transport protein, called divalent metal transporter-1 (DMT-1) or Nramp2, is expressed on the luminal surface of villus cells and its expression is up-regulated by iron deficiency[34,35]. We have observed that HFE protein is highly expressed in the crypt cells of human duodenum[12,19], and is physically associated with TfR at this site[12]. Based on this foundation, we have developed a working hypothesis concerning the mechanism by which HFE protein modulates dietary iron absorption[33]. We propose that normal HFE protein facilitates the uptake of plasma iron by the TfR-mediated pathway in duodenal crypt cells, and that mutant HFE protein lacks this facilitating effect thereby decreasing the regulatory iron pool in crypt cells. A decrease in the regulatory iron pool can increase the binding of iron regulatory protein to iron-responsive elements in certain mRNAs: this could result in an increase in the apical expression of DMT-1 in daughter villus enterocytes, thus increasing dietary iron absorption. This hypothesis is supported by the recent observations that HH patients[36] and *HFE* –/– mice[33] demonstrate an increase in duodenal DMT-1 mRNA levels. The availability of *HFE* –/– and C282Y/C282Y mice will allow the steps in this working hypothesis to be tested experimentally.

DIAGNOSIS OF HEREDITARY HAEMOCHROMATOSIS

The diagnosis of HH should be considered in: symptomatic individuals with clinical features suggestive of HH, first-degree relatives of HH patients, and individuals with abnormal iron on screening[1,2,10]. Delayed diagnosis most often results when a physician does not consider HH as a possibility, incorrectly thinking that it is a rare disorder. Once considered, fasting transferrin saturation (serum iron divided by total iron binding capacity or transferrin × 100%) and ferritin levels should be obtained; both of these will be elevated in a symptomatic patient. Transferrin saturation should be obtained in the fasting state since serum iron levels have a diurnal variation and can be increased following a meal. Unfortunately, the sensitivity and specificity of transferrin saturation and ferritin levels become problematic when young individuals are being evaluated or when patients have abnormal iron studies in the context of other diseases. Up to 30% of women with HH below the age of 30 years may have a normal transferrin saturation[1], and in the absence of HH, serum iron studies (predominantly ferritin) can be abnormal in about 40–50% of patients with chronic viral hepatitis, non-alcoholic steatohepatitis, or alcoholic liver disease[1]. Additionally, because ferritin is an acute phase reactant, other inflammatory disorders (e.g. rheumatoid arthritis) and various neoplastic diseases (e.g. lymphoma, other cancers) can cause elevated serum ferritin levels in the absence of iron overload. Thus, serum iron studies alone produce many false-positive and false-negative results in predicting iron stores, and reliance on these studies by themselves for diagnosis of HH can result in errors of diagnosis. The development of a widely available genetic test for the C282Y and H63D mutations of *HFE* has already contributed to better characterization of those patients with underlying liver disease and abnormal serum iron studies. Nonetheless, in the absence of any other medical illness, the combination of an elevated transferrin saturation and an elevated ferritin level is approximately 90% sensitive and specific for the diagnosis of HH[1]. However, it must be remembered that all that may be required is a transferrin saturation of >45% and a ferritin of >200 ng/ml in a young woman. It is not necessary to have a transferrin saturation of 90% to 100% or a ferritin of greater than 1000 ng/ml.

Currently, if either the fasting transferrin saturation or ferritin level is elevated, regardless of what has led to it being obtained, genetic testing for *HFE* mutations should be performed and a liver biopsy (especially in patients >40 years old) should be considered to evaluate hepatic iron loading and fibrosis[1]. The liver biopsy should be processed for histochemical iron staining (Perls' Prussian blue stain) and biochemical determination of hepatic iron concentration (HIC) with calculation of the hepatic iron index. Additionally, liver biopsy can provide an assessment of the degree of fibrosis and whether or not cirrhosis or other histological abnormalities such as steatosis are present. From a prognostic standpoint, the presence of fibrosis and/or cirrhosis is important to establish, and the risk of hepatocellular cancer is significantly increased in those who have established cirrhosis. Histologically, iron deposition is found in higher levels in periportal (zone 1) hepatocytes with a periportal to pericentral gradient, and Kupffer cells have little or no iron deposition. Without early diagnosis and treatment patients can progress to micronodular cirrhosis and liver failure. In symptomatic patients, the HIC will typically be >10 000 μg/g dry weight (normal <1500 μg/g dry weight) and values as high as 40 000 μg/g can be seen[1]. In patients with alcoholic siderosis or with secondary iron overload related to chronic viral hepatitis or nonalcoholic steatohepatitis, the HIC is usually not higher than 10 000 μg/g. With the diagnosis of younger patients with earlier HH because of family studies or use of genetic screening tests, HIC levels at the time of diagnosis can be as low as 3000 μg/g.

While the genetic test is now the gold standard for establishing the diagnosis of HH, the hepatic iron index (HII) has been a helpful criterion for diagnosing HH and for distinguishing heterozygotes and patients with alcoholic liver disease with secondary iron overload from homozygotes[37]. The HII is based upon a concept that patients with HH have a progressive increase in HIC with age, whereas heterozygotes for HH or patients with various forms of secondary iron overload do not have a progressive increase with age; however, recent studies have challenged the concept that HIC increases with age[38,39]. Nonetheless, the HII is calculated by taking the HIC (converted to μmol iron/g dry weight) and dividing by the patient's age (in years). Numerous studies from around the world have shown that a HII > 1.9 is consistent with a diagnosis of homozygous HH. The HII is not meant to be used in patients with parenteral (or transfusional) iron overload. However, recent studies have shown that as many as 15% of patients with HH (identified by genetic testing) will have a HII < 1.9[40]. As additional experience with genotyping and early diagnosis is obtained, it is anticipated that there will be a substantial proportion of patients with a HII < 1.9 who are homozygous for the genetic defect.

Whether a liver biopsy needs to be performed in all HH patients is controversial. Most hepatologists consider liver biopsy in this setting a relatively minor and safe outpatient procedure that gives definitive information about hepatic iron levels and fibrosis that has prognostic significance. Other physicians consider that an elevated transferrin saturation (or ferritin level) and a positive genetic test provide sufficient information, and that therapeutic phlebotomy can be initiated on these grounds alone[8]. The rationale for this approach is that phlebotomy is relatively harmless and that the amount of excess total body iron can be estimated from the number of phlebotomies required to normalize serum ferritin levels (<50 ng/ml) and transferrin saturation (<50%) (based on 500 ml of blood containing about 250 mg iron). However, there is concern that without a liver biopsy, the presence of hepatic cirrhosis may be missed in some HH patients. Recent results suggest that the age of the patient may be used as a criterion to determine whether liver biopsy should be performed[40]. In individuals less than 40 years of age identified by genetic testing (C282Y homozygote) and without any clinical evidence of liver disease, it may be appropriate to proceed with therapeutic phlebotomy without performing a liver biopsy. In this setting, it is unlikely that the patient will have cirrhosis or a significant increase in hepatic fibrosis. It is hoped that future studies will ascertain the proportion of the individuals with *HFE* mutations that have phenotypic expression of iron overload, and will establish criteria for performing liver biopsy in HH patients.

SUMMARY

Our understanding of several aspects of HH has greatly expanded over the last few years with the identification and cloning of the HH gene (*HFE*), the introduction of a commercially available genetic test for the C282Y and H63D mutations, and a new understanding of the normal physiology and pathophysiology of the HFE protein. It is anticipated that these advances will eventually lead to population screening with earlier and more accurate diagnosis of HH, and the prevention of cirrhosis and other iron-induced toxicity in HH patients by timely treatment with phlebotomy.

REFERENCES

1. Bacon BR. Hereditary hemochromatosis. In: Bacon BR, Di Bisceglie AM, eds. Liver Disease. Diagnosis and Management. New York: Churchill Livingstone, 2000: pp. 140–9.
2. Eijkelkamp EJ, Yapp TR, Powell LW. HFE-associated hereditary hemochromatosis. Can J Gastroenterol. 2000;14:121–5.
3. Simon M, Bourel M, Genetet B, Fauchet R. Idiopathic hemochromatosis. Demonstration of recessive transmission and early detection by family HLA typing. N Engl J Med. 1977;297:1017–21.
4. Feder JN, Gnirke A, Thomas W, Tsuchihashi Z, Ruddy DA, Basava A et al. A novel MHC class I-like gene is mutated in patients with hereditary haemochromatosis. Nature Genet. 1996;13:399–408.
5. Bacon BR, Powell LW, Adams PC, Kresina TF, Hoofnagle JH. Molecular medicine and hemochromatosis: At the crossroads. Gastroenterology. 1999;116:193–207.
6. Andrews NC, Levy JE. Iron is hot: An update on the pathophysiology of hemochromatosis. Blood. 1998;92:1845–51.
7. Feder JN. The hereditary hemochromatosis gene (HFE): A MHC class I-like gene that functions in the regulation of iron homeostasis. Immunol Res. 1999;20:175–85.
8. Felitti VJ, Beutler E. New developments in hereditary hemochromatosis. Am J Med Sci. 1999;318:257–68.

9. Bacon BR, Schilsky ML. New knowledge of genetic pathogenesis of hemochromatosis and Wilson's disease. Adv Intern Med. 1999;44:91–116.
10. Brandhagen DJ, Fairbanks VF, Batts KP, Thibodeau SN. Update on hereditary hemochromatosis and the *HFE* gene. Mayo Clin Proc. 1999;74:917–21.
11. Lebron JA, Bennett MJ, Vaughn DE, Chirino AJ, Snow PM, Mintier GA et al. Crystal structure of the hemochromatosis protein HFE and characterization of its interaction with transferrin receptor. Cell. 1998;93:111–23.
12. Waheed A, Parkkila S, Saarnio J, Fleming RE, Zhou XY, Tomatsu S et al. Association of HFE protein with transferrin receptor in crypt enterocytes of human duodenum. Proc Natl Acad Sci USA. 1999;96:1579–84.
13. Parkkila S, Waheed A, Britton RS, Bacon BR, Zhou XY, Tomatsu S et al. Association of the transferrin receptor in human placenta with HFE, the protein defective in hereditary hemochromatosis. Proc Natl Acad Sci USA. 1997;94:13198–202.
14. Feder JN, Tsuchihashi Z, Irrinki A, Lee VK, Mapa FA, Morikang E et al. The hemochromatosis founder mutation in HLA-H disrupts β2-microglobulin interaction and cell surface expression. J Biol Chem. 1997;272:14025–8.
15. Waheed A, Parkkila S, Zhou XY, Tomatsu S, Tsuchihashi Z, Feder JN et al. Hereditary hemochromatosis: Effects of C282Y and H63D mutations on association with β2-microglobulin, intracellular processing, and cell surface expression of the HFE protein in COS-7 cells. Proc Natl Acad Sci USA. 1997;94:12384–9.
16. Gross CN, Irrinki A, Feder JN, Enns CA. Co-trafficking of HFE, a nonclassical major histocompatibility complex class I protein, with the transferrin receptor implies a role in intracellular iron regulation. J Biol Chem. 1998;273:22068–74.
17. de Sousa M, Reimao R, Lacerda R, Hugo P, Kaufmann SH, Porto G. Iron overload in β2-microglobulin-deficient mice. Immunol Lett. 1994;39:105–11.
18. Santos M, Schilham MW, Rademakers LH, Marx JJ, de Sousa M, Clevers H. Defective iron homeostasis in β2-microglobulin knockout mice recapitulates hereditary hemochromatosis in man. J Exp Med. 1996;184:1975–85.
19. Parkkila S, Waheed A, Britton RS, Feder JN, Tsuchihashi Z, Schatzman RC et al. Immunohistochemistry of HLA-H, the protein defective in patients with hereditary hemochromatosis, reveals unique pattern of expression in gastrointestinal tract. Proc Natl Acad Sci USA. 1997;94:2534–9.
20. Bastin JM, Jones M, O'Callaghan CA, Schimanski L, Mason DY, Townsend AR. Kupffer cell staining by an HFE-specific monoclonal antibody: Implications for hereditary haemochromatosis. Br J Haematol. 1998;103:931–41.
21. Feder JN, Penny DM, Irrinki A, Lee VK, Lebron JA, Watson N et al. The hemochromatosis gene product complexes with the transferrin receptor and lowers its affinity for ligand binding. Proc Natl Acad Sci USA. 1998;95:1472–7.
22. Lebron JA, Bjorkman PJ. The transferrin receptor binding site on HFE, the class I MHC-related protein mutated in hereditary hemochromatosis. J Mol Biol. 1999;289:1109–18.
23. Lebron JA, West AP Jr, Bjorkman PJ. The hemochromatosis protein HFE competes with transferrin for binding to the transferrin receptor. J Mol Biol. 1999;294:239–45.
24. Bennett MJ, Lebron JA, Bjorkman PJ. Crystal structure of the hereditary haemochromatosis protein HFE complexed with transferrin receptor. Nature. 2000;403:46–53.
25. Ponka P. Cellular iron metabolism. Kidney Int. 1999;69(suppl):S2–11.
26. Roy CN, Penny DM, Feder JN, Enns CA. The hereditary hemochromatosis protein, HFE, specifically regulates transferrin-mediated iron uptake in HeLa cells. J Biol Chem. 1999;274:9022–8.
27. Salter-Cid L, Brunmark A, Li Y, Leturcq D, Peterson PA, Jackson MR, Yang Y. Transferrin receptor is negatively modulated by the hemochromatosis protein HFE: Implications for cellular iron homeostasis. Proc Natl Acad Sci USA. 1999;96:5434–9.
28. Corsi B, Levi S, Cozzi A, Corti A, Altimare D, Albertini A, Arosio P. Overexpression of the hereditary hemochromatosis protein, HFE, in HeLa cells induces an iron-deficient phenotype. FEBS Lett. 1999;460:149–52.
29. Riedel HD, Muckenthaler MU, Gehrke SG, Mohr I, Brennan K, Herrmann T et al. HFE downregulates iron uptake from transferrin and induces iron-regulatory protein activity in stably transfected cells. Blood. 1999;94:3915–21.
30. Zhou XY, Tomatsu S, Fleming RE, Parkkila S, Waheed A, Jiang J et al. HFE gene knockout produces mouse model of hereditary hemochromatosis. Proc Natl Acad Sci USA. 1998;95:2492–7.

31. Bahram S, Gilfillan S, Kuhn LC, Moret R, Schulze JB, Lebeau A, Schumann K. Experimental hemochromatosis due to MHC class I HFE deficiency: Immune status and iron metabolism. Proc Natl Acad Sci USA. 1999;96:13312–17.
32. Levy JE, Montross LK, Cohen DE, Fleming MD, Andrews NC. The C282Y mutation causing hereditary hemochromatosis does not produce a null allele. Blood. 1999;94:9–11.
33. Fleming RE, Migas MC, Zhou X, Jiang J, Britton RS, Brunt EM et al. Mechanism of increased iron absorption in murine model of hereditary hemochromatosis: increased duodenal expression of the iron transporter DMT1. Proc Natl Acad Sci USA. 1999;96:3143–8.
34. Gunshin H, Mackenzie B, Berger UV, Gunshin Y, Romero MF, Boron WF et al. Cloning and characterization of a mammalian proton-coupled metal-ion transporter. Nature. 1997;388:482–8.
35. Fleming MD, Trenor CC 3rd, Su MA, Foernzler D, Beier DR, Dietrich WF, Andrews NC. Microcytic anaemia mice have a mutation in Nramp2, a candidate iron transporter gene. Nature Genet. 1997;16:383–6.
36. Zoller H, Pietrangelo A, Vogel W, Weiss G. Duodenal metal-transporter (DMT-1, NRAMP-2) expression in patients with hereditary haemochromatosis. Lancet. 1999;353:2120–3.
37. Bassett ML, Halliday JW, Powell LW. Value of hepatic iron measurements in early hemochromatosis and determination of the critical iron level associated with fibrosis. Hepatology. 1986;6:24–9.
38. Adams PC, Deugnier Y, Moirand R, Brissot P. The relationship between iron overload, clinical symptoms, and age in 410 patients with genetic hemochromatosis. Hepatology. 1997;25:162–6.
39. Olynyk JK, Luxon BA, Britton RS, Bacon BR. Hepatic iron concentration in hereditary hemochromatosis does not saturate or accurately predict phlebotomy requirements. Am J Gastroenterol. 1998;93:346–50.
40. Bacon BR, Olynyk JK, Brunt EM, Britton RS, Wolff RK. HFE genotype in patients with hemochromatosis and other liver diseases. Ann Intern Med. 1999;130:953–62.

21
Haemochromatosis: natural course and therapy

W. STREMMEL, S. G. GEHRKE and T. HERRMANN

CLASSIFICATION OF HAEMOCHROMATOSIS

Iron overload states are subdivided into haemochromatosis and aquired iron overload syndromes. The term haemochromatosis is synonymous with the terms hereditary haemochromatosis and primary iron overload. Haemochromatosis affects approximately 1 in 400 Caucasians, with an estimated carrier frequency of 1 in 10 individuals[1]. Thus it represents one of the most common inherited diseases overall. The disease occurs worldwide, but is most common among individuals of northern European descent, particularly those of Celtic origin[2].

HFE-related hereditary haemochromatosis (C282Y homozygosity; C282Y/H63D compound heterozygosity) is the most common form of hereditary haemochromatosis. HFE-related haemochromatosis is uncommon in indigenous populations of Africa, Central and South America, Eastern Asia, and the Pacific Islands[3]. Other, non-HFE related forms are the adult form of non-HFE related hereditary haemochromatosis[4,5], juvenile haemochromatosis[6,7] and neonatal iron overload[8,9]. A special form is the autosomal dominant haemochromatosis found on the Solomon Islands[10].

In juvenile haemochromatosis, severe iron overload and organ failure occur early, between 15 and 30 years of age, with a high frequency of cardiac disease and hypogonadism. The mode of inheritance is autosomal recessive. The locus maps to the long arm of chromosome 1[11]. Neonatal haemochromatosis presents with hepatic failure in newborn infants due to severe iron overload in the liver. Affected newborns show liver cirrhosis and cardiac disease; they usually die in the early neonatal period. About 100 cases of neonatal haemochromatosis have been reported. The genetic basis has not yet been identified.

COURSE AND CLINICAL SPECTRUM OF HAEMOCHROMATOSIS

In haemochromatosis increased duodenal iron absorption leads to a positive iron balance and accumulation of excess body iron. Only specific organs are affected by

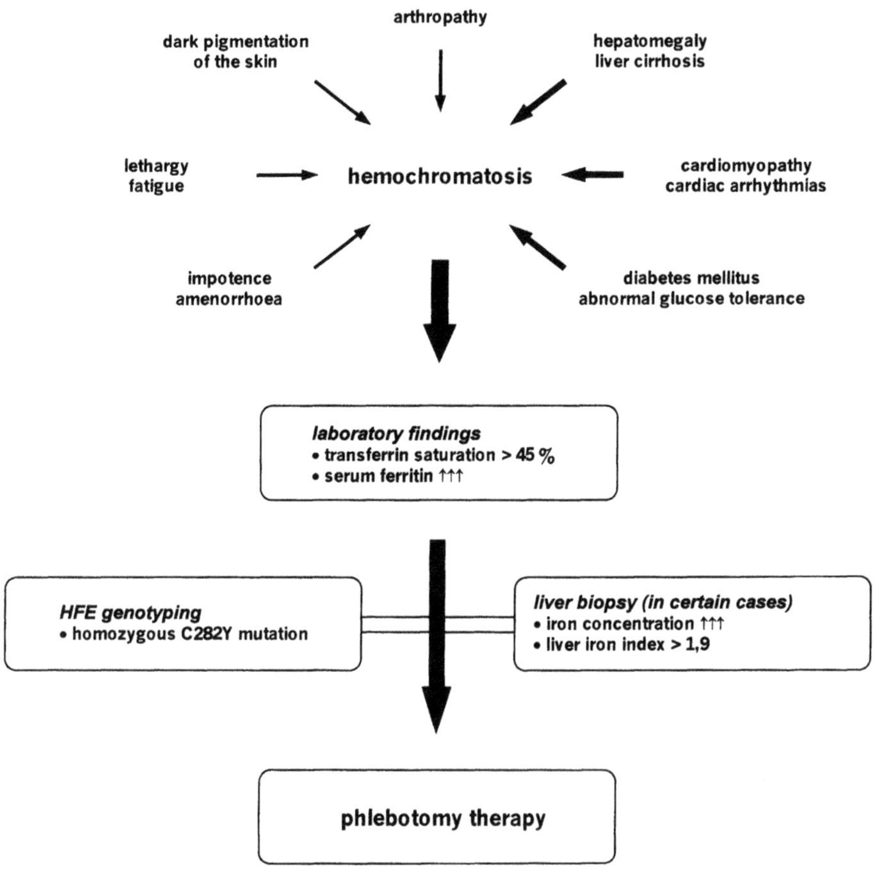

Figure 1 Clinical spectrum and therapy of haemochromatosis.

the iron overload. Those include liver and pancreas and to a lesser extent endocrine glands, particularly the pituitary, as well as heart, skin and joints[12]. Liver cirrhosis, diabetes mellitus, hypogonadism, cardiomyopathy, skin pigmentation, and arthropathy are the most frequent manifestations of the disease (Fig. 1).

First symptoms can be observed at the age of 20 to 40 years in men and after the menopause in women, respectively[12]. The course of the disease is usually less severe in women than in men. Typically, the symptoms and pathologic abnormalities occur in different states of the disease. Weakness and arthralgia are early signs, while liver cirrhosis, diabetes mellitus and cardiomyopathy occur in advanced disease. Hepatomegaly, skin pigmentation and impotence may occur as early or delayed signs. The development of liver cirrhosis and of diabetes mellitus are closely related.

Deaths caused by hepatocellular carcinoma (about 280 times increased), cardiomyopathy, liver cirrhosis, and diabetes mellitus (each about 10–15 times increased) are significantly more frequent compared with the normal population[13]. The two major causes of death in haemochromatosis patients are complications of liver cirrhosis (including hepatocellular carcinoma) and of cardiomyopathy[13]. In a former study[14] 82% of untreated patients died within 5 years after diagnosis. In a recent study[13] the mortality of treated patients within 5 years was 7%.

In the course of haemochromatosis, specific patterns of morphological changes and functional impairment are observed in different organs. The parenchymal deposits of iron in livers of patients with haemochromatosis consist of ferritin and haemosiderin. In early stages these deposits are found in the periportal parenchymal cells, in more advanced stages also in the bile duct epithelium[15]. In parallel with the increasing iron deposition, perilobular fibrosis and liver cirrhosis develop. Hepatocellular carcinoma is observed in about 30% of cirrhotic patients after 20–30 years, even after removal of excess body iron stores by phlebotomy[12]. Iron deposits in the pancreas are predominantly localized in the exocrine parenchyma, where they are associated with the development of tissue fibrosis. However, exocrine pancreas insufficiency is a rare clinical feature. On the other hand, the accumulation of iron in the B-cells of the endocrine pancreas leads to cell damage and contributes to the diabetes mellitus observed in haemochromatosis patients[12]. In addition to impaired insulin secretion, there is an almost obligatory insulin resistance[16], which is, in contrast to the destruction of the B-cells, often reversible after therapeutic iron depletion.

A typical clinical feature is the dark pigmentation of the skin, which is mainly caused by an increased melanin synthesis in the cells of the basal layer. The pigmentation is particularly pronounced in areas which are exposed to the sun and on nipples, perineum, inner sides of the hands and scars[15].

Another cell type which selectively accumulates iron in haemochromatosis is the gonadotropic cell of the pituitary gland. Iron-induced cell damage leads to impaired secretion of FSH and LH, which results in the clinical manifestation of hypogonadotropic hypogonadism with impotence in males and amenorrhoea in females. Despite secondary low testosterone levels in male patients, peripheral sexual hormone metabolism remains unaltered[16]. Thus, certain testosterone preparations (e.g. testosterone enantate) can be used for substitution therapy, without enhanced conversion to estrogens.

Clinically relevant iron deposition in the heart is observed in about 15% of patients. Those deposits are more extensive in ventricular than in atrial myocardium. The ensuing haemodynamic derangement is generally a dilated cardiomyopathy, rarely a myocardial restriction[17].

Arthropathy develops in 25–30% of patients at any stage of the disease[18]. The small joints of the hands (2nd and 3rd metacarpophalangeal joints) are the first joints to be involved. Histologically, deposits of iron are observed around the synovial lining cells of joints, and calcium pyrophosphate crystals may be seen within deposits of calcium embedded in the synovial tissue. A progressive polyarthritis involving wrists, hips, and knees may ensue. Radiological signs are subchondral sclerosis and cystic changes, loss of articular cartilage, diffuse demineralization, hypertrophic bone proliferation and calcification of the synovium.

THERAPY

The aim of therapy is the depletion of body iron stores, which is most efficiently achieved by repeated phlebotomies[19]. Under therapy the different symptoms of the disease improve to different extents (Fig. 2). Arthralgia can worsen under therapy; fatigue and arthralgia can even occur under therapy. Initially, 500 ml of whole blood (equivalent to approximately 250 mg of iron) in men and 400 ml in women, respectively, should be withdrawn every week. In advanced haemochromatosis it takes about 1.5 years until the iron stores are depleted. The most suitable parameter to quantify the body iron stores under therapy is the serum ferritin. Treatment should be continued weekly until the serum ferritin level is <50 μg/l. During this period, haemoglobin should be checked every week, and ferritin every 1–2 months. When the serum ferritin level has fallen below 50 μg/l, the frequency of phlebotomies has to be reduced. Due to the genetically determined increase of iron absorption, phlebotomy has to be continued for the rest of the patient's life, otherwise iron reaccumulates: lifelong maintenance therapy requires 4–12 phlebotomies/year. During maintenance therapy, serum ferritin should be monitored once a year.

There is no need for an iron-free or iron-reduced diet in the therapy of haemochromatosis. However, a recent study showed that regular consumption

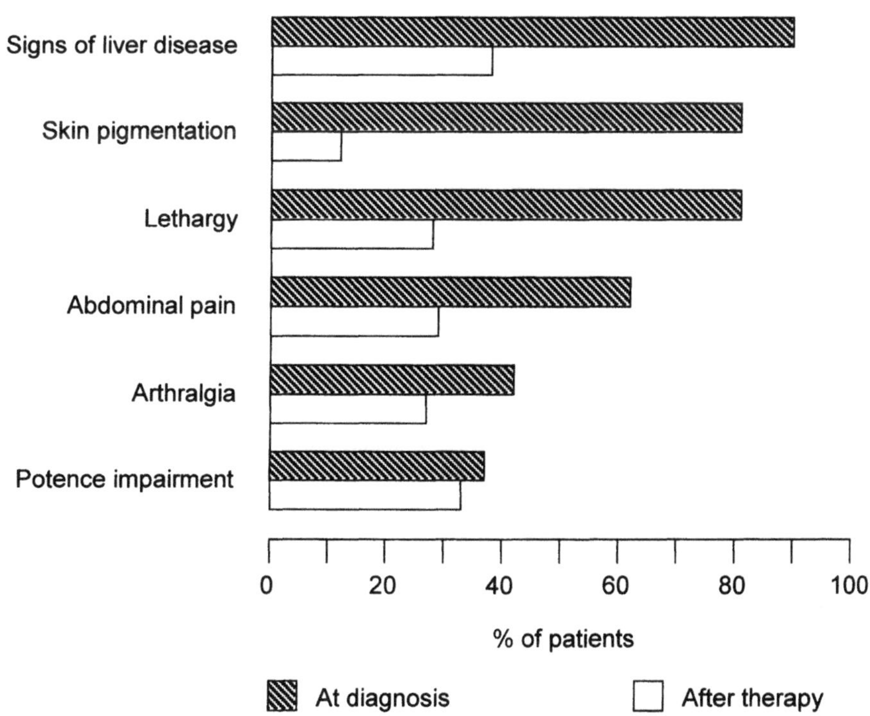

Figure 2 Influence of phlebotomy therapy on symptoms of haemochromatosis (modified from Ref. 19).

of black tea can reduce the number of phlebotomies that are required in the maintenance therapy by about one-third[20].

Iron chelation therapy with desferoxamine should be restricted to patients in whom phlebotomies are not feasible, i.e. patients with marked heart insufficiency or with secondary iron overload and anaemia[15]. The chelator binds iron in serum and tissues and is eliminated through bile and urine. Due to its short half-life of only 5–10 min, desferoxamine has to be given continuously by subcutaneous infusion for 12–24 h/day, 5–7 days/week. Neurological, ophthalmological and otological impairments are the most frequent side effects. Desferoxamine therapy is more expensive, less efficient and causes more side effects than phlebotomy.

The only available treatment for end-stage liver disease is liver transplantation. Compared with other chronic liver diseases, the success of liver transplantation in haemochromatotic liver disease seems to be worse[21–23].

The symptoms and pathological abnormalities in haemochromatosis improve to different extents after therapeutic iron depletion. Fatigue, abdominal pain, hepatomegaly, elevation of serum transaminases and skin pigmentation usually respond well to therapy. Abnormal glucose tolerance or non-insulin-dependent diabetes usually improve under removal of iron, while insulin-dependent diabetes mellitus cannot be reversed. Signs of cardiomyopathy and liver fibrosis may improve under treatment, while impotence usually does not. Destructive arthropathy and liver cirrhosis are always irreversible[13].

PROGNOSIS

The prognosis of untreated haemochromatosis is poor[14]. Occurrence of complications and prognosis depend on the amount of iron excess and on the point at which iron accumulation is interrupted by phlebotomy. The life expectancy of patients without liver cirrhosis and diabetes mellitus at the time of therapy initiation is normal[13]. In patients with liver cirrhosis, survival is improved by phlebotomy. Thus, early diagnosis and therapy are most important in haemochromatosis.

REFERENCES

1. Feder J, Gnirke W, Thomas W, Tsuchihashi Z, Ruddy DA, Basava A et al. A novel MHC class I-like gene is mutated in patients with hereditary haemochromatosis. Nature Genet. 1996;13:399–408.
2. Smith BN, Kantrowitz W, Grace ND, Greenberg MS, Patton TJ, Ookubo R et al. Prevalence of hereditary hemochromatosis in a Massachusetts corporation: is Celtic origin a risk factor? Hepatology. 1997;25:1439–46.
3. Bacon BR, Powell LW, Adams PC, Kresina TF, Hoofnagle JH. Molecular medicine and hemochromatosis: at the crossroads. Gastroenterology. 1999;116:193–207.
4. Carella M, D'Ambrosio L, Totaro A, Grifa A, Valentino M, Piperno A et al. Mutation analysis of the HLA-H gene in Italian hemochromatosis patients. Am J Hum Genet. 1997;60:828–32.
5. Shaheen NJ, Bacon BR, Grimm IS. Clinical characteristics of hereditary hemochromatosis patients who lack the C282Y mutation. Hepatology. 1998;28:526–9.
6. Kaltwasser JP, Schalk K, Werner E. Juvenile hemochromatosis. Ann NY Acad Med. 1988;28:526–9.

7. Camaschella C, Roetto A, Cicilano M, Pasquero P, Bosio S, Gubetta L et al. Juvenile and adult hemochromatosis are distinct genetic disorders. Eur J Hum Genet. 1997;5:371–5.
8. Goldfischer S, Grotsky HW, Chang C-H, Berman EL, Richert RR, Karmarkar SD et al. Idiopathic neonatal iron storage involving the liver, pancreas, heart, and endocrine and exocrine glands. Hepatology. 1981;1:58–64.
9. Silver MM, Beverley DW, Valberg LS, Cutz E, Phillips MJ, Shaheed WA. Perinatal hemochromatosis: clinical, morphologic, and quantitative iron studies. Am J Pathol. 1987;128:538–54.
10. Eason RJ, Adams PC, Aston CE, Searle J. Familial iron overload with possible autosomal dominant inheritance. Aust NZ J Med. 1990;20:226–30.
11. Roetto A, Totaro A, Cazzola M, Cicilano M, Bosio S, D'Ascola G et al. Juvenile hemochromatosis locus maps to chromosome 1q. Am J Hum Genet. 1999;64:1388–93.
12. Niederau C, Fischer R, Sonnenberg A, Stremmel W, Trampisch HJ, Strohmeyer G. Survival and causes of death in cirrhotic and noncirrhotic patients with primary hemochromatosis. N Engl J Med. 1985;313:1256–62.
13. Niederau C, Fischer R, Pürschel A, Stremmel W, Häussinger D, Strohmeyer G. Long-term survival in patients with hereditary hemochromatosis. Gastroenterology. 1996;110:1107–19.
14. Bomford A, Williams R. Long term results of venesection therapy in idiopathic haemochromatosis. Q J Med. 1976;45:611–23.
15. Stremmel W, Riedel HD, Niederau C, Strohmeyer G. Pathogenesis of genetic haemochromatosis. Eur J Clin Invest. 1993;23:321–9.
16. Stremmel W, Niederau C, Berger M, Kley HK, Krüskemper HL, Strohmeyer G. Abnormalities in estrogen, androgen, insulin metabolism in idiopathic hemochromatosis. Ann NY Acad Sci. 1988;526:209–23.
17. Dabestani A, Child JS, Henze E, Perlof JK, Schon H, Figueroa WG et al. Primary hemochromatosis: anatomic and physiologic characteristics of the cardiac ventricles and their response to phlebotomy. Am J Cardiol. 1984;54:153–9.
18. Hamilton EBD, Bomford AB, Laws JW, Williams R. The natural history of arthritis in idiopathic hemochromatosis: progression of the clinical and radiologic features over ten years. Q J Med NS. 1982;199:321–9.
19. Stremmel W, Niederau C, Strohmeyer G. Therapie der Hämochromatose. Dtsch Med Wschr. 1993;118:267–9.
20. Kaltwasser JP, Werner E, Schalk K, Hansen C, Gottschalk R, Seidl C. Clinical trial on the effect of regular tea drinking on iron accumulation in genetic haemochromatosis. Gut. 1998;43:699–704.
21. Kilpe VE, Krakauer H, Wren RE. An analysis of liver transplantation experience from 37 transplant centers reported to Medicare. Transplantation. 1993;56:554–61.
22. Kowdley KV, Hassanein T, Kaur S, Farrell FJ, Van Thiel DH, Keffe EB et al. Primary liver cancer and survival in patients undergoing liver transplantation for hemochromatosis. Liver Transpl Surg. 1995;1:237–41.
23. Farrell FJ, Nguyen M, Woodley S, Imperial JC, Garcia-Kennedy R, Man KM et al. Outcome of liver transplantation in patients with hemochromatosis. Hepatology. 1994;20:404–10.

22
Wilson disease: pathogenesis and diagnosis

P. FERENCI

PATHOGENESIS

Understanding of the pathogenesis of Wilson disease has markedly increased since the discovery of the disease causing gene defect in 1993.

The Wilson disease gene (ATP7B)

The Wilson disease gene was identified on chromosome 13[1–4]. It codes for a copper transporting P-type ATPase, ATP7B. Its functionally important regions are six copper binding domains, a transduction domain involved in the transduction of the energy of ATP hydrolysis to cation transport, a cation channel and phosphorylation domain, an ATP-binding domain and eight hydrophobic regions predicted to span the cell membrane. More than 100 mutations[4] occurring throughout the whole gene have been documented so far. Some are associated with a severe liver disease very early in life, other mutations appear to be less severe, with disease appearance in mid-adulthood.

Copper is an essential component of important enzymes such as ceruloplasmin, lysyl oxydase, superoxyde dismutase, cytochrome C, tyrosinase and DOPA-β-monooxygenase. On the other hand, excess copper is toxic to many tissues, and intracellular copper homeostasis is, therefore, carefully controlled. Dietary copper intake (about 1–4 mg/day) far exceeds the trace amounts required: most ingested copper is taken up by the liver. Cellular copper transport processes are required by all organisms for correct utilization in cell biochemical processes and avoidance of the toxicity of copper excess[5]. Metallothionein-bound copper is non-toxic. Several metals, including zinc, can induce metallothionein synthesis. Metallothionein is a cytosolic, low molecular weight, cystein-rich, metal binding protein. The copper stored in metallothionein can be used for protein synthesis in the Golgi compartment or can be incorporated in lysosomes and transported to the bile canaliculus, where it is excreted into the bile. ATP7B is involved in both processes. ATP7B requires a copper chaperone protein as it is major source for copper, probably HAH1[6]. Hepatic expression of

ATP7B revealed a single 165 kDa protein[7], which by immunofluorescence was present only in hepatocytes and localized predominantly to the trans-Golgi network, and exclusively in this compartment under low hepatic copper concentrations[8]. Others found the WND protein to be present in two forms, the 160 kDa and the 140 kDa products. The 160 kDa product was located in the trans-Golgi network[9], the 140 kDa product in mitochondria[10]. The WND protein may function in the copper transport coupled with the synthesis of ceruloplasmin, and the Golgi apparatus is the likely site for WND protein to manifest its function[11]. Although hepatic copper concentration had no effect on the steady-state levels of the Wilson's disease protein, copper administration in vivo resulted in redistribution of this protein to a cytoplasmic vesicular compartment localized toward the hepatocyte canalicular membrane. This post-translational mechanism of copper homeostasis in vivo is consistent with the proposed function of the Wilson's disease protein in holocaeruloplasmin biosynthesis and biliary copper excretion.

The function of the WND protein was studied by expressing wild-type and mutant Wilson cDNAs in a Menke's copper transporter-deficient mottled fibroblast cell line defective in copper export[9] or in a yeast complementation assay based on the ability of ATP7B to complement the high-affinity iron-uptake deficiency of the yeast mutant ccc2[12]. Expression of the Wilson cDNA rescued the mottled phenotype, as evidenced by a reduction in copper accumulation and restoration of cell viability. In contrast, expression of an H1069Q mutant Wilson cDNA did not rescue the mottled phenotype, and immunofluorescence studies showed that this mutant Wilson protein was localized in the endoplasmic reticulum. Pulse-chase analysis demonstrated a 5-fold decrease in the half-life of the H1069Q mutant compared with the wild-type protein. Further experiments suggested that a temperature-sensitive defect in protein folding followed by degradation constitutes the molecular basis of Wilson disease in patients harbouring the H1069Q mutation. The H1069Q missense mutation is the most common mutation in WD and is found in up to 95% of patients of East European origin.

Pathogenesis of liver disease in Wilson disease

Because hepatic uptake of dietary copper in not saturable, hepatic copper accumulation can easily be induced. Toxicity of copper, however, depends on its molecular association and subcellular localization rather than on its concentration in the liver. Excess copper in tissues leads to the production of free radicals and to DNA cleavage. Probably the greatest source of damage is through the production of free radicals. Copper overload particularly affects mitochondrial respiration and causes a decrease in cytochrome C activity[13]. Damage to mitochondria is an early pathological effect in the liver. Hepatocellular damage due to increased lipid peroxidation and abnormal mitochondrial respiration was shown both in copper-loaded dogs and in patients with Wilson disease[14]. The mechanism(s) triggering copper-induced lipid peroxidation are unknown, but it is conceivable that hepatic copper accumulation renders patients with Wilson disease susceptible to any oxidative stress.

Pathogenesis of CNS disease in Wilson disease

The precise role of ATP7B in the brain is unknown. Immunohistochemical localization of ATP7B was visualized in rat brain and was intense in neuronal cells of the hippocampal formation, olfactory bulbs, cerebellum, cerebral cortex and nuclei in the brain stem in which high amounts of copper and cuproenzymes, dopamine β-hydroxylase and Cu,Zn-superoxide dismutase (Cu,Zn-SOD) were detected[15]. ATP7B may play a key role in neurotransmission of the catecholamine pathway and in preventing brain tissue from injury by superoxide radicals to regulate the cellular Cu concentration and/or activities of cuproenzymes related to neurotransmissions and a free radical metabolism. It is also reasonable to assume that neurotoxicity due to abnormal copper accumulation or irregular regulation of cuproenzymes in the critical brain regions by mutation of the ATP7B gene leads to neurological failure in Wilson disease. Copper may be directly toxic to neurons or may exert its effects by selective inhibition of brain MAO-A[16]. Phenotypic expression of neurological disease may be influenced by subtypes of apolipoprotein E. WD patients with the normal subtype $\epsilon3/\epsilon3$ develop symptoms 5–10 years later than those with other subtypes[17].

DIAGNOSIS

The diagnosis of Wilson disease is based on clinical findings and laboratory abnormalities (see Table 1) and can be made if two of the following symptoms are present[18]: Kayser–Fleischer rings, typical neurological symptoms and low serum caeruloplasmin levels.

Table 1 Routine tests for diagnosis of Wilson disease

Test	*Typical finding*	*False-negative*	*False-positive*
Serum caeruloplasmin	decreased	normal levels in patients with marked hepatic inflammation overestimation by immunological assay	low levels in: – malabsorption – acaeruloplasminaemia – liver insufficiency – heterozygotes
24 h urinary copper	>100 μg/dl	normal: – incorrect collection – children without liver disease	increased: – hepatocellular necrosis – contamination
Serum free copper	>10 μg/dl	normal if caeruloplasmin overestimated by immunological assay	
Hepatic copper	>250 μg/g dry weight	due to regional variation – in patients with active liver disease – in patients with regenerative nodules	cholestatic syndromes
Kayser–Fleischer rings by slit lamp	present	– in up to 40% of patients with hepatic Wilson disease – in most asymptomatic siblings	primary biliary cirrhosis

Patients with neurological disease

In a patient presenting with typical neurological symptoms and having Kayser–Fleischer rings the diagnosis is straightforward. No additional tests are required and routine laboratory parameters just confirm the diagnosis. Kayser–Fleischer rings are rarely absent in neurologically symptomatic patients. However, there are a few well documented cases of neurologic Wilson disease without demonstrable Kayser–Fleischer rings[19]. In such patients diagnosis is usually made by a low serum caeruloplasmin level. Brain magnetic resonance imaging is useful to document the extent of changes in the central nervous system[20]. Auditory evoked brain stem potentials are helpful to document the degree of functional impairment and the improvement by decoppering treatment[21].

Patients with liver disease and haemolytic anaemia

Diagnosis is far more complex in patients presenting with liver diseases. None of the commonly used parameters alone allows a certain diagnosis of Wilson disease. Usually a combination of various laboratory parameters is necessary to firmly establish the diagnosis. Kayser–Fleischer rings may be absent in up to 50% of patients with Wilsonian liver disease[22].

Routine laboratory parameters of liver disease

In general, transaminases are only mildly increased. Deep jaundice combined with mild elevation of liver enzymes in non-surgical patients should raise the suspicion for fulminant Wilson disease. Sometimes alkaline phosphatase activities are low, and an alkaline phosphatase: total bilirubin ratio below 2.0 has been claimed to provide 100% sensitivity and specificity to diagnose Wilsonian fulminant liver failure[23], but the usefulness of this test was not confirmed in larger series[24].

Serum caeruloplasmin

Serum caeruloplasmin is decreased in most patients with neurological Wilson disease, but is in the low normal range in up to 45% of patients with hepatic disease[22]. On the other hand, even a low caeruloplasmin level is not diagnostic for Wilson disease in the absence of Kayser–Fleischer rings. It may be low in familial hypocaeruloplasminaemia, in severely malnourished subjects, and in heterozygous carriers of the Wilson disease gene[25]. Thus, in patients with liver disease a normal caeruloplasmin level cannot exclude, nor is a low level sufficient to make the diagnosis of, Wilson disease.

Serum copper

Serum copper values parallel those of caeruloplasmin and are frequently low in patients with Wilson disease. Patients with fulminant Wilson disease and/or haemolytic anaemia may even have markedly increased levels. Most of the copper in serum is bound to ceruloplasmin, and under normal conditions less than 5% circulates as free copper. The free copper concentration can be calculated by subtracting from the total copper concentration the ceruloplasmin-bound copper (ceruloplasmin times 3.3). An increased free copper level (>10 μg/dl) is considered as a useful diagnostic test for Wilson disease.

Urinary copper excretion

Urine copper excretion is markedly increased in Wilson disease (88% in our study)[22], but its usefulness in clinical practice is limited. The estimation of urinary copper excretion may be misleading due to incorrect collection of 24 h urine volume or to copper contamination. In presymptomatic patients urinary copper excretion may be normal. On the other hand urinary copper excretion is also increased in any disease with extensive hepatocellular necrosis. The 24 h urinary copper excretion after challenge with 500 mg D-penicillamine was the most accurate single diagnostic test in children with Wilson disease[26], but even after D-penicillamine copper excretion was not elevated in 10% of the tested patients.

Hepatic copper content

Hepatic copper content is increased in most patients with Wilson disease and usually exceeds 250 μg/g dry weight (normal: up to 50). In the absence of other tests suggestive for abnormal copper metabolism, diagnosis of Wilson disease cannot be made based on an increased hepatic copper content alone. Patients with chronic cholostatic diseases, neonates and young children and possibly also subjects with exogenous copper overload have hepatic copper concentration >250 μg/g. Hepatic copper content may be normal or borderline in about 10% of patients with unquestionable Wilson disease due to sampling given great regional differences in hepatic copper distribution, especially in the cirrhotic liver[27].

Liver biopsy

Liver biopsy findings are non-specific and not directly helpful in making the diagnosis of Wilson disease. Liver pathology includes early changes such as fatty intracellular accumulations, which often proceed to marked steatosis. At later stages, hepatic inflammation with portal and periportal lymphocytic infiltrates, presence of necrosis and of fibrosis may be indistinguishable from other forms of hepatitis. Some patients have cirrhosis without any inflammation. The detection of focal copper stores by the Rhodanin stain is a pathognomic feature of Wilson disease but is only present in the minority of patients[28].

The ultrastructural abnormalities include pathological changes of mitochondria and peroxisomes. Hepatocellular mitochondria are pleomorphic, with varying combinations of abnormalities including enlargement, bizarre shapes, increased matrix density, separation of the normally apposed inner and outer membranes, widened intercristal spaces, enlarged granules, and crystalline, vacuolated, or dense inclusions. Sometimes peroxisomes are enlarged and contain a granular or flocculent matrix of varying electron density.

Radiocopper test

The basis of this test are the biphasic plasma kinetics of copper after an oral dose of ^{64}Cu[29]. Initially, labeled copper is taken up by the liver and is completely removed from the serum. Later, the label reappears bound to caeruloplasmin. This second peak is absent in Wilson disease patients. The test is only useful in patients and siblings with caeruloplasmin levels in or close to the normal range. There is a considerable overlap between affected patients and heterozygotes.

Family screening

Once diagnosis of Wilson disease is made in an index patient evaluation of his family is mandatory. The likelihood of finding a homozygote among siblings is 25%, among children 0.5%. Testing of second degree relatives is only useful if the gene was found in one of the immediate members of his/her family. No single test is able to identify affected siblings or heterozygote carriers of the Wilson disease gene with sufficient certainty. Today, mutation analysis is the only reliable tool for family screening.

Mutation analysis

Direct mutation analysis

Because of the many mutations direct molecular genetic diagnosis of Wilson disease is difficult. Furthermore, most patients are compound heterozygotes (i.e. carry two different mutations). Screening for mutations is typically done by single-strand conformation polymorphism analysis. This approach is quite useful as research tool, but impractical for clinical diagnosis. In contrast, using allele-specific probes, direct mutation diagnosis is rapid and helpful, if a mutation occurs with a reasonable frequency in the population. In Central Europe, the H1069Q mutation is present in 60–90% of Wilson disease patients, and a direct test for this mutation is useful[30]. Eventually, a multiplex PCR for the most frequent mutations in Wilson disease should make direct mutation analysis for diagnosis feasible.

Haplotype analysis

Because of the complexity in identifying the many mutations in Wilson disease, haplotypes can be used to screen for mutations and to examine asymptomatic siblings of index patients. A number of highly polymorphic microsatellite markers have been described that closely flank the gene and are highly variable: D13S316, D13S314, D13S301, D13S133[31]. Where the markers are different at each locus in a patient, testing of at least one parent/or child of the patient is necessary to obtain the haplotype. The identification of unusual haplotypes can lend support, but is not sufficient to confirm the diagnosis of Wilson disease. Haplotype analysis and restriction fragment length polymorphism of flanking genes proved to be very useful for prenatal testing and firm diagnosis of affected siblings in Wilson disease families[32,33].

An algorithm for diagnosis of Wilson disease

A diagnostic algorithm is suggested in Fig. 1. In the absence of typical clinical findings, measurement of hepatic copper content is mandatory in every patient with unexplained elevations of liver enzymes and some abnormal parameters of

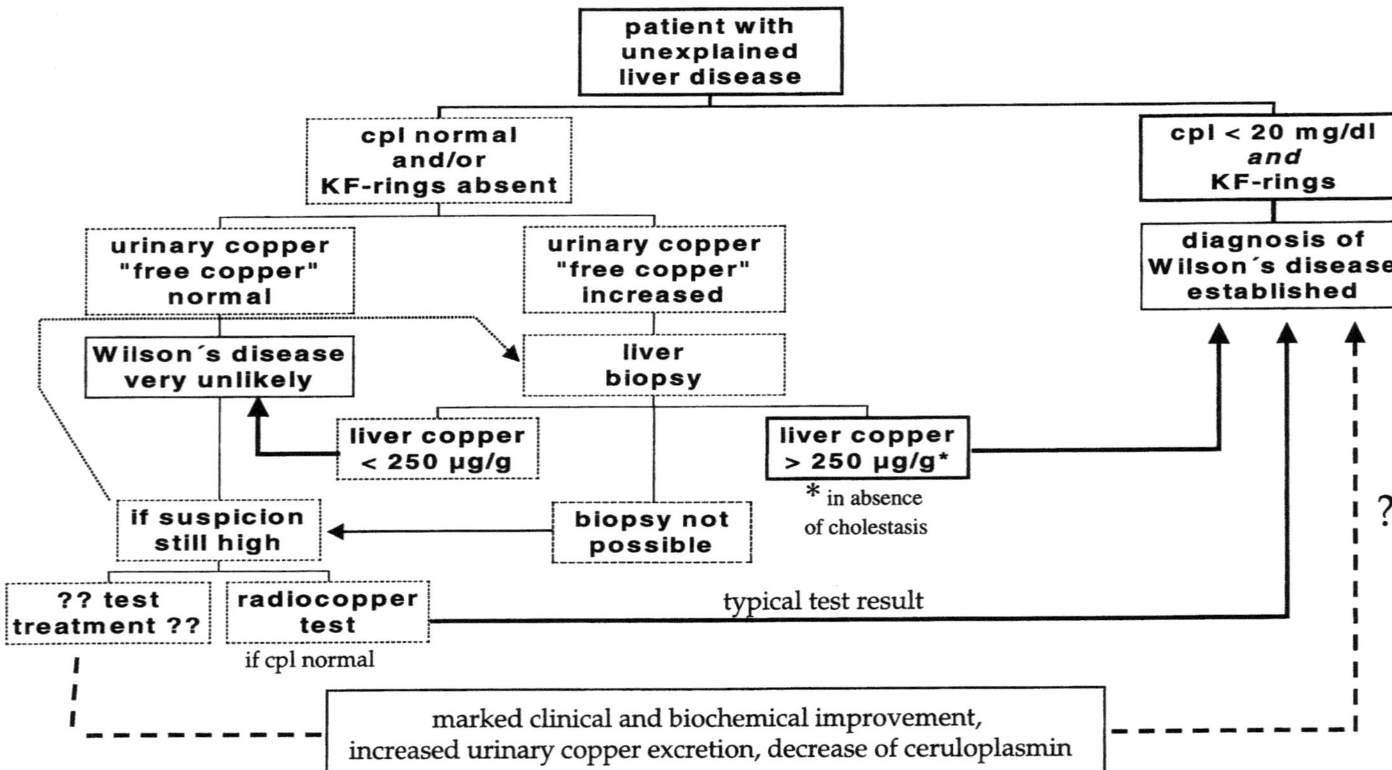

Figure 1 Flow diagram for diagnosis of Wilson disease (according to Ref. 22).

copper metabolism. Furthermore, if suspicion is high, patients with caeruloplasmin levels in the normal range should be referred for a radiocopper test or PCR based mutation analysis. In selected patients with unclear findings or in whom a liver biopsy cannot be performed, a test treatment with decoppering agents can be initiated for a period of 6–12 months.

REFERENCES

1. Petrukhin K, Fischer SG, Pirastu M, Tanzi RE, Chernov I, Devoto M et al. Mapping, cloning and genetic characterization of the region containing the Wilson disease gene. Nature Genet. 1993;5:338–43.
2. Petrukhin KE, Lutsenko S, Chernov I, Ross BM, Kaplan JH, Gilliam TC. Characterization of the Wilson disease gene encoding a P-type copper transporting ATPase: genomic organization, alternative splicing, and structure/function predictions. Hum Mol Genet. 1994;3:1647–56.
3. Tanzi RE, Petrukhin K, Chernov I, Pellequer JL, Wasco W, Ross B et al. The Wilson disease gene is a copper transporting ATPase with homology to the Menkes disease gene. Nature Genet. 1993;5:344–50.
4. Thomas GJ, Forbes JR, Roberts EA, Walshe JM, Cox DW. The Wilson disease gene: spectrum of mutations and their consequences. Nature Genet. 1995;9:210–17.
5. McArdle HJ, Bingham MJ, Summer K, Ong TJ. Copper metabolism in the liver. Adv Exp Med Biol. 1999;448:29–37.
6. Klomp LW, Lin SJ, Yuan DS, Klausner RD, Culotta VC, Gitlin JD. Identification and functional expression of HAH1, a novel human gene involved in copper homeostasis. J Biol Chem. 1997;272:9221–6.
7. Schaefer M, Hopkins RG, Failla ML, Gitlin JD, Hepatocyte-specific localization and copper-dependent trafficking of the Wilson's disease protein in the liver. Am J Physiol. 1999;276:G639–46.
8. Nagano K, Nakamura K, Urakami KI, Umeyama K, Koiwai K, Hattori S et al. Intracellular distribution of the Wilson's disease gene product (ATPase7B) after in vitro and in vivo exogenous expression in hepatocytes from the LEC rat, an animal model of Wilson's disease. Hepatology. 1998;27:799–807.
9. Payne AS, Kelly EJ, Gitlin JD. Functional expression of the Wilson disease protein reveals mislocalization and impaired copper-dependent trafficking of the common H1069Q mutation. Proc Natl Acad Sci USA. 1998;95:10854–9.
10. Lutsenko S, Cooper MJ. Localization of the Wilson's disease protein product to mitochondria. Proc Natl Acad Sci USA. 1998;95:6004–9.
11. Terada K, Nakako T, Yang XL, Iida M, Aiba N, Minamiya Y et al. Restoration of holoceruloplasmin synthesis in LEC rat after infusion of recombinant adenovirus bearing WND cDNA. J Biol Chem. 1998;273:1815–20.
12. Forbes JR, Cox DW. Functional characterization of missense mutations in ATP7B: Wilson disease mutation or normal variant? Am J Hum Genet. 1998;63:1663–74.
13. Sokol RJ, Devereaux MW, O'Brien K, Khandawala RA, Loehr JP. Abnormal hepatic mitochondrial respiration and cytochrome oxidase activity in rats with long-term copper overload. Gastroenterology. 1993;105:178–87.
14. Sokol RJ, Twedt D, McKim JM Jr, Devereaux MW, Karrer FM, Kam I et al. Oxidant injury to hepatic mitochondria in patients with Wilson's disease and Bedlington terriers with copper toxicosis. Gastroenterology. 1994;107:1788–98.
15. Saito T, Okabe M, Hosokawa T, Kurasaki M, Hata A, Endo F et al. Immunohistochemical determination of the Wilson Copper-transporting P-type ATPase in the brain tissues of the rat. Neurosci Lett. 1999;266:13–16.
16. Leung TK, Lim L, Lai JC. Differential effects of metal ions on type A and type B monoamine oxidase activities in rat brain and liver mitochondria. Metab Brain Dis. 1992;7:139–46.
17. Schiefermeier M, Kollegger H, Madl C, Polli C, Oder W, Kühn HJ et al. The impact of apolipoprotein E genotypes on phenotypic expression of Wilson's disease. Brain. 2000;123:585–590.
18. Sternlieb I. Perspectives on Wilson‘s disease. Hepatology. 1990;12:1234–9.

19. Demirkiran M, Jankovic J, Lewis RA, Cox DW. Neurologic presentation of Wilson disease without Kayser–Fleischer rings. Neurology. 1996;46:1040–3.
20. van Wassenaer-van Hall HN, van den Heuvel AG, Algra A, Hoogenraad TU, Mali WP. Wilson disease: findings at MR imaging and CT of the brain with clinical correlation. Radiology. 1996;198:531–6.
21. Grimm G, Madl Ch, Katzenschlager R, Oder W, Ferenci P, Gangl A. Detailed evaluation of brain dysfunction in patients with Wilson's disease. EEG Clin Neurophysiol. 1992;82:119–24.
22. Steindl P, Ferenci P, Dienes HP, Grimm G, Pabinger I, Madl Ch et al. Diagnosis of Wilson's disease in patients with liver disease without neurological symptoms – comparison with other clinical presentations. Gastroenterology. 1997;113:212–18.
23. Willson RA, Clayson KJ, Leon S. Unmeasurable serum alkaline phosphatase activity in Wilson's disease associated with fulminant hepatic failure and hemolysis. Hepatology. 1987;7:613–15.
24. Sallie R, Katsiyiannakis L, Baldwin D, Davies S, O'Grady J, Mowat A et al. Failure of simple biochemical indices to reliably differentiate fulminant Wilson's disease from other causes of fulminant liver failure. Hepatology. 1992;16:1206–11.
25. Cauza E, Maier-Dobersberger Th, Kaserer K, Kramer L, Ferenci P. Plasma ceruloplasmin as screening test for Wilson's disease. J Hepatol. 1997;27:358–62.
26. Da Costa CM, Baldwin D, Portmann B, Lolin Y, Mowat AP, Mieli-Vergani G. Value of urinary copper excretion after penicillamine challenge in the diagnosis of Wilson's disease. Hepatology. 1992;15:609–15.
27. McDonald JA, Snitch P, Painter D, Hensle W, Gallagher ND, McCaughan GW. Striking variability of hepatic copper levels in fulminant hepatic failure. J Gastroenterol Hepatol. 1992;7:396–8.
28. Ludwig J, Moyer Th P, Rakela J. The liver biopsy diagnosis of Wilson's disease. Am J Clin Pathol. 1994;102:443–6.
29. Sternlieb I, Scheinberg IH. The role of radiocopper in the diagnosis of Wilson's disease. Gastroenterology. 1979;77:138–42.
30. Maier-Dobersberger Th, Ferenci P, Polli C, Balac P, Dienes HP, Kaserer K et al. The His1069Gln mutation in Wilson's disease: detection by a rapid PCR-test, clinical course, and liver biopsy findings. Ann Intern Med. 1997;127:21–6.
31. Cox DW. Molecular advances in Wilson disease. In: Progress in Liver Disease, Vol. X, 1996: pp. 245–63.
32. Maier-Dobersberger Th, Rack S, Granditsch G, Korninger L, Steindl P, Mannhalter Ch, Ferenci P. Diagnosis of Wilson's disease in an asymptomatic sibling by DNA linkage analysis. Gastroenterology. 1995;109:2015–18.
33. Vidaud D, Assouline B, Lecoz P, Cadranel JF, Chappuis P. Misdiagnosis revealed by genetic linkage analysis in a family with Wilson disease. Neurology. 1996;46:1485–6.

23
Wilson disease: natural course and therapeutic strategies

J. L. GOLLAN

Almost 90 years ago the London neurologist Samuel Alexander Kinnier Wilson defined the familial syndrome of progressive lenticular degeneration associated with cirrhosis. Impressive advances have been achieved in the elucidation of the biochemical and clinical features, and in the management of patients, as well as in the cloning of the Wilson disease gene 7 years ago; however, understanding of the pathogenic defect and the pathobiology of the disease is still incomplete.

GENETICS AND PATHOGENESIS

The gene for Wilson disease is distributed worldwide, and the disorder has been demonstrated in virtually all races. Current estimates indicate that the prevalence of the disease is approximately 1 in 30 000 live births, with an incidence ranging from 15 to 30 per million. The gene frequency varies between 0.3 and 0.7%, corresponding to a heterozygote carrier rate of slightly greater than 1 in 100. In 1993, a candidate gene for Wilson disease (WND) was reported independently by several different groups of investigators, using positional cloning strategies[1–3]. The WND gene (designated ATP7B) consists of a transcript of approximately 7.5 kb, which is expressed primarily in liver, kidney and placenta. The full-length cDNA sequence of the WND gene[1–3] predicts a 1411 amino acid protein, which is a member of the cation-transporting P-type ATPase subfamily, highly homologous to the Menke's disease gene product and the copper transporting ATPase (cop A) found in copper resistant strains of *Enterococcus hirae*. From sequence analysis of the cDNA, the WND protein is predicted to possess a metal binding domain (containing five binding sites), an ATP binding domain, a cation channel and phosphorylation region, and a transduction domain responsible for the conversion of the energy of ATP hydrolysis to cation transport.

To date, some 100 unique mutations in the Wilson disease gene have been identified, the majority of which are single base transversions or deletions.

The most common WND mutation (His 1069 Glu) may account for some 40% of cases, but approximately half of all mutations occur only rarely in any population[4]. The wide spectrum of clinical manifestations in Wilson disease has raised the question of whether variability exists at the molecular level. The fact that Wilson disease is linked to chromosome 13 markers in all populations studied suggests that there is a single genetic locus for the disease, and it has been postulated that different mutations at that locus may explain the clinical variability, although this concept remains controversial. Indeed, physiological studies employing the LEC rat, an animal model of Wilson disease, reveal that a single gene mutation may inhibit copper transport at more than one location within the cell. Thus, the variety of mutations identified in the Wilson disease gene potentially may affect copper transport to varying degrees, and at different cellular sites[5]. However, detailed genetic and epidemiological studies suggest that the variability in clinical expression observed in Wilson disease patients may not be solely a consequence of allelic heterogeneity, since marked differences in presentation, age of onset and disease course have been observed in family members who have inherited two identical (mutant) alleles.

It is postulated that the harmful effects of excess copper are mediated by the generation of free radicals, which deplete cellular stores of glutathione and oxidize lipids, enzymes and cytoskeletal proteins. Indeed, it has been shown that a number of intracellular systems are disrupted by elevated copper concentrations, including organellar membranes (e.g. mitochondrial), DNA, microtubules, and various enzymes and proteins, although the principal cellular target of copper toxicity is still unknown. In the earliest stages of hepatocellular injury, ultrastructural abnormalities involving the mitochondria endoplasmic reticulum, peroxisomes and nuclei all have been identified[6]. These changes, in conjunction with diminished activity of mitochondrial enzymes, may be important steps in the pathophysiological events leading to lipid peroxidation and triglyceride accumulation in the hepatocyte[6].

Wilson disease patients exhibit impaired biliary excretion of copper, which is believed to be the fundamental cause of the copper overload. The prompt reversal of abnormal copper metabolism in Wilson disease patients following orthotopic liver transplantation confirms that the primary defect resides in the liver. It has been proposed that the Wilson disease gene product is responsible for copper excretion from the liver cell, either across the canalicular (apical) membrane of the hepatocyte or more likely into a subcellular compartment that ultimately communicates with the bile canaliculus[3]. The latter is consistent with a trans-Golgi network-related defect underlying the diminished biliary excretion and systemic accumulation of copper observed in patients with Wilson disease[7]. In an animal model of Wilson disease, the Long–Evans Cinnamon (LEC) rat, excessive hepatic copper accumulation occurs in the setting of diminished biliary excretion. These rodents exhibit impaired entry of copper into lysosomes, with normal delivery of lysosomal copper to the bile[8]. The LEC rat is a mutant strain of the Long–Evans rat, which spontaneously develops fulminant hepatitis at 3–4 months of age, resulting in a 40% mortality rate. Surviving animals manifest chronic liver disease, low serum caeruloplasmin levels, and increased copper concentrations in the liver. Thus, the LEC rat shares key clinical, biochemical and histologic features with Wilson disease, and the recent availability of this animal model will continue to provide new insight into the pathogenesis of the human disorder.

CLINICAL FEATURES

The biochemical defect which leads to the accumulation of copper in Wilson disease is present at birth; however, clinical symptoms rarely are observed before the age of 5 years. The initial signs of Wilson disease generally are detected in older children, adolescents and young adults. Patients typically present with hepatic and/or neurological dysfunction. In a large series of patients[9], the initial clinical manifestations were hepatic in 42%, neurological in 34%, psychiatric in 10%, haematological in 12% and renal in 1%. Less commonly, patients present with skeletal, cardiac, ophthalmological, endocrinological or dermatological symptoms (Table 1). Approximately 25% of patients have involvement of two or more organ systems at initial evaluation, although, with the advent of more aggressive screening, there has been a substantial increase in the number of asymptomatic patients diagnosed.

HEPATIC DISEASE

Hepatic involvement in Wilson disease tends to manifest at a younger age (mean 8–12 years) than does neurological dysfunction, and is non-specific, mimicking the features of a variety of acute and chronic liver diseases. Three major clinical patterns of liver disease are observed: cirrhosis, chronic hepatitis and fulminant hepatic failure. In the early asymptomatic phase, or in the presence of inactive cirrhosis, liver tests may be normal or only minimally elevated. In the majority of cases, hepatic injury develops insidiously and, if untreated, pursues a relentless course to cirrhosis.

Table 1 Clinical manifestations of Wilson disease

Hepatic	–	cirrhosis, chronic hepatitis, fulminant hepatic failure
Ophthalmological	–	Kayser–Fleischer rings, sunflower cataracts
Neurological	–	bradykinesia, rigidity, tremor, ataxia, dyskinesia, dysarthria, seizures
Psychiatric	–	behavioral disturbances, cognitive impairment, affective disorder, psychosis
Hematological	–	haemolysis, coagulopathy
Renal	–	renal tubular defects, diminished glomerular filtration, nephrolithiasis
Cardiovascular	–	cardiomyopathy, arrhythmias, conduction disturbances, autonomic dysfunction
Musculoskeletal	–	osteomalacia, osteoporosis, degenerative joint disease
Gastrointestinal	–	cholelithiasis, pancreatitis, spontaneous bacterial peritonitis
Endocrinological	–	amenorrhoea, spontaneous abortion, delayed puberty, gynecomastia
Dermatological	–	azure lunulae, hyperpigmentation, acanthosis nigricans

An estimated 5–30% of patients with Wilson disease exhibit clinical, biochemical and histologic features similar to those observed in chronic hepatitis[10,11]. The diagnosis may be overlooked in these patients, since a significant percentage, almost 50% in one series[10], have no evidence of neurologic dysfunction or Kayser–Fleischer rings on ophthalmological examination. Serum caeruloplasmin levels also may be normal in the setting of severe hepatic inflammation. It has been estimated that Wilson disease represents the underlying aetiology in 5% of patients with idiopathic chronic hepatitis under 35 years of age[11]. A distinctive feature of Wilsonian chronic hepatitis is the relatively modest elevations of serum aminotransferase levels in the presence of severe hepatocellular necrosis and inflammation[11].

Wilson disease occasionally manifests as fulminant hepatic failure. These patients may be indistinguishable from individuals with virus-induced hepatic necrosis, and many of the biochemical tests used to establish the diagnosis of Wilson disease are abnormal in patients with other forms of fulminant hepatic failure[12]. The clinical features most suggestive of fulminant Wilsonian hepatitis include the presence of intravascular haemolysis, splenomegaly and Kayser–Fleischer rings. Biochemical markers indicative of Wilson disease include relatively mild elevations in serum transaminases, despite massive hepatic necrosis, hyperbilirubinaemia with normal or low alkaline phosphatase levels, and a markedly elevated serum copper concentration[12]. The serum level of aspartate aminotransferase (AST) typically is higher than that of alanine aminotransferase (ALT), as a result of the associated haemolysis. Although uncommonly observed in Wilsonian fulminant hepatic failure, Kayser–Fleischer rings are not pathognomonic, since they occasionally are seen in patients with other cholestatic hepatic diseases. The presence of severe coagulopathy and hypercupriuria are not useful in distinguishing Wilsonian from non-Wilsonian hepatic failure[12]. Liver biopsy with measurement of quantitative copper may be helpful, although deranged clotting function may preclude this procedure or necessitate the transjugular approach. If a biopsy specimen is obtained, histological evidence of cirrhosis (predominantly micronodular) in a young patient with fulminant hepatitis is suggestive of Wilson disease, as is an elevated hepatic copper content.

Wilson disease patients with acute hepatic failure tend to be young and to have a fulminant clinical course, with survival generally no longer than days to weeks unless hepatic transplantation is performed[12,13]. Medical treatment is frequently unsuccessful, particularly when the disorder is associated with haemolysis and renal insufficiency. It should be noted, however, that there are reports of recovery from Wilsonian chronic hepatitis, with acute hepatic failure, on medical therapy alone. Even when transplantation is unavailable, it remains imperative to make the diagnosis of Wilson disease for the purpose of aggressive medical therapy and family screening.

HEPATIC PATHOLOGY

Abnormal liver histology is usually evident in biopsy specimens obtained in the first decade of life from asymptomatic Wilson disease patients. The earliest changes detectable on light microscopy include glycogen deposition in the nuclei of periportal hepatocytes, and moderate fatty infiltration. The lipid droplets, which are composed of triglycerides, progressively increase in number and size, in some cases resembling the steatosis induced by ethanol. Ultrastructural abnormalities in liver cells may co-exist with or even precede the changes observed by light microscopy. Hepatocyte mitochondria typically exhibit heterogeneity in size and shape, with increased matrix density, separation of the normally apposed inner and outer mitochondrial membranes, widened intercristal spaces, and an array of vacuolated and crystalline inclusions within the matrix. Although similar isolated abnormalities may be observed in other pathological conditions, the occurrence of several of these anomalies in the same mitochondrion appears to be specific for patients with early Wilson disease. The mitochondrial changes generally become less pronounced or disappear after several years of therapy with D-penicillamine, indirectly supporting the notion that these abnormalities are a consequence of copper toxicity. Over time, the ultrastructural abnormalities found in early Wilson disease usually regress as the liver disease progresses to fibrosis and, ultimately, cirrhosis.

The histochemical staining of liver biopsy specimens for copper is of little diagnostic value in patients with Wilson disease. This is due to the fact that during the initial stages of copper accumulation the metal is distributed diffusely in the cytoplasm, and is frequently undetectable by rhodamine or rubeanic acid staining. Orcein, which is believed to stain polymerized metallothionein sequestered in lysosomes, exhibits a characteristic granular pattern in only 50% of patients with early Wilson disease. As the disease becomes more advanced, copper is sequestered within hepatocyte lysosomes and is detectable by routine histochemical techniques, even though tissue concentrations actually are lower than in earlier stages of the disorder. In contradistinction to Wilson disease, other conditions in which hepatic copper is elevated (e.g. primary biliary cirrhosis, sclerosing cholangitis, biliary atresia, intrahepatic cholestasis of childhood, Indian childhood cirrhosis, idiopathic copper toxicosis, and the normal neonate) are nearly always associated with stainable copper. Due to the insensitivity of copper staining techniques, time-dependent changes in the distribution of copper within the liver cell, heterogeneity of hepatic copper deposition, and the lack of specificity of hepatocyte copper granules, histochemical staining for copper is unreliable in establishing the diagnosis of Wilson disease.

The rate of progression of the liver histology from fatty infiltration to cirrhosis is variable, although it tends to occur by one of two general processes, either with or without hepatic inflammation. Some Wilson disease patients develop a histological picture that is indistinguishable from chronic hepatitis[10,11]. Pathological features include mononuclear cell infiltrates, which consist mainly of lymphocytes and plasma cells, piecemeal necrosis extending beyond the limiting plate, parenchymal collapse, bridging hepatic necrosis and fibrosis. If untreated, this may evolve into macronodular cirrhosis or progress rapidly to fulminant hepatitis. The development of cirrhosis also may occur in the absence of significant parenchymal inflammatory infiltrate or necrosis. It is notable that the majority of Wilson disease patients have evidence of fibrosis on liver biopsy, despite widely varying levels and patterns of hepatic inflammation and injury.

Hepatocellular carcinoma is uncommonly associated with Wilson disease, in contrast to haemochromatosis. It has been proposed that the diminished cancer risk is due to the relative dearth of an inflammatory component in the pathogenesis of Wilsonian cirrhosis. Indeed, animal studies suggest that copper may exert a protective effect against the development of malignancy. On the other hand, LEC rats exhibit a high incidence of hepatocellular carcinoma in the setting of marked hepatic copper accumulation[14], and this neoplastic potential is effectively abrogated by the administration of D-penicillamine. These observations have led to speculation that the low incidence of hepatocellular carcinoma in Wilson disease patients may be attributable to chelation therapy, since long-term survival is uncommon in untreated patients.

DIAGNOSTIC SCREENING

The diagnostic approach to Wilson disease must be tailored according to the clinical presentation. It must be emphasized that, in the absence of definitive DNA haplotype analysis, the diagnosis of Wilson disease should not be based on the results of an individual laboratory test, and can only be established in the setting of confirmatory clinical and biochemical data. Patients with neurological or psychiatric manifestations should undergo slit-lamp examination of the eyes and determination of serum caeruloplasmin. The documentation of Kayser–Fleischer rings and a low serum caeruloplasmin concentration is sufficient to establish the diagnosis, which can be confirmed by the presence of an increased 24 h urinary copper excretion. In the absence of DNA haplotype analysis, a liver biopsy with quantification of hepatic copper is essential if Kayser–Fleischer rings are absent (in order to exclude the possibility that the patient is heterozygous for the gene), or if caeruloplasmin levels are normal (as occurs in up to 15% of cases).

In patients who present primarily with hepatic dysfunction, the diagnosis may be difficult[15], since caeruloplasmin levels may be falsely elevated and ophthalmological findings absent. It is imperative that biochemical screening for Wilson disease be performed in all patients under 40 years of age who have clinical or histological findings compatible with chronic hepatitis, and in whom autoimmune and viral hepatitis have been excluded. In patients with a high index of suspicion, a serum caeruloplasmin concentration should be obtained, urinary copper excretion measured, and a liver biopsy performed (providing no contraindication exists). In the rare circumstance where the diagnosis remains in doubt, a radiolabelled copper study may be confirmatory or, if feasible, haplotype analysis performed.

It is imperative that all first-degree relatives be screened, particularly siblings. Wilson disease may be clinically silent even in the presence of significant organ damage; hence, a delay in the diagnosis or in the initiation of therapy may lead to irreversible hepatic and/or neurological injury. Biochemical screening of children should not be performed before 3–4 years of age. The evaluation should consist of a careful history and physical examination, serologic tests of liver function, a slit-lamp examination of the eyes, and a serum caeruloplasmin level, with liver biopsy and quantitative hepatic copper determination and/or DNA linkage analysis being reserved for diagnostic dilemmas. Once the diagnosis of presymptomatic Wilson disease is established, lifelong chelation therapy should be initiated immediately.

TREATMENT

Diet

The ubiquitous presence of copper in most foodstuffs makes stringent dietary copper restriction impractical. It still is suggested that patients avoid frequent ingestion of foods with a high copper content, such as liver, chocolate, nuts, mushrooms, legumes and shellfish. The use of deionized or distilled water is recommended if the copper content of the patient's home drinking water exceeds 0.2 ppm, particularly during initial therapy. The use of domestic water softeners should be avoided, since these may substantially increase copper concentration.

Pharmacological therapy

Penicillamine

Over the past three decades, it has been well-documented that oral D-penicillamine results in complete reversal or alleviation of hepatic, neurological and psychiatric abnormalities in most patients with Wilson disease, and this drug still remains the gold standard therapy for this disorder. The key to a successful outcome is early diagnosis and treatment, since clinical disease can be prevented indefinitely in asymptomatic patients, provided that they adhere to continuous maintenance therapy. Some individuals demonstrate a dramatic response within weeks of initiating D-penicillamine, while others may exhibit no clinical improvement, or even temporary neurological deterioration, for several months.

The precise mechanisms of action of D-penicillamine remains controversial. Although the logic for the use of this drug in the treatment of Wilson disease is based on its in vitro copper chelating properties, there is conflicting evidence regarding the ability of penicillamine to decopper the liver and other organs. It also has been proposed that D-penicillamine detoxifies the liver by sequestering intracellular copper in an innocuous state, either through the direct formation of copper complexes or by the induction of metallothionein synthesis. The fulminant decompensation observed in previously compliant patients who discontinue D-penicillamine therapy for a relatively brief period of time offers support for this hypothesis. Other postulated mechanisms of action of D-penicillamine include inhibition of collagen cross-linking, enhancement of intracellular levels of reduced glutathione, and suppression of inflammation via effects on leukotriene and prostaglandin metabolism.

The standard dose of D-penicillamine is 1–2 g daily given orally in four divided doses 30 min before meals, although as much as 4 g/day can be administered to critically ill patients for brief periods of time. It is best taken on an empty stomach since food reduces its absorption. Most of the excess liver copper appears to be mobilized within the initial year of therapy, with urinary copper excretion approaching 2–5 mg/day during this period. After several years of treatment, urinary copper levels decline (to 0.5–1.0 mg daily), as hepatic copper concentrations approach normal levels. When symptoms have largely abated and a stable clinical course has been achieved, the maintenance dose of D-penicillamine in adults may be reduced to 1 g daily. Liver function test abnormalities may persist for a year or more after the initiation of appropriate treatment. As they subside, a corresponding resolution of hepatic histologic abnormalities is observed, although regression of hepatic fibrosis and portal hypertension is less impressive.

A syndrome of acute deterioration has been described following the initiation of D-penicillamine therapy in as many as 20% of Wilson disease patients presenting with neurological symptoms. If observed, worsening of neurological dysfunction tends to occur within the first 4 weeks of therapy, and generally only in those patients who present with nervous system involvement, although the rare occurrence in asymptomatic patients has been reported. The cause of this exacerbation of neurological manifestations remains conjectural. However, the exacerbation of neurological sequelae associated with the initiation of treatment does not appear to be unique to penicillamine, as it also has been noted with all other forms of chelation therapy, including trientine. The dose of D-penicillamine should be reduced to 250 mg/day in any patient who exhibits an exacerbation of neurological symptoms following initiation of therapy. The dose should then be increased by 250 mg/day every 4–7 days until a urinary copper concentration of at least 1 and preferably 2 mg/day is attained. Indeed, it is prudent to introduce D-penicillamine in a low initial dose in all asymptomatic Wilson disease patients, or in those individuals presenting with mild symptomatology. Despite early clinical deterioration, continued treatment is mandatory in order to achieve subsequent improvement. Recent studies with thiomolybdates (see below) suggest that this may be an alternative approach in patients who exhibit neurologic deterioration with initial D-penicillamine therapy.

A variety of adverse effects of D-penicillamine have been recognized[9,16], although serious complications necessitating discontinuation of the drug are infrequent. Thus, D-penicillamine has been demonstrated to be effective and safe for use in the treatment of Wilson disease, and remains the first-line drug in this disorder.

Trientine

Trientine (triethylene tetramine dihydrochloride) was introduced in 1969 as an alternative chelating agent for cases in which serious toxic reactions to D-penicillamine occur. It has been well-established that 1–2 g administered orally in three divided doses induces a negative copper balance and produces clinical improvement. As with penicillamine, trientine should be administered prior to meals. The exact mechanism of action of this drug remains unknown, although it has been shown to enhance urinary copper excretion and to decrease intestinal copper absorption. Unlike D-penicillamine, trientine causes the serum copper concentration to rise during cupriuresis, suggesting that the two agents may mobilize copper from different systemic pools. Most of the toxic side-effects necessitating conversion from D-penicillamine to trientine typically subside while on trientine. The exception is elastosis perforans serpiginosa, which may progress in some patients. Sideroblastic anaemia is the major side-effect attributed to this medication. Although trientine appears to cause minimal toxicity, it has less cupriuretic effect than D-penicillamine and, hence, is currently not recommended as primary therapy.

Zinc

The principal mode of action of zinc is believed to be via the induction of intestinal metallothionein synthesis, which results in the sequestration of copper in intestinal epithelial cells, thereby enhancing fecal copper excretion and preventing absorption into the portal circulation. Zinc also may directly exhibit a protective effect in hepatocytes by inducing the synthesis of metallothionein in these cells. A minimum of 75 mg zinc sulphate or zinc acetate per day, administered in two divided doses between meals, appears to maintain neutral or negative copper balance, although most studies have administered 50 mg thrice daily. Side-effects of oral zinc include headaches and gastrointestinal upset, the incidence of which may be reduced by the use of zinc acetate, rather than zinc sulphate. Although long-term follow up is limited, major complications have not been reported with the use of zinc in patients with Wilson disease.

Due to the slower onset of action than is seen with other chelating agents, zinc is not recommended for the initial treatment of symptomatic Wilson disease. In fact, most of the published experience with zinc therapy has been in patients who previously had been decoppered with D-penicillamine. It has been suggested that zinc may be useful for presymptomatic or pregnant patients, as well as for maintenance therapy in individuals who have previously been de-coppered with chelating drugs. However, there are data indicating that hepatic copper may continue to accrue in some Wilson disease patients treated with zinc alone[16]. Additionally, long-term follow up studies are needed to determine whether the de-coppered state is sustained with zinc therapy, and to monitor for untoward side-effects. Based on the information currently available, oral zinc should be used as therapy in the rare patients who develop intolerance to both D-penicillamine and trientine. Whether a synergistic effect occurs with zinc in combination with a chelating agent has not been demonstrated; hence, the basis for concomitant administration of penicillamine or trientine and zinc is not established, and awaits the outcome of clinical trials.

Thiomolybdates

Thiomolybdates appear to lower systemic copper levels by complexing lumenal copper, and thereby inhibiting intestinal absorption. In addition, the portion of the drug that is systemically absorbed may bind excessive serum copper and render it less available for cellular uptake, ultimately resulting in the removal of copper from intracellular stores. Moreover, in contrast to penicillamine and trientine, thiomolybdates exhibit a higher affinity for copper than metallothionein in vitro, suggesting that this drug may be able to more effectively remove copper from the cell. Limited studies of ammonium tetrathiomolybdate (60–100 mg daily in two divided doses) in Wilson disease patients in whom D-penicillamine and/or trientine was poorly tolerated or ineffective have demonstrated the drug to be highly successful in lowering hepatic copper concentrations[16]. Additional trials have supported the efficacy and safety of ammonium tetrathiomolybdate in the initial treatment of Wilson disease, and have further suggested that this medication is less prone to precipitate the neurological decompensation observed with other chelating agents[17]. Although initial results appear promising, thiomolybdates have caused bone marrow suppression. Further experience is warranted before this drug can be recommended for routine use.

Long-term management

Patients with Wilson disease require careful supervision during the first several months of therapy to ensure adequate copper excretion, and to monitor for the potential development of early adverse reactions to D-penicillamine. It is suggested that a physical examination be performed and a 24 h urinary copper excretion, complete blood count, urinalysis, and renal and liver function tests be checked on a weekly basis for the first 4–6 weeks following the initiation of chelation therapy. Bimonthly evaluations are then recommended through the first year, followed by at least yearly examinations thereafter. Lifelong therapy, without interruption, is essential in all patients. Cessation of therapy may result in rapid and irreversible hepatic and neurologic deterioration. In a study of 11 patients who discontinued treatment, eight died of fulminant hepatitis after an average period of only 2.6 years without treatment. Thus, it is imperative that an alternative agent be administered to any patient who is unable to continue D-penicillamine due to adverse effects[18].

Liver transplantation

Despite advances in medical therapy, significant mortality rates are still observed in specific subsets of patients with Wilson disease. These individuals, in whom orthotopic liver transplantation has proven most successful, generally present with acute fulminant hepatic failure associated with haemolysis and hypercupraemia (either as the initial presentation or following poor compliance with medical therapy), or with advanced cirrhosis and hepatic insufficiency, unresponsive to an adequate trial of chelation therapy and supportive measures. In the absence of severe hepatic disease, liver transplantation is not generally recommended for the management of refractory extrahepatic manifestations, such as neurological deterioration. In a series of 55 patients with Wilson disease who underwent hepatic transplantation, a 79% 1-year survival, and overall survival rate of 72% at 3 months to 20 years was reported[19]. In a more recent study of 45 patients, 73% survived more than 5 years after transplantation, and 10 of the 13 surviving patients showed neurological improvement[20]. Transplant recipients uniformly manifest complete reversal of the underlying defects in copper metabolism, and exhibit significant improvement in most symptoms and signs of the disease.

REFERENCES

1. Bull PC, Thomas GR, Rommens JM et al. The Wilson's disease gene is a putative copper transporting P-type ATPase similar to the Menkes gene. Nature Genet. 1993;5:327–37.
2. Petrukhin K, Fischer SG, Pirastu M et al. Mapping, cloning and genetic characterization of the region containing the Wilson disease gene. Nature Genet. 1993;5:338–43.

3. Tanzi RE, Petrukhin K, Chernov J et al. The Wilson disease gene is a copper transporting ATPase with homology to the Menkes disease gene. Nature Genet. 1993;5:344–50.
4. Shah AB, Chernov I, Zhand HT et al. Identification and analysis of mutations in the Wilson's disease gene (ATP7B): Population frequencies, genotype-phenotype correlation, and functional analyses. Am J Hum Genet. 1997;61:317–28.
5. Schilsky ML. Identification of the Wilson's disease gene: clues for disease pathogenesis and the potential for molecular diagnosis. Hepatology. 1994;20:529–33.
6. Sternlieb I. Perspectives on Wilson's disease. Hepatology. 1990;12:1234–9.
7. Hung IH, Suzuki M, Yamaguchi Y et al. Biochemical characterization of the Wilson disease protein and functional expression in the yeast *Saccharomyces cerevisiae*. J Biol Chem. 1997;272:21461–6.
8. Schilsky ML, Stockert RJ, Sternlieb I. Pleiotropic effect of the LEC mutation: a rodent model of Wilson's disease. Am J Physiol. 1994;266:G907–13.
9. Sternlieb I, Scheinberg IH. Wilson's disease. In: Wright R, Millward-Sadler GH, Alberti KGMM et al, eds. Liver and Biliary Disease. London: W.B. Saunders, 1985;949–61.
10. Scott J, Gollan JL, Samourian S et al. Wilson's disease, presenting as chronic active hepatitis. Gastroenterology. 1978;74:645–51.
11. Schilsky ML, Scheinberg IH, Sternlieb I. Prognosis of Wilsonian chronic active hepatitis. Gastroenterology. 1991;100:762–7.
12. McCullough AJ, Fleming R, Thistle JL et al. Diagnosis of Wilson's disease presenting as fulminant hepatic failure. Gastroenterology. 1983;84:161–7.
13. Mowat AP. Liver disorders in children: the indications for liver replacement in parenchymal and metabolic diseases. Transplant Proc. 1987;19:3236–41.
14. Sokol RJ. At long last: An animal model of Wilson's disease. Hepatology. 1994;20:533–5.
15. Schilsky ML, Sternlieb I. Overcoming obstacles to the diagnosis of Wilson's disease. Gastroenterology. 1997;113:350–3.
16. Gollan JL, Gollan TJ. Wilson Disease in 1998: Genetic, diagnostic and therapeutic aspects. J Hepatol. 1998;28:28–36.
17. Brewer GJ, Johnson V, Dick RD et al. Treatment of Wilson disease with ammonium tetrathiomolybdate. II. Initial therapy in 33 neurologically affected patients and follow-up with zinc therapy. Arch Neurol. 1996;53:1017–25.
18. Scheinberg IH, Jaffe ME, Sternlieb I. The use of trientine in preventing the effects of interrupting penicillamine therapy in Wilson's disease. N Engl J Med. 1987;317:209–13.
19. Schilsky ML, Scheinberg IH, Sternlieb I. Liver transplantation for Wilson's disease: Indications and outcome. Hepatology. 1994;19:583–7.
20. Eghtesad B, Nezakatoo N, Geraci L et al. Liver transplantation for Wilson's disease: A single-center experience. Liver Transplant Surg. 1999;5:467–74.

24
Alpha-1-antitrypsin deficiency: pathogenesis and diagnosis

J. H. TECKMAN

BACKGROUND

PIZZ alpha-1-antitrypsin ($\alpha 1$AT) deficiency is an autosomal recessive genetic disease in which the frequency of homozygotes is approximately 1 in 1500–3500 live births in North American and European populations[1]. It is the most common genetic cause of liver disease in children, the most common genetic disease that necessitates liver transplantation in children, and can also cause chronic liver disease, hepatocellular carcinoma and premature pulmonary emphysema in adults[1,2]. $\alpha 1$AT is predominantly synthesized in the liver and is then secreted into the serum and extracellular fluid, although it is also expressed in a variety of extrahepatic cell types including enterocytes and macrophages[3–5]. The contribution of the liver to systemic circulating $\alpha 1$AT is illustrated by the observation that serum $\alpha 1$AT phenotype converts to the donor liver type following orthotopic liver transplantation.

The $\alpha 1$AT gene is 12.2 kb in size and is located on chromosome 14q. The gene contains five exons that encode an approximately 55 kDa polypeptide of 395 amino acids[6]. Post-translational modifications involve the addition of three asparagine-linked complex carbohydrate side chains. $\alpha 1$AT is the archetype of the serpin (serine protease inhibitor) family of structurally related proteins, although not all members of the family appear to act as anti-proteases. Wild-type $\alpha 1$AT M functions as an inhibitor of neutrophil elastase, cathepsin G, and proteinase 3, among other proteases, all of which are released by activated neutrophils during the host response to inflammation[6]. In this way, $\alpha 1$AT appears to be physiologically important in protecting the lungs and other host tissues from inflammation-induced damage[1,4].

MECHANISM OF DEFICIENCY

The Z mutation of the $\alpha 1$AT gene is a single base pair substitution encoding the amino acid substitution of lysine for glutamic acid at codon 342[7]. During bio-

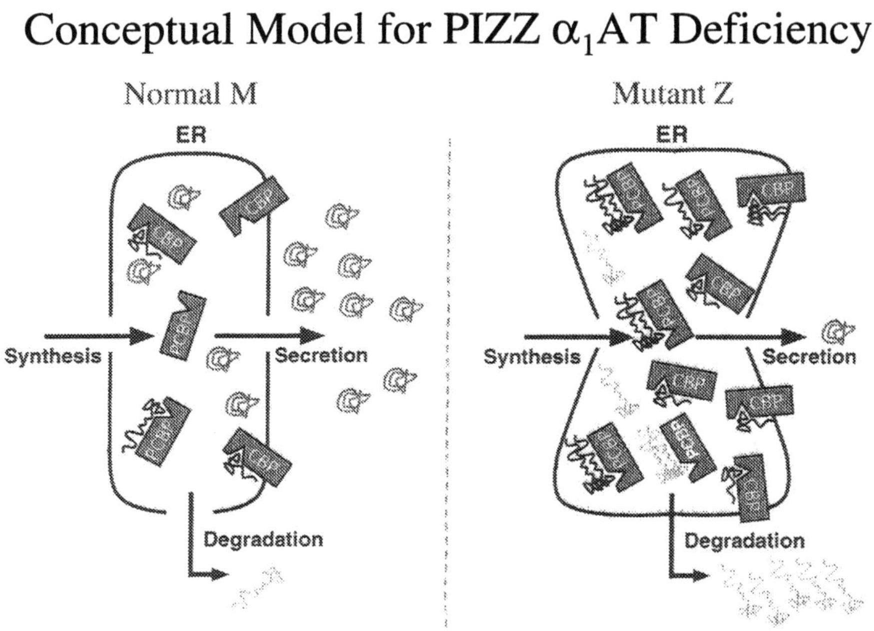

Figure 1 Conceptual model for PIZZ α 1-antitrypsin deficiency. Two types of ER molecular chaperones, polypeptide chain-binding proteins (PCBP) and membrane-associated calcium-binding proteins (CBP) are shown as hatched bars. The nascent α1AT molecules that are unfolded are shown as dark, long wavy lines, and those with mature folding are shown as light, tightly knotted lines. In individuals with the normal α1AT M gene, the normal α1AT M molecule enters the secretory pathway (ER) in an unfolded state. Interaction with PCBP and CBP chaperones facilitate folding into a mature state, allowing for the dissociation from PCBP and CBP in a form competent for secretion. A very small proportion of the normal α1ATM molecules are unable to fold into the mature state and are directed into degradation pathways. In the individual with the mutant α1ATZ gene, only a small proportion of the nascent α1ATZ protein molecules are able to attain the mature folding in the ER that permits secretion. Some of the mutant α1ATZ molecules polymerize. There is a net accumulation of Z molecules within an engorged ER. Greater numbers of improperly folded α1ATZ molecules are directed into degradative pathways.

genesis, the nascent polypeptide chain is translated on a ribosome and then translocated into the lumen of the endoplasmic reticulum (ER). In the ER the nascent polypeptide binds to a family of proteins known as chaperones that are part of the cellular quality control apparatus[1]. These chaperones, many of which are members of the heat shock/stress protein family, assist nascent polypeptides in folding into their final conformations (Fig. 1). Chaperones of the quality control pathway are also involved in directing fully folded proteins to continue along the secretory pathway or retaining improperly folded, abnormally assembled or mutant proteins within the ER. Abnormal proteins retained within the ER by the quality control apparatus are ultimately directed into a series of protein degradation pathways to prevent damage to the cell or to the surrounding tissues.

Interestingly, the α1ATZ mutant polypeptide folds unusually slowly in the ER and assumes an abnormal conformation[4,8]. Studies have shown this abnormal

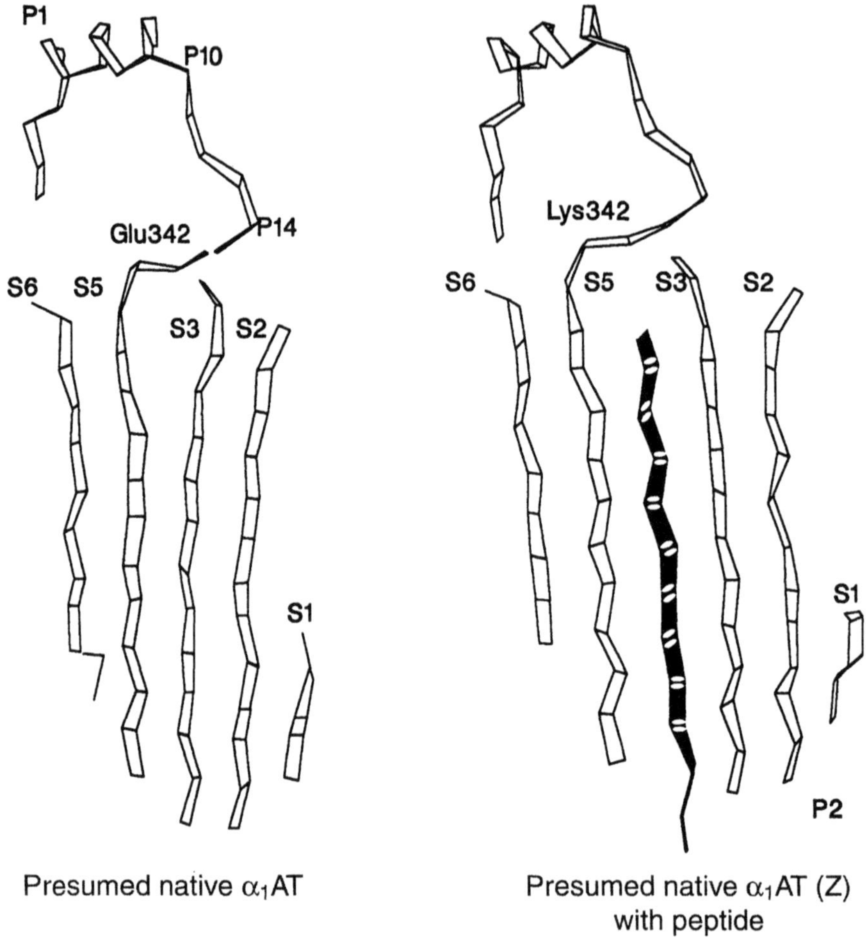

Figure 2 Ribbon diagrams of the A sheet and reactive-site loop of α1AT. On the left is shown native, wild type α1ATM. In the reactive-site loop residues are numbered P1, P10, and P14 from the reactive-site methionine P1. The β-helices of the A sheet are referred to as S1–S6. The position of glutamate 342 at the base of the reactive-site loop is indicated. There is a gap in the A-sheet between S3 and S5. On the right is shown native, mutant α1ATZ. The amino acid substitution of lysine at position 342 is shown at the base of the reactive-site loop. The dark structure in the space between S3 and S5 represents the reactive-site loop of a neighboring α1ATZ molecule inserted into the gap. (Adapted from Carrell RW, Evans DL, Stein DE. Nature. 1991;353:576 and from Lomas DA, Evans DL, Finch JT, Carrell RW. Nature. 1992;357:605.)

conformation is associated with altered binding to ER chaperone proteins[9]. Studies have also shown that α1ATZ molecules can aggregate by the loop–sheet insertion mechanism, in which the reactive site loop portion of the peptide forms a projection that fits into a gap in the surface of a neighboring α1ATZ molecule (Fig. 2)[10–12]. The Z mutation of the α1ATZ molecule is at the base of the reactive site loop apparently leading to increased mobility of this portion of the molecule. α1ATZ aggregation has been shown to occur spontaneously, although it may increase during minor cellular perturbations such as an increase in temperature. It is possible that an increase in patient body temperature during a period of systemic inflammation would increase this tendency in vivo. This effect is sometimes referred to as polymerization rather than aggregation, although no peptide bonds are actually formed between the neighbouring molecules. Electron microscopic analysis of liver biopsy specimens from PIZZ α1AT deficient individuals have confirmed the presence of aggregated α1ATZ in human hepatocytes and circulating in the serum[10–12].

The vast majority of mutant α1ATZ molecules synthesized are retained within the ER rather than being secreted leading to the decreased, 10–15% of normal, α1AT serum level observed in PIZZ patients[1]. ER retention has been observed for α1ATZ in all cell types examined, not only hepatocytes, and site directed mutagenesis studies have proven that the Z mutation alone is sufficient to trigger ER retention[6,8,13,14]. However, the specific mechanism of ER retention and the exact contributions of the quality control apparatus and/or aggregation are still unclear. Molecular mutagenesis studies indicate that additional mutations in the α1ATZ molecule designed to inhibit aggregation do decrease the rate of ER retention of the molecule. However, these studies have been criticized in that any change in the conformation of the molecule brought on by the new mutations could not only alter aggregation but also could alter chaperone protein binding. Changes in chaperone binding could in turn affect retention by a mechanism unrelated to aggregation. In addition, many other mutant proteins have been described with abnormal conformations that do not aggregate and are still retained in the ER at high rates by the quality control apparatus. The CFTRΔf508 molecule is one such example[15]. A number of researchers have attempted to decrease retention and improve secretion of α1ATZ by using the presence of molecules specially designed to disrupt aggregation. To date, these attempts have been unsuccessful. Further investigation will be needed to fully understand the molecular mechanism(s) of ER retention of mutant α1ATZ.

MECHANISMS OF INJURY

The ER retention of mutant α1ATZ and the resulting low serum levels are thought to be directly related to the development of premature pulmonary emphysema in adults due to inadequate serum defence of lung parenchyma against proteolytic attack[1,6,7]. However, the mechanism of liver injury in α1AT deficiency has been more difficult to understand. Studies in several strains of mice transgenic for the human α1ATZ gene have demonstrated the development of liver injury even though these mice have normal levels of their endogenous murine anti-elastases[16–18]. Therefore, these studies rule out the possibility that the liver injury in α1AT deficiency is related to deficient serum anti-elastase activity. Liver abnormalities described in various α1ATZ transgenic mice include neonatal liver disease, the development of hepatic fibrosis, and liver cancer later in life, all of which are similar to various aspects of the human disease.

Other authors have suggested that an abnormal host immune response against liver antigens causes liver injury based on the observation that peripheral blood lymphocytes from PIZZ infants are cytotoxic for isolated hepatocytes[19]. However, this is more likely a non-specific effect since lymphocytes from PIMM infants with the neonatal hepatitis syndrome and a similar degree of liver injury are also cytotoxic for isolated hepatocytes in some reports. One study suggested an increase in the HLA DR3-DW25 haplotype in PIZZ patients with liver disease, although there was no difference found in class II MHC expression[20,21]. No further evidence has come to light to support a connection between $\alpha 1$ATZ associated liver disease and HLA type.

The only explanation for the development of liver injury in $\alpha 1$AT deficiency, which is supported by significant experimental evidence, is the accumulation theory. This theory states that it is the chronic accumulation of the abnormal, mutant $\alpha 1$ATZ molecule retained within the ER of hepatocytes that leads to liver injury. However, it has been difficult to reconcile this theory to descriptions from a number of studies, including the prospective population based Swedish study by Sveger and colleagues of the extremely wide range of clinical liver injury[1,2,6,22,23]. Some PIZZ individuals develop life threatening liver disease as infants, some individuals develop hepatocellular carcinoma as adults, but most patients never develop significant liver damage. Therefore, other genetic and/or environmental factors are thought to also be involved in the development of liver disease. One factor described in a series of studies by Perlmutter and colleagues is that patients susceptible to liver injury appear to have inefficient intracellular degradation of the mutant $\alpha 1$ATZ protein retained within the ER[9]. Inefficient intracellular degradation of the accumulated $\alpha 1$ATZ would lead to a greater net

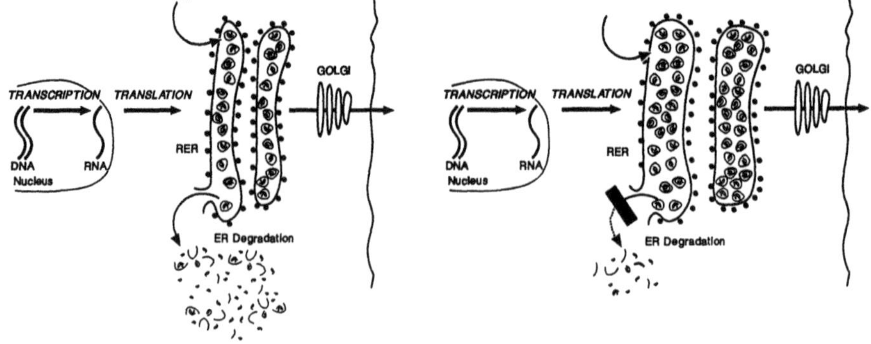

Figure 3 The difference in ER degradation of $\alpha 1$ATZ protein in liver disease protected versus liver disease susceptible hosts. Schematic representations of protein transcription/translation, secretion, ER retention, and ER degradation within hepatocytes are shown. The block in ER degradation in the susceptible hosts is represented by the dark bar.

burden of the presumably toxic $\alpha 1$ATZ within the ER and a greater tendency for liver injury (Fig. 3).

Detailed investigations of the cellular mechanisms by which proteins retained within the ER are degraded have revealed that several possible proteolytic pathways may be involved[9,24,25]. There is also evidence to suggest that genetically determined abnormalities in specific steps of these degradation pathways could be responsible for susceptibility to liver injury in individual patients and family groups. One important mechanism for ER protein degradation has been shown to involve the proteasome proteolytic complex present in the cytoplasm. The proteasome attacks polypeptides that have been flagged for degradation by the attachment of chains of ubiquitin molecules, and proteasome function serves many important degradative and regulatory needs within the cell. In the case of $\alpha 1$ATZ molecules retained within the ER lumen, it has been shown that binding to the ER lumenal tail of the transmembrane molecular chaperone, calnexin, followed by ubiquitination of the cytoplasmic portion of the calnexin molecule leads to proteasomal degradation of the $\alpha 1$ATZ-calnexin-ubiquitin complex (Fig. 4). Further analysis has also revealed that alternative pathways to the proteasome, independent of ubiquitination, can also be traversed by $\alpha 1$ATZ

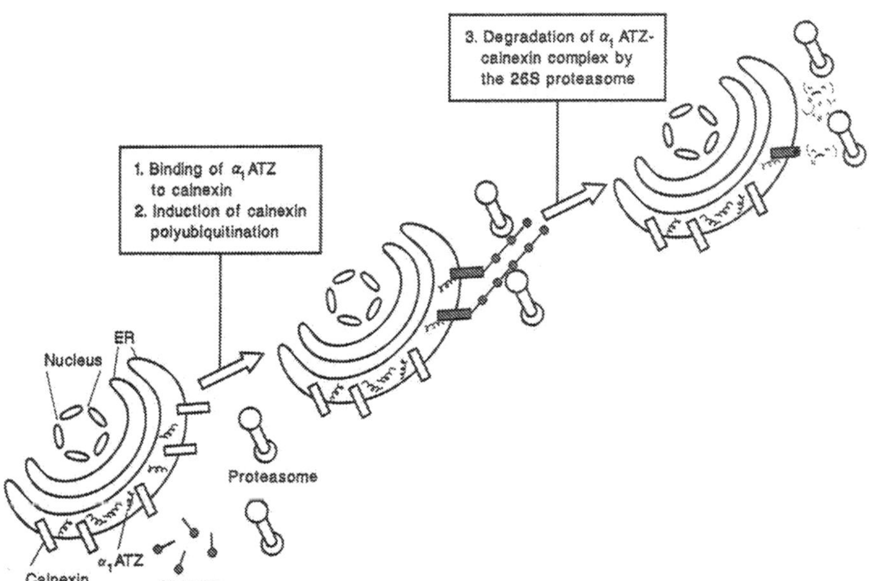

Figure 4 The working model for the degradation of $\alpha 1$ATZ retained in the ER by the ubiquitin-dependent proteasome pathway. $\alpha 1$ATZ molecules are shown as wavy lines within the ER lumen. Calnexin is shown as an open bar in the ER membrane; when it is bound to $\alpha 1$ATZ and ubiquitinated, calnexin is shown as a dark bar. Ubiquitin molecules are shown as solid circles with stems that form chains when attached to calnexin. The proteasome complex is shown as open, tubular structures. In step 1, $\alpha 1$ATZ molecules retained within the ER lumen bind to the chaperone, calnexin. In step 2, the abnormal conformation of the bound $\alpha 1$ATZ molecule presumably induces a signal and results in the ubiquitination of the cytoplasmic tail of calnexin. In step 3, the proteasome degrades the transmembrane $\alpha 1$ATZ-calnexin-ubiquitin trimolecular complex.

molecules retained within the ER. Preliminary evidence from several investigators also suggests non-proteasomal mechanisms for the ER associated degradation of α1ATZ, although the exact pathways and enzymes involved are still being elucidated.

Despite strong evidence that accumulation of α1ATZ within hepatocytes is damaging to the cell and that inefficient degradation of the retained molecules leading to increased net retention is associated with the potentiation of liver injury, the exact mechanism by which cell damage occurs is still unknown. Cellular stress response pathways have been identified that appear to be activated by a burden of unfolded protein within the ER. Two of the best known are the unfolded protein response and the ER overload state[1,4,6,24]. It has been hypothesized that these pathways are designed to assist the cell in coping with acute stress, perhaps in the same way as the heat shock response. However, it is possible that a chronic burden of accumulated α1ATZ within the ER leads to repeated or continuous activation of these pathways that is then damaging to the hepatocyte.

Many investigators have tried to identify environmental factors that might contribute to the pathogenesis of liver disease in α1AT deficiency, although to date, no firm associations have been made[1,2,6,26]. Some researchers have proposed that viral hepatitis infection may be an important environmental factor in the development of liver injury in α1AT deficiency. However, reports of increased prevalence of viral hepatitis in PIZZ patients with liver disease have not been consistent across all reports and have been weakened by referral center bias[27]. Interestingly, both hepatitis B and hepatitis C viruses encode polypeptides that are retained within the ER and may play a role in the pathogenesis of the hepatocellular injury in these infections. The consequences of ER retention of α1ATZ in the presence of retained viral proteins, while interesting to contemplate, has not yet been investigated. Some authors have suggested that episodes of fever during systemic infections or inflammatory illness could exacerbate the intracellular accumulation of α1ATZ due to increased aggregation, as has been shown with increased temperature in vitro[10–12]. However, no systematic examination of this hypothesis has been made in PIZZ patients. Despite continuing investigation, the specific cellular mechanism by which the accumulated α1ATZ causes direct hepatocellular injury is still unknown.

DIAGNOSIS

The diagnosis of PIZZ α1AT deficiency is established by phenotype (PI-type) analysis of the α1AT protein present in a sample of the patient's serum as determined by isoelectric focusing or by agarose gel electrophoresis at acid pH[1,4,6]. Although reliable and acknowledged as the gold standard for diagnosis in experienced hands, isoelectric focusing is technically difficult, and therefore is best performed in specialty labs with significant experience with the technique. Determination of a patient's total serum α1AT level should not be the sole basis for the diagnosis. α1AT is an acute phase reactant and therefore even PIZZ individuals can transiently increase their baseline total serum levels during periods of inflammation. However, determination of total serum α1AT levels and

PI typing of family members are supplemental tests that may be required to fully differentiate homozygous ZZ patients from patients who are compound heterozygotes with null or other disease associated alleles. If available, examination of liver biopsy specimens may support the diagnosis by revealing the characteristic periodic acid – Schiff (PAS)-positive, diastase-resistant globules present within hepatocytes, which represent the intracellular accumulations of α1ATZ protein. However, liver biopsy is not necessary to establish the diagnosis, and the diagnosis should not rest on the presence or absence of these characteristic globules. Many reports indicate that the globules may be absent in very young PIZZ infants, that the globules are often not present within all hepatocytes in an affected liver, and that globules with a similar appearance can sometimes be seen in the livers of normal, PIMM individuals with other types of liver disease[4,28]. In the future, analysis of genomic DNA by polymerase chain reaction may become a rapid and sensitive technique for the detection of specific α1AT alleles in clinical practice, screening and prenatal diagnosis. However at present, direct molecular DNA testing is only a research tool.

The diagnosis of PIZZ α1AT deficiency associated liver disease should be considered in any child with unexplained conjugated hyperbilirubinaemia, symptoms of cholestasis, hypertransaminasaemia, cirrhosis, or the neonatal hepatitis syndrome. The diagnosis should also be considered in older children or adults with unexplained persistently elevated transaminases, cirrhosis, hepatocellular carcinoma, or other evidence of chronic liver disease. The phenotyping of siblings or other family members of newly diagnosed patients is often considered so that other deficient individuals can be identified and urgently cautioned against cigarette smoking. Smoking has been clearly shown to dramatically increase the risk of premature pulmonary emphysema in α1AT deficient adults, although smoking is not related to the pathogenesis of liver disease.

In summary, PIZZ α1AT deficiency is a relatively common genetic disease that can be associated with a wide range of clinical presentations. The majority of individuals appear to be protected from liver disease, while a few may develop chronic liver disease as children or adults. The hepatocellular injury is associated with the retention of the mutant α1ATZ protein within the ER of hepatocytes, although other factors including genetic determinants of the intracellular quality control system, polymerization, and the cellular response to accumulation may modulate the effect of the injury.

REFERENCES

1. Teckman JH, Dongfeng Q, Perlmutter DH. Molecular pathogenesis of liver disease in α1-antitrypsin deficiency. Hepatology. 1996;24:1504–16.
2. Mowat AP. Alpha-1-antitrypsin deficiency (PiZZ): features of liver involvement in childhood. Acta Paediatr Suppl. 1994;393:13–17.
3. Carlson JA, Rogers BB, Sifers RN, Hawkins HK, Finegold MJ, Woo SLC. Multiple tissues express alpha$_1$-antitrypsin in transgenic mice and man. J Clin Invest. 1988;82:26–36.
4. Perlmutter DH. Alpha-1-antitrypsin deficiency. Semin Liver Dis. 1998;18:217–25.
5. Perlmutter DH, Cole FS, Kilbridge P, Rossing TH, Colten HR. Expression of the α1-proteinase inhibitor gene in human monocytes and macrophages. Proc Natl Acad Sci USA. 1985;82:795–9.
6. Cox, DW. Alpha-1-antitrypsin deficiency. In: Scriver CR, Beautt AL, Sly WS, Valle D, eds. The Metabolic Basis of Inherited Disease, 6th edn. New York: McGraw-Hill, 1989: pp. 2409–37.

7. Owen MC, Carrell RW. Alpha-1-antitrypsin: sequence of the Z variant tryptic peptide. FEBS Lett. 1976;79:247–9.
8. Yu M-H, Lee KN, Kim J. The Z type variation of human α1-antitrypsin causes a protein folding defect. Nature Struct Biol. 1995;2:363–7.
9. Wu Y, Whitman I, Molmenti E, Moore K, Hippenmeyer P, Perlmutter DH. A lag in intracellular degradation of mutant α1-antitrypsin correlates with the liver disease phenotype in homozygous PiZZ α1-antitrypsin deficiency. Proc Natl Acad Sci USA. 1994;91:9014–18.
10. Lomas DA, Evans DL, Finch JJ, Carrell RW. The mechanism of Z α1-antitrypsin accumulation in the liver. Nature. 1992;357:605–7.
11. Lomas DA, Finch JT, Seyama K, Nukiwa T, Carrell RW. α1-Antitrypsin S_{iiyama} ($Ser^{53} \rightarrow$ Phe): Further evidence for intracellular loop-sheet polymerization. J Biol Chem. 1993;268:15333–5.
12. Lomas DA, Elliott PR, Sidhar SK, Foreman RC, Finch JT, Cox DW et al. α1-antitrypsin M_{malton} ($Phe^{52\text{-deleted}}$) forms loop-sheet polymers in vivo: Evidence for the C-sheet mechanism of polymerization. J Biol Chem. 1995;270:16864–74.
13. Perlmutter DH, Kay RM, Cole FS, Rossing TH, Van Thiel D, Colten HR. The cellular defect in α1-proteinase inhibitor deficiency is expressed in human monocytes and xenopus oocytes injected with human liver mRNA. Proc Natl Acad Sci USA. 1985;82:6918–21.
14. Qu D, Teckman JH, Perlmutter DH. Review: α1-antitrypsin deficiency associated liver disease. J Gastroenterol Hepatol. 1997;12:404–16.
15. Kartner N, Augustinas O, Jensen TJ, Naismith AL, Riordan JR. Mislocalization of ΔF508 CFTR in cystic fibrosis sweat gland. Nature Genet. 1992;1:321–7.
16. Ali R, Perfumo S, della Rocca C, Amicone L, Pozzi L, McCullagh P et al. Evaluation of a transgenic mouse model for alpha-1-antitrypsin (AAT) related liver disease. Ann Hum Genet. 1994;58:305–20.
17. Dycaico MJ, Grant SG, Felts K, Nichols WS, Geller SA, Hager JH et al. Neonatal hepatitis induced by alpha-1-antitrypsin: a transgenic mouse model. Science. 1988;242:1409–12.
18. Geller SA, Nichols WS, Dycaico MJ, Felts KA, Sorge JA. Histopathology of alpha-1-antitrypsin liver disease in a transgenic mouse model. Hepatology. 1990;121:40–7.
19. Mondelli M, Mieli-Vergani G, Eddleston ALWF, Williams R, Mowat AP. Lymphocyte cytotoxicity to autologous hepatocytes in alpha-1-antitrypsin deficiency. Gut. 1984;25:1044–9.
20. Lobo-Yeo A, Senaldi G, Portmann R, Mowat AP, Mieli-Vergani G, Vergani D. Class I and class II major histocompatibility complex antigen expression on hepatocytes: A study in children with liver disease. Hepatology. 1990;12:224–32.
21. Povey S. Genetics of α1-antitrypsin deficiency in relation to neonatal liver disease. Mol Biol Med. 1990;7:161–2.
22. Sveger T. Liver disease in α1-antitrypsin deficiency detected by screening of 200 000 infants. N Engl J Med. 1976;294:1316–21.
23. Sveger T, Eriksson S. The liver in adolescents with α1-antitrypsin deficiency. Hepatology. 1995;22:514–17.
24. Qu D, Teckman J, Omura S, Perlmutter DH. Degradation of a mutant secretory protein, α_1-antitrypsin Z, in the endoplasmic reticulum requires proteasome activity. J Biol Chem. 1996;271:22791–5.
25. Teckman J, Perlmutter DH. The role of ubiquitin in the proteasomal degradation of mutant α1-antitrypsin Z in the endoplasmic reticulum. Am J Physiology (in press).
26. Labrune P, Odievre M, Alagille D. Influence of sex and breastfeeding on liver disease in alpha-1-antitrypsin deficiency. Hepatology. 1989;10:122.
27. Propst T, Propst A, Dietze O, Judmaier G, Braunsteiner H, Vogal W. High prevalence of viral infections in adults with homozygous and heterozygous α1-antitrypsin deficiency and chronic liver disease. Ann Intern Med. 1992;117:641–5.
28. Qizilbash A, Young-Pong O. Alpha-1-antitrypsin liver disease differential diagnosis of PAS-positive, diastase-resistant globules in liver cells. Am J Clin Pathol. 1983;79:697–702.

25
Alpha-1-antitrypsin deficiency: natural course and therapeutic strategies

S. ERIKSSON

INTRODUCTION

The major clinical correlates in α_1-antitrypsin deficiency (AAT-D) are emphysema, chronic liver disease (CLD) and vasculitic disorders[1]. AAT-D is a prevalent genetic disorder among Caucasians of European descent. Classical severe AAT-D, PiZZ is present in 0.06% of Scandinavians and heterozygous, intermediate AAT-D in 5% of these populations. However, the condition seems to be widely underdiagnosed. Even in countries with relatively high detection rates such as Sweden and Denmark, only 20–25% of homozygous PiZZ individuals have been diagnosed. The failure to diagnose AAT-D may be explained in several ways; it is a relatively new entity, the phenotypic expression is variable and an unknown proportion, perhaps 25–30%, live a completely normal life span. The large number of undiagnosed individuals and severe ascertainment bias contributes to difficulties in defining the natural history. The neonatal screening for AAT-D undertaken in Sweden from 1972 to 1974 and the prospective follow-up of the AAT-D children dramatically improved our understanding of the early onset liver disease (LD) in AAT-D[2]. The prospective studies of the 125 Swedish PiZZ newborns identified by screening 200 000 neonates provide an estimate for risk of liver disease. A majority of these individuals had abnormal liver function tests (LFT) that tended to normalize with increasing age, only 15% developed clinically overt neonatal disease. Of these at least two-thirds recovered from liver damage. Up to age 20 only 3% of all PiZZ children developed cirrhosis[3]. The continued long-term follow-up of the Swedish cohort will finally define the natural history of AAT-D. Today, however, very limited and non-biased information concerning the final outcome in AAT-D is available. Most published series are hospital-based and dominated by lung cases (referred to as index cases). Never-smokers are generally under-represented, resulting in an over-representation of fatalities caused by respiratory insufficiency. In an attempt to improve knowledge of the natural history we analysed the cause of death in AAT-D in a defined population (the City of Malmö, Sweden) characterized by both high detection and autopsy rates.

NATURAL COURSE

Cause of death in AAT-D

In our recent retrospective study of cause of death in all fatalities due to AAT-D (only PiZZ) in the City of Malmö from 1962 to 1997, 41 cases were identified. Autopsy was performed in 37 cases (88%). The male/female ratio was 20/21; 44% were never-smokers. Notes from all relevant clinics, autopsy protocols and death certificates were scrutinized to establish the main and contributory causes of death in each individual case. Records were also analysed with respect to incidence of other diseases such as hypertension, diabetes, myocardial infarction and other atherosclerotic manifestations.

The Malmö AAT-D cohort is unique from several points of view. It represents an effort to systematically trace and register all patients with a diagnosis of severe AAT-D, PiZZ, in one defined population of close to a quarter of a million (mean 242 000), and also follow up these with well standardized autopsies. The expected number of PiZZ-cases can be estimated at 58 (96 600/1700). Of these 58, 41 cases (40 adults and one child), or 70% of all cases, had been medically recognized. The figures are based on the well-established PiZZ-frequency of 1/1700 in the adult Swedish population[1] and on the total number of deaths during the 35 year study period (1962–97). The high detection and autopsy rates (70 and 88% respectively) and a complete access to medical records makes the cohort, although small, the best available at present for estimates of the natural history and final outcome in AAT-D. The cohort included only one child (2.5%) who died from cirrhosis at an early age. This figure is in agreement with data from the prospective Swedish series[3], indicating that the early prognosis in AAT-D-related neonatal hepatitis is more favourable than previously reported.

Mean age at death in the series as a whole was 63 years, a modestly reduced survival rate when compared to the background non-Pi-Z population. However, there was, as expected and in agreement with many previous studies[4,5], a marked survival disadvantage in ex-smokers, 56 years, as compared to never-smokers, 73 years ($p < 0.01$) (Fig. 1).

Liver disease

The most impressive finding was the predominant role of cirrhosis-related mortality, especially in the elderly never-smokers (Fig. 1). Cirrhosis and its complications was the main cause of death in 12/41 and occurred in 14/41, but in only 2/23 smokers as compared to 12/17 never-smokers ($p < 0.001$). Hepatocellular carcinoma occurred in five cirrhotic livers but was not seen in any non-cirrhotic liver. In five of 14 cases of cirrhosis the diagnosis had not been suspected *intra vitam* but was based on autopsy findings. Hepatitis B and C markers had been analysed in the majority of cirrhotic cases but were negative in all. Table 1

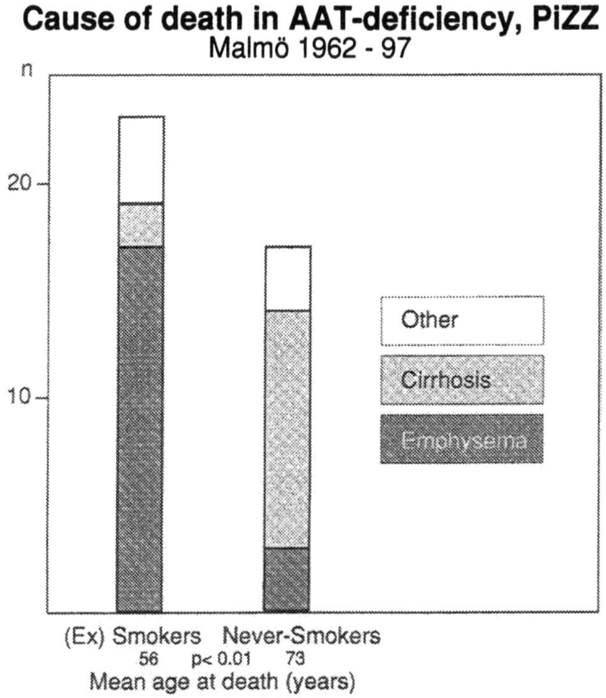

Figure 1 Cause of death in AAT deficiency.

Table 1 Liver histopathology at autopsy in 37 PiZZ cases

	Smokers (22)	*Never-smokers (15)*	*All (37)*
Cirrhosis	2* $p < 0.001$	11**	13
Hepatocellular carcinoma	0	5	5
Fibrosis	4	0	4
Steatosis	3	3	6
Normal	14	3	17

* In one case alcohol + hemochromatosis
Hepatitis B and C markers absent
** Severe, refractory encephalopathy in two.

summarizes the histopathological findings at autopsy (n = 37). In addition to cirrhosis and HCC, fibrosis and severe steatosis were frequent findings.

It is obvious that the incidence of cirrhosis in AAT-D has been underestimated. The figure of 5% mentioned in a recent WHO-report[6] is much too low. It seems realistic to estimate the total risk at 30–40%, in agreement with previous Swedish studies[7]. It is evident that cirrhosis should be regarded as a complication of greater age, predominantly occurring in those AAT-deficient individuals who have not smoked, and have therefore survived without developing severe emphysema. Cirrhosis in AAT-deficiency may occur at any age but it is important to realise that the peak incidence is to be expected in the elderly never-smoker.

Other diseases

Multisystemic vasculitis and/or nephropathy

No case of vasculitic disease but two cases of nephropathy were observed. One was a male who died from complications of a bleeding duodenal ulcer, an interstitial nephropathy with accumulation of PAS-positive material, possibly PiZ-protein in tubular cells. The other was a female dying from haemorrhagic pneumonia where a glomerulopathy was found.

Aneurysmal disease

No case of aneurysmal disease (abdominal aorta or intracerebral) was observed.

Pancreatic endocrine tumours

Two cases of pancreatic endocrine tumours, one benign and one malignant, were noted.

Diabetes and atherosclerotic diseases

In the series as a whole there was a notable absence of diabetes, hypertension and atherosclerotic complications.

The association between the presence of the PiZ-allele and c-ANCA positive vasculitic disorders has been repeatedly documented[8]. The absence of vasculitic cases in the present cohort does not argue against this concept, but merely stresses the rarity of such an association in homozygous AAT-D[9]. The same holds true for both aortic abdominal and intracranial aneurysms[10].

The association between AAT-D and pancreatic endocrine tumours has not previously been reported. Considering the rarity of such tumours the appearance of two such cases in the Malmö cohort seems less likely to be a matter of chance, but more probably related to pancreatic islet cell hyperplasia. Islet cell hyperplasia, first described in 1983 by Ray et al.[11], is a universal feature of AAT-D. An accumulation of aggregated Z-AAT in islet cells may provoke a sequential development of hyperplasia → benign → malignant tumours. The function of hyperplastic islets in AAT-D deserves further study. One may speculate that islet cell hyperplasia confers a metabolic advantage. This explains the apparent low incidence of diabetes, hypertension and atherosclerotic complications in this condition.

Risk of liver disease in AAT-D (PiMZ, PiSZ) heterozygotes

Heterozygous carriers of a single dose of the mutant PiZ-gene are common, close to 5%, in Europe. Their relative risk of developing CLD has been controversial. Most investigators have analysed hospital-based cohorts and results may be influenced by assignment bias. Only one prospective population-based study has been published[12]. Among 25 000 Italian newborns, IEF identified 833 PiMZ children (3.3%). A mainly self-limiting subclinical liver involvement was present in 20% of these children. The results of a long-term follow-up are awaited with interest.

As expected, PAS-D-positive inclusion bodies are less abundant in biopsies from heterozygotes than from homozygotes, indicating a less pronounced formation of hepatotoxic Z-polymers. The presence of additional factors such as chronic viral infections may therefore be necessary to provoke liver disease in heterozygotes. A large Austrian study suggested that CLD in patients with heterozygous deficiency might be associated with a high prevalence of HBV or HCV infection. The infection rather than the deficiency alone was suggested to be the cause of liver disease[13]. PiZ homozygosity does not seem to be associated with an increased prevalence of viral infection[14,15].

Another recent analysis provided further evidence of an association of heterozygous PiZ AAT deficiency with end stage liver disease of several aetiologies, but not HCV infection alone[16]. These authors concluded that the association with some types of CLD (i.e. HCV and alcohol liver disease) but not others (i.e. autoimmune hepatitis) supports the concept that exaggeration of the retention of AAT may be the pathogenetic mechanism involved.

The risk of end-stage LD in heterozygotes can be roughly estimated by using recently published data from the Mayo Clinic[17], where 14 homozygotes had been transplanted between 1985 and 1995. The heterozygote prevalence in the referral population is 3%. According to Hardy–Weinberg's law, the homozygote prevalence is 1/4000. In other words, heterozygotes are 120 times more frequent than homozygotes. Had the risk of end-stage LD been identical in hetero- and homozygotes, $14 \times 120 = 1680$ heterozygotes would have been referred. The actual figure was 50. In this population the risk of developing end-stage LD is thus

$$\frac{50 \times 100\%}{1680} = 3\%,$$

i.e. less than $^{1}/_{10}$th of the risk in homozygotes.

Liver carcinoma in AAT-D

Repeated autopsy-based studies in PiZ homozygotes have clearly demonstrated a propensity to malignant transformation in AAT deficiency-related cirrhosis[7,15,18]. Hepatocellular carcinoma (HCC) has been documented at autopsy in approximately one-third of cirrhotic livers. Cholangiocarcinoma has been seen only in a minority of these cases[7]. The high incidence of malignant transformation in the Swedish PiZ-homozygotes seems to be independent of such risk factors as alcoholism or chronic viral (B and/or C) infection and has been regarded as a consequence of the cirrhosis per se, combined with the putative carcinogenic effect of retained mutant Z-AAT in liver cells. The pivotal role of aggregated Z AAT is underlined by findings in the Z-AAT-transgenic mouse, an important model of human malignancy. These high copy lineage mice have shown a sequential development of PAS-positive inclusions, chronic hepatitis, preneoplastic nodules and, finally, HCC[19]. Although the underlying molecular alterations are unknown, it seems possible that retained Z AAT even in the heterozygous PiZ carrier may have a carcinogenic effect. In fact, early Swedish[20] and more recent Austrian[21] and American[16,17] studies underline the propensity of PiZ heterozygotes to develop both cirrhosis and HCC. The role of coincidental chronic viral infections in this setting, however, requires further study. Interestingly, viral markers were absent in the majority of 13 PiZ-positive (by a PiZ-specific monoclonal antibody) German patients with primary liver carcinoma, appearing in non-cirrhotic liver tissue and demonstrating a considerable morphological heterogeneity[22].

THERAPEUTIC STRATEGIES

Population-based screening for AAT-D

Advice against smoking in order to retard emphysema development is at present the only preventive measure likely to prolong survival in AAT-D patients. Early detection of AAT-D, before definite smoking habits have been established, is essential. It is imperative that all first-degree relatives be screened, particularly siblings.

Although AAT-D belongs to the group of genetic conditions where population-based screening is motivated, it is important to realise that the inherited trait per se is not an overt disease, but rather a disease susceptibility. An unknown proportion, perhaps 25–30%, mainly non-smoking AAT-deficient individuals, can probably live a normal life-span. The propensity for cigarette smokers to develop premature emphysema is the predominant clinical problem. Except for organ transplantation there is no effective treatment for either established emphysema or liver disease. Consequently, primary prevention by non-smoking is an excellent and effective therapeutic alternative. Given the relatively modest results of anti-smoking advice in the Swedish prospective study, considering the adverse psychosocial reactions described[23] and the general recommendation that screening should be undertaken as close as possible to the age when prevention may be realistic, screening ages other than the neonatal have to be considered. If general screening for AAT-D is to be resumed, it may be recommended to focus on adolescents aged 12–15 years, i.e. before definite smoking habits have been established. The programme should be based on voluntariness, confidentiality and informed consent[23]. Screening for AAT-D in adolescents could easily be combined with DNA-based voluntary screening for other frequent, inherited conditions like hemochromatosis, familial hypercholesterolemia and Factor V deficiency, all traits where the clinical expression could be modified by early preventive measures. Such a programme, however, demands a screening organization, guarantees for future medical surveillance and psychological support and clear rules concerning insurance coverage of affected individuals. In any population-based screening program including AAT-D, not only the PiZ-allele frequency, but also the smoking frequency must be considered, when estimating the cost—benefit ratio.

Targeted screening for AAT-D

A targeted testing programme can bring many AAT-deficient individuals to medical attention. The World Health Organization (WHO) has recommended that all patients with COPD and adolescents with asthma be tested for AAT-D.

The WHO recommendations also include patients with chronic liver disease[6], at any age. It is obvious that testing should also be performed in patients with PR-3 positive vasculitic syndromes[8].

Specific therapy

Replacement therapy with infusions of purified human AAT has been used in emphysema patients to raise plasma levels and retard rapid emphysema progress. Although no strictly randomized trials are yet available both European and American data[24,25] suggest that a subgroup of patients with modestly severe emphysema may benefit from such treatment. There is no evidence that such therapy is of any value in AAT-related liver disease.

Gene therapy has a great future potential but is not at present a feasible alternative in AAT-D. Zern et al.[26] recently reported on a dual approach to the two predominant pathophysiological problems. Using a Simian virus-40 based vector and specific ribozymes they managed not only to achieve an effective expression of the normal gene, but also to suppress the expression of the Z-protein. This dual approach thus has the potential to prevent both lung and liver disease.

Transplantation is the last resort in end-stage lung disease in AAT-D. Notably, there may be an increased risk of hepatocellular carcinoma following immune-suppressive therapy in lung-transplanted AAT-deficient recipients.

Most AAT-D patients are seen in chest clinics, where a regular assessment of liver function by simple tests (aminotransferases, GT and alkaline phosphates) should be performed, at least on the elderly. Even modest elevations of enzymes should alert the physician to exclude concomitant hemochromatosis, autoimmunity and/or chronic viral infection in these patients. Liver biopsy is only indicated for staging of liver disease. Ultrasonography is a preferable form of surveillance when cirrhosis and its complications, including malignant transformation, are suspected.

In end-stage liver disease orthotopic liver transplantation provides a new source of plasma AAT. The recipient assumes the donor's phenotype and plasma level. The indications for transplantation are essentially those for end-stage liver disease of any type. AAT-D is the most frequent genetic cause of liver disease in childhood and is the most common metabolic error for which liver transplantation is indicated. In children dismal prognostic factors include severity of jaundice, LFT abnormalities, histopathology and in some reports male sex. Five years' survival approaches 90%[27,28]. The majority of transplanted adult AAT-deficient patients are heterozygotes with cirrhosis and portal hypertension[16,17,29].

Prevention of AAT aggregation in hepatocytes

Any factor that increases the net balance of abnormally aggregated Z AAT in the ER would theoretically predispose an accentuated liver cell injury and vice versa. During episodes of inflammation and fever, the formation of Z-polymers is likely to overwhelm the capacity of the degradative pathway, thereby promoting hepatocellular damage. Bouts of pyrexia should be prevented[30].

In vitro, the polymerization rate of PiZ AAT is also markedly stimulated by hydrophobic bile acids, such as lithocholic and 3β-hydroxy-5-cholenoic acids, both monohydroxy acids with hepatotoxic and cholestatic properties. An excessive formation of such acids during fetal life via the cholesterol 27-hydroxylase pathway may therefore contribute to the development of neonatal hepatitis in AAT deficiency[31]. In this setting, ursodeoxycholic treatment may be of benefit.

The proteasome inhibitor lactacystin prevents intracellular degradation of Z AAT in transfected hamster ovary (CHO) cells. The inhibition is associated with a partial restoration of vesicular transport. Altering the fate of a mutant protein may thus be an option in the treatment of diseases associated with misfolded proteins[32]. Butyric acid derivates such as 4-phenyl-butyrate affect glycosylation and transport in the ER. It has been used in cystic fibrosis patients to normalize trafficking of the cystic fibrosis transmembrane conductane regulator resulting in normalisation of chloride transport[33]. In CHO models it seems to diminish intracellular accumulation and increase vesicular transport (Brantly, personal communication).

Rapid progress in the understanding of the polymerization and transport processes in AAT-D opens exciting possibilities for rational drug design to block the protein–protein interaction and polymer formation and thus to prevent both lung and liver disease.

ACKNOWLEDGEMENTS

Supported by grants from the Swedish Heart and Lung Foundation.

REFERENCES

1. Eriksson S, Elzouki A-N. α_1-Antitrypsin deficiency. In: Powell LW, ed. Baillière's Clinical Gastroenterology. International Practice and Research: Hereditary Diseases of the Liver. Baillière Tindall, 1998;12:257–73.
2. Sveger T. The natural history of liver disease in α_1-antitrypsin deficient children. Acta Paediatr Scand. 1988;2:847–51.
3. Sveger T, Eriksson S. The liver in adolescents with α_1-antitrypsin deficiency. Hepatology. 1995;22:514–17.
4. Larsson C. Natural history and life expectancy in severe alpha 1-antitrypsin deficiency, PiZ. Acta Med Scand. 1978;204:345–51.
5. Seersholm N, Kok-Jensen A, Dirksen A. Survival of patients with severe alpha 1-antitrypsin deficiency with special reference to non-index cases. Thorax. 1994;49:695–8.
6. Stoller JK, Dodge JA, Boulyjenkov V et al. α_1-Antitrypsin deficiency: memorandum from a WHO-meeting. Bull WHO. 1997;75:397–415.
7. Eriksson S. α_1-Antitrypsin deficiency in liver cirrhosis in adults. Acta Med Scand. 1987;221:461–7.
8. Esnault VLM, Audrain MAP, Sesbüe R. Alpha-1-antitrypsin phenotyping in ANCA-associated diseases: one of several arguments for protease/antiprotease imbalance in systemic vasculitis. Exp Clin Immunogenet. 1997;14:206–13.
9. Mazodier P, Elzouki A-N, Segelmark M, Eriksson S. Systemic necrotizing vasculitides in severe α_1-antitrypsin deficiency. Q J Med. 1996;89:599–611.
10. St. Jean P, Hart B, Webster M, Steed D, Adamson J, Powell J, Ferrell R. Alpha-1-antitrypsin deficiency in aneurysmal disease. Hum Hered. 1996;46:92–7.
11. Ray MB, Zumwalt R. Islet-cell hyperplasia in genetic deficiency of alpha-1-proteinase inhibitor. Am J Clin Pathol. 1986;85:681–7.
12. Pittschieler K. Heterozygotes and liver involvement. Acta Paediatr. 1994;83(Suppl 393):21–3.
13. Propst T, Propst A, Dietze O, Judmaier G, Braunsteiner H, Vogel W. High prevalence of viral infection in adults with homozygous and heterozygous alpha$_1$-antitrypsin deficiency and chronic liver disease. Ann Intern Med. 1992;117:641–5.

14. Qu D, Teckman JH, Perlmutter DH. α_1-Antitrypsin deficiency associated liver disease. J Gastroenterol Hepatol. 1997;12:404–16.
15. Elzouki A-N, Eriksson S. Risk of hepatobiliary disease in adults with severe α_1-antitrypsin deficiency (PiZZ); is chronic viral hepatitis B or C an additional risk factor for cirrhosis and hepatocellular carcinoma? Eur J Gastroenterol Hepatol. 1996;8:989–94.
16. Eigenbrodt ML, McCashland TM, Dy RM, Clark JC, Galati J. Heterozygous α_1-antitrypsin phenotypes in patients with end stage liver disease. Am J Gastroenterol. 1997;92:602–6.
17. Graziadei IW, Joseph JJ, Wiesner RH, Therneau TM, Batts KP, Porayko MK. Increased risk of chronic liver failure in adults with heterozygous α_1-antitrypsin deficiency. Hepatology. 1998;28:1058–63.
18. Eriksson S, Carlson J, Velez R. Risk of cirrhosis and hepatocellular carcinoma in alpha$_1$-antitrypsin deficiency. N Engl J Med. 1986;314:736–9.
19. Geller SA, Nichols WS, Kim S, Tolmachoff T, Lee S, Dycaico MJ et al. Hepatocarcinogenesis is the sequel to hepatitis in Z#2 α_1-antitrypsin transgenic mice: histopathological and DNA ploidy studies. Hepatology. 1994;19:389–97.
20. Carlson J, Eriksson S. Chronic 'cryptogenic' liver disease and malignant hepatoma in intermediate α_1-antitrypsin deficiency identified by a PiZ specific monoclonal antibody. Scand J Gastroenterol. 1985;20:835–42.
21. Propst T, Propst A, Dietze O, Judmaier G, Braunsteiner H, Vogel W. Prevalence of hepatocellular carcinoma in alpha-1-antitrypsin deficiency. J Hepatol. 1994;21:1006–11.
22. Zhou H, Fischer H-P. Liver carcinoma in PiZ alpha-1-antitrypsin deficiency. Am J Surg Pathol. 1998;22:742–8.
23. Thelin T, Sveger T, McNeil TF. Primary prevention in a high-risk group: smoking habits in adolescents with homozygous alpha-1-antitrypsin deficiency. Acta Paediatr. 1996;85:1207–12.
24. Seersholm N, Wencker M, Banik N, Viskum K, Dirksen A, Kok-Jensen A, Konietzko N. Does α_1-antitrypsin augmentation therapy slow the annual decline in FEV_1 in patients with severe hereditary α_1-antitrypsin deficiency? Eur Respir J. 1997;10:2260–3.
25. The Alpha-1-Antitrypsin Deficiency Registry Study Group. Survival and FEV_1 decline in individuals with severe deficiency of α_1-antitrypsin. Am J Respir Crit Care Med. 1998;158:49–59.
26. Zern MA, Ozaki I, Duan L, Pomerantz R, Liu S-L, Strayer DS. A novel SV40-based vector successfully transduces and expresses an alpha 1-antitrypsin ribozyme in a human hepatoma-derived cell line. Gene Ther. 1999;6:114–20.
27. Filipponi F, Soubrane O, Labrousse F, Devictor D, Bernard O, Valayer J, Houssin D. Liver transplantation for end-stage liver disease associated with alpha-1-antitrypsin deficiency in children: pretransplant natural history, timing and results of transplantation. J Hepatol. 1994;20:72–8.
28. Esquivel CO, Vincente D, Van Thiel D, Gordon R, Marsh W, Makowka L et al. Orthotopic liver transplantation for alpha-1-antitrypsin deficiency: an experience in 29 children and ten adults. Transplant Proc. 1987;19:3798–802.
29. Vennarecci G, Gunson BK, Ismail T, Hübscher G, Kelly DA, McMaster P et al. Transplantation for end stage liver disease related to alpha 1 antitrypsin. Transplantation. 1996;61:1488–95.
30. Lomas DA, Evans DLI, Finch JT, Carrell RW. The mechanism of Z α_1-antitrypsin accumulation in the liver. Nature. 1992;357:605–7.
31. Gerbod MC, Janciauskiene S, Jeppsson J-O, Eriksson S. The in vitro effect of lithocholic acid on the polymerization properties of PiZ alpha-1-antitrypsin. Arch Biochem Biophys. 1998;351:167–74.
32. Novoradovskaya N, Lee JH, Yu Z-X, Ferrans VJ, Brantly M. Inhibition of intracellular degradation increases secretion of a mutant form of α_1-antitrypsin associated with profound deficiency. J Clin Invest. 1998;101:2693–701.
33. Rubenstein RC, Zeitlin PL. A pilot clinical trial of oral sodium 4-phenylbutyrate (buphenyl) in ΔF508-homozygous cystic fibrosis patients. Partial restoration of nasal epithelial CFTR function. Am J Respir Crit Care Med. 1998;157:484–90.

26
The porphyrias: pathogenesis and diagnosis

U. GROSS and M. O. DOSS

INTRODUCTION

Porphyrias are metabolic diseases which develop out of either inherited or acquired disturbance of haem biosynthesis (Table 1). They are characterized by an overproduction of haem precursors in liver and bone marrow. Thus, porphyrias are differentiated into hepatic and erythropoietic, depending on the main site of expression of the enzymatic defect. Eight enzymes are involved in haem biosynthesis. With exception of δ-aminolevulinic acid (ALA) synthase, the first

Table 1 Hereditary enzyme defects in the haem biosynthetic pathway as determinants of porphyrias

Enzymes	*Metabolites*	*Porphyrias*
	Glycine + Succinyl-CoA	
δ-Aminolevulinic acid synthase	↓	Sideroblastic anaemia
	δ-Aminolevulinic acid	
Porphobilinogen synthase*	↓	Doss porphyria**
	Porphobilinogen	
Porphobilinogen deaminase	↓	Acute intermittent porphyria**
	Hydroxymethylbilane	
Uroporphyrinogen III synthase	↓	Morbus Günther
	Uroporphyrinogen	
Uroporphyrinogen decarboxylase	↓	Porphyria cutanea tarda
	Coproporphyrinogen	
Coproporphyrinogen oxidase	↓	Hereditary coproporphyria**
	Protoporphyrinogen	
Protoporphyrinogen oxidase	↓	Porphyria variegata**
	Protoporphyrin	
Ferrochelatase	↓	Erythropoietic protoporphyria
	Haem	

* Synonym: δ-Aminolevulinic acid dehydratase
** Acute hepatic porphyrias

enzyme with rate-limiting function, each sequence of haem biosynthesis correlates with a specific form of porphyria.

Hepatic porphyrias are differentiated into acute and non-acute (chronic) types. On principle, porphyrias are characterized by a specific enzyme deficiency which has been recognized at all seven steps of the haem biosynthetic pathway, from porphobilinogen (PBG) synthase (ALA dehydratase) up to ferrochelatase. Primary enzyme defects represent partial deficiencies, because a complete enzyme deficiency along the haem pathway is not compatible with life; however, an inherited enzyme defect in the homozygous state may, under rare conditions, approach a nearly total deficiency as has been observed in Morbus Günther and ALA dehydratase defect porphyria[1].

CLASSIFICATION AND ENZYME DEFICIENCIES

Acute porphyrias are classified as acute intermittent porphyria (AIP), variegate porphyria, hereditary coproporphyria and an acute porphyria with PBG synthase deficiency[1–4]. Lead poisoning is regarded as an acute toxic or toxogenetic erythrohepatic porphyria[2]. Acute hepatic porphyrias develop an analogous intermittent acute clinical syndrome with abdominal-neurological-mental and cardiovascular symptoms in all four types[1,2,4]. In addition, skin symptoms can occur in variegate porphyria (VP) and hereditary coproporphyria (HCP), but are observed in only about one-third of clinically overt cases in Middle Europe.

On the basis of an analogous clinical acute syndrome in all four types of acute porphyrias, these porphyrias can be rationally classified by relating their specific enzyme deficiency in the haem biosynthetic chain: type 1, PBG synthase deficiency; type 2, PBG deaminase (hydroxymethylbilane synthase); type 3, coproporphyrinogen oxidase; and type 4, protoporphyrinogen oxidase deficiency. About 85% of acute porphyrias are associated with the classical acute intermittent porphyria with PBG deaminase deficiency (Table 2). With the exception of the PBG synthase-deficient porphyria, acute hepatic porphyrias result from an autosomal dominant genetic trait.

Exceptional homozygous states of autosomal dominant acute hepatic porphyrias were observed in AIP, in HCP[5], in a special mutant of HCP designated as harderoporphyria[6,7], and also in VP[8,9]. A previously unrecognized form of porphyria has

Table 2 Prevalence

Porphyria cutanea tarda (1 : 25 000)
Acute intermittent porphyria (1 : 50 000)
Protoporphyria (1 : 100 000)
Porphyria variegata
Hereditary coproporphyria
Congenital erythropoietic porphyria (Günther's disease)
Hepatoerythropoietic porphyria
ALAD deficiency porphyria (Doss porphyria)

been identified in a large family in Chester in the UK; it is characterized by dual enzyme deficiency with reduced activity of both uroporphyrinogen synthase and protoporphyrinogen oxidase[10]. Co-existent VP and porphyria cutanea tarda (PCT) have been reported from Cape Town[11]: about 40% of patients with this dual porphyria suffered from acute symptoms of variegata. This dual porphyria was also observed in patients from Germany and India[12]. A new dual porphyria with the combination of AIP and PCT was described by the author[13].

DIAGNOSTIC STRATEGY IN PORPHYRINOLOGY

Diagnosis of overt porphyria requires metabolite studies. Enzyme tests, both in AIP and PCT (PBG deaminase and uroporphyrinogen decarboxylase), do not establish that the actual clinical findings are due to an acute or chronic hepatic porphyria. The enzyme deficiency itself is not the factor causing illness: decreased enzyme activity reflects only that the patient carries an enzyme mutation. As clinical experience shows, only in a minority of genetically affected family members does the mutation lead to disease expression. This holds for genetically affected family members in AIP, HCP, and VP as well as in PCT and erythropoietic protoporphyria (EPP). In establishing the diagnosis of porphyria under clinical circumstances one has to start with metabolite studies: urinary porphyrin precursors and porphyrins if an acute porphyria syndrome is suspected, urinary porphyrins if PCT is suspected, and blood porphyrins if EPP is suspected. In PCT red cell uroporphyrinogen decarboxylase studies should follow to differentiate between hereditary and non-hereditary forms.

For the acute porphyrias, there is little doubt that in the future DNA analysis will be the method of choice to detect presymptomatic carriers, and consequently to improve the prevention of the acute clinical expression of these porphyrias[14].

ACUTE INTERMITTENT PORPHYRIA

Molecular genetics of acute intermittent porphyria

AIP is an autosomal dominant disorder resulting from a partial deficiency of PBG deaminase (E.C. 4.3.1.8) activity. In AIP more than 130 different mutations have been identified to date[15]; more than half of these are single-base substitutions and a quarter of them consist of small insertions or deletions[16]. A one-base-pair insertion in exon 14 of the PBG deaminase gene of a native North American family with AIP was observed. This mutation shifts the reading frame of mRNA and generates a premature stop codon[17]. Founder effects of single mutations from selected geographic areas have been reported[18–20].

Steady-state mRNA levels of the PBG deaminase gene were analysed in eight patients with AIP. The levels of the mutant transcripts showed large variations independent of the CRIM class, the location of the mutation or the clinical phenotype[21]. The molecular pathogenesis and laboratory diagnosis by molecular methods in AIP has been discussed extensively by Petersen et al.[22].

An association between AIP and hepatocellular carcinoma was reported. However, the PBG deaminase gene does not function as a tumour suppressor gene. Intrinsic aberrations in AIP, including reduced haem synthesis and endogenous oxidative damage to DNA, may incite carcinogenic mutations in the genome of liver cell[23].

The non-erythroid subtype of AIP

The PBG deaminase gene shows that two different isoenzymes may be coded by a single gene. Such a single gene with two different promotors produces two different mRNAs, which differ in their 5′ end[24]. With respect to PBG deaminase activity in erythrocytes three different groups can be distinguished. In Germany 87% of the observed gene carriers with AIP show a lowered PBG deaminase activity, 8% exhibit an activity within an intermediate range and 5% have a normal activity in erythrocytes[25]. The subtype of AIP with normal PBG deaminase activity in the erythrocytes was first described in Finland[26].

The variant of AIP in which patients have normal erythroid activity, but half-normal activity of the housekeeping isoenzyme, resulted from three different splicing defects located in the intron 1 donor splice site. The mutations entailed in the activation of a cryptic splice site 67 bp downstream in intron 1, leading to a frameshift and a premature stop codon in exon 4[27].

An animal model for acute porphyria

Studies of the pathogenesis of porphyric neuropathy have been hampered by lack of an experimental model. Nowadays it can be studied in transgenic mice with a partial deficiency of PBG deaminase. These animals imitate acute porphyria through the induction of hepatic ALA synthase by drugs. They develop impairment of motor coordination and muscle weakness[28]. The data from PBG deaminase-deficient mice suggest that multiple mechanisms interact in causing the neurological symptoms: these are ALA interaction with GABA receptors, altered tryptophan metabolism, and haem depletion in nerve cells[29].

Molecular dysregulation and the disorder–disease process

Acute hepatic porphyrias (Table 1) are considered to be molecular regulatory diseases in contrast to non-acute, chronic hepatic porphyria, clinically appearing as porphyria cutanea tarda, which is always associated with liver injury[2]. Porphyrins do not accumulate in the liver in acute porphyrias, whereas in chronic hepatic porphyrias they do. Thus, chronic hepatic porphyria (i.e. PCT) is a porphyrin accumulation disease, comparable to congenital erythropoietic porphyria (CEP), whereas acute hepatic porphyrias are haem pathway dysregulation diseases, characterized in general by induction of the ALA synthase in the liver. More than 90% of all acute hepatic porphyrias are in the latent, subclinical phase; the essential diagnostic goal is the recognition of hepatic porphyria in the latent phase.

In the disorder–disease progression of AIP, four phases can be differentiated:

(1) The enzyme deficiency alone or the genetic phase;
(2) a compensated latent phase with slight to moderate increase of metabolite excretion, but without clinical symptoms;

Table 3 Acute hepatic porphyrias as pharmacogenetic diseases

Genetic factor in haem synthesis	*→ Drug action*	*→ Metabolic response*	*→ Clinical response*
Relative enzyme deficiency 'Regulatory' haem decreased	Induction of ALA synthase	Increase of ALA, PBG & porphyrins	Acute porphyria symptoms

(3) the decompensated latent phase with a remarkable increase of porphyrin precursor and porphyrin excretion;
(4) and the phase of the acute syndrome.

A relationship has been established between the extent of haem precursor excretion and acute symptoms and the probability of clinical precipitation[2]. Because in the first place drugs are disease-inducing factors, acute hepatic porphyrias are priorly classed as pharmacogenetic diseases (Table 3).

The enzyme deficiency (Table 1) itself is not the factor causing illness in acute hepatic porphyrias. Hereditary enzyme deficiencies lead to a destabilization of the haem control over hepatic ALA synthase (Table 4). ALA synthase is regulated by endogenous haem and glucose and can also be repressed by exogenous glucose and haem. A decrease of regulatory liver haem, for example by drugs, is followed by an induction of the initial enzyme. This mechanism is considered to be a counter-regulatory modulation compensating for the specific enzyme deficiency; by this means porphyrinogen synthesis should be maximized, providing sufficient hepatic haem biosynthesis. Furthermore, derepression of ALA synthase will be stimulated by high porphyrinogen substrate loss from

Table 4 Pathogenesis of hereditary acute hepatic porphyrias and the porphyria disease process

Mutation → hereditary gene defect →
Fault in enzyme biosynthesis →
Modified enzyme with lowered activity →
Destabilisation of haem control on ALA synthase →
Susceptible inductivity of the hepatic key enzyme by
Porphyrinogenic substances and/or conditions →
Induction of hepatic ALA synthase →
Metabolic expression →
Increase of ALA, PBG and porphyrins →
Secondary limiting function of PBG deaminase →
Induction of ALA synthase →
Excessive overproduction of haem precursors →
Clinical expression →
Abdominal-neurological-cardiovascular-psychiatric syndrome

hepatocytes[30]. After inducing ALA synthase, ALA and PBG will be overproduced, but their metabolic conversion into porphyrinogens is principally limited by the secondary controlling sequence of PBG deaminase[31]. This limiting function of hepatic PBG deaminase explains the simultaneous increase of porphyrin precursors (ALA and PBG) in all three types of dominant acute porphyrias in the acute clinical syndrome[2], although in coproporphyria and variegata a primary disturbance of PBG deaminase does not exist (Table 1). The limitation of haem synthesis by PBG deaminase under the compensatory pressure of metabolic counter-regulation seems to be the dominant molecular factor for the clinical expression of the acute porphyria disease condition[32,33]. By inducing ALA synthase, counter-regulation becomes a new pathogenic event. Enhanced porphyrinogen synthesis is then modulated by the limiting function of PBG deaminase. These dynamic features characterize acute porphyrias as molecular dysregulatory diseases. By means of glucose and/or haem compounds the induction of ALA synthase is reversed. Thus, this therapeutic approach can be called a regulatory treatment in contrast to the other known symptomatic measures.

Disease expression

In 100 acute porphyria patients the following triggering factors were noted: drugs and alcohol were factors in 54% of patients, followed in frequency by fasting and alcohol, premenstrual manifestation, oestrogens, anticonvulsant treatment, several infections and stress. In this context two issues in clinical porphyrinology demand examination: the pathogenesis of neuropsychiatric symptoms[34,35] and the wide individual variability in biochemical and clinical expression of porphyria disease, including unexplainable individual differences in porphyrinogenic response with regard to a similar enzyme deficiency[1–3]. Recently, acute porphyria has been considered as a condition of a permanent system overload of oxidative stress, with long-term effects on hepatic and renal tissue, and with instances of periodic overload of free radicals giving rise to acute neurological involvement[36]. Experimental studies argue in favour of ALA-triggered oxidative stress in the brain accompanied by iron metabolism alterations and GABAergic receptor damage, which may be implicated in the neuropsychiatric manifestations of the aforementioned porphyrias[37].

The clinical response includes a wide variety of symptoms and signs. Abdominal and extremity pain, paresthesias, constipation, tachycardia, peripheral neuropathy and mental confusion, dark urine and hypertension are the most frequent. Consequently this interdisciplinary clinical complexity can lead to the potential erroneous diagnoses shown in Table 5 and arranged according to their abdominal-neurological psychiatric and cardiovascular aspects.

Diagnostic approach

Diagnosis of the clinical stage of acute hepatic porphyrias depends on increase of urinary porphyrin precursors (ALA and PBG), as well as of urinary porphyrins, analysed by specific chromatographic procedures (thin-layer or high pressure liquid chromatography). For differential diagnoses faecal porphyrins should be investigated simultaneously. The diagnostic strategy for acute porphyrias can be established in four consecutive steps (Table 6).

Table 5 Acute hepatic porphyrias: possible erroneous diagnoses

Abdominal	*Neurologic-psychiatric*	*Cardiovascular*
Acute abdomen	Neurosis	Hypertonus
Ileus	Depression	Myocardial infarction
Pancreatitis	Psychosis, schizophrenia	Angina pectoris
Cholelithiasis, cholecystitis	Polyneuritis	Myocarditis
Appendicitis	Landry paralysis	Orthostatic dysregulation
Peritonitis	Guillain-Barré syndrome	Circulatory failure
Gastritis	Epilepsy	
Ulcus ventriculi, duodeni	Alcohol intoxication	
Nephrolithiasis	Apoplexy	
Pyelonephritis	Poliomyelitis	
Hepatitis	Lead intoxication	
Alcohol liver syndrome	Thallium intoxication	
Ulcerative colitis	Polyarthritis	
Crohn's disease	Arteritis temporalis	
Chilaiditi syndrome		
Familial mediterranean fever		
Periarteritis nodosa	Hyperthyreosis	
Tube pregnancy		
Adnexitis		
Mesenterial vein thrombosis		
Angina abdominalis		
Hyperlipidaemia		

Table 6 A four-step diagnostic strategy for acute hepatic porphyria

Step 1	Bedside screening – PBG & porphyrins – suspicion of acute hepatic porphyria Clinical conclusion: Omission of porphyrinogenic drugs and initiation of glucose infusions
Step 2	Porphobilinogen & porphyrins by chromatography – confirmation of the general diagnosis of acute porphyria
Step 3	Specific differentiation of urinary and fecal metabolites, PBG deaminase and PBG synthase in red cells – Type diagnosis of acute hepatic porphyrias: acute intermittent porphyria, porphyria variegata, hereditary coproporphyria and PBG synthase defect porphyria
Step 4	Family studies: metabolites, enzymes and mutations

For rapid bedside or laboratory screening of urinary metabolites the Hoesch test for PBG and a fluorescence test for porphyrins (adsorbed onto talc) are convenient. Total urinary porphyrins can also be approximately detected by use of second-derivative spectroscopy. Positive results in the qualitative tests for PBG and porphyrins are such certain signs of acute porphyria that clinical procedures may be started, such as omission of porphyrinogenic drugs[34,38] and glucose infusions[33]. The first diagnostic step, screening for PBG and for porphyrins, is followed by step two: specific determination of PBG and porphyrins by ion-exchange column chromatography. Positive results confirm the general diagnosis of acute hepatic porphyria (Table 6).

In step three, a specific chromatographic differentiation of urinary precursors, urinary and faecal porphyrins by ion-exchange, thin-layer and/or high-pressure liquid chromatography is necessary and should be completed by enzyme studies in red cells. The evaluation of these indices allows the special porphyria diagnosis for clinical and scientific requirements as well as for an individual-risk interpretation and prophylaxis. As a fourth step, family studies of enzyme deficiencies and mutations for the recognition of gene carriers and individuals in the latent phases are recommended.

The confirmation of an acute porphyria diagnosis by specific biochemical studies is necessary, and, last but not least, asking for a second opinion is essential in order to clarify observations of acute hepatic porphyria for differential diagnostic and clinical purposes. An acute porphyria syndrome is excluded by normal porphyrin precursor and porphyrin excretion. In cases with slight to moderate increase of urinary coproporphyrin, but with normal PBG and normal fecal porphyrin excretion, we are dealing with a secondary coproporphyrinuria[1,2], a disorder without clinical relevance concerning porphyrin metabolism (see Table 7). Metabolic borderline constellations of excretory parameters should be evaluated and interpreted by an experienced consiliarius.

The determination of the parameters compiled in Table 6 allows a differential diagnosis of acute hepatic porphyrias: ALA, PBG, uro- and coproporphyrin in urine, copro- and protoporphyrin in faeces; and protoporphyrin as well as the enzymes PBG synthase and PBG deaminase in red cells. During the acute syndrome the urinary findings in the three autosomal dominant porphyrias are very similar. Faecal coproporphyrin is increased in coproporphyria, and protoporphyrin in protoporphyria. Four different mutant classes were identified in Finnish families with AIP[39]. However, it must be stressed that enzyme investigations are not necessary for the diagnosis of acute porphyria in the clinical stage. Urinary and faecal metabolites are the fundamental markers and indicators of an overt porphyria and of both disease progression and disease improvement[2].

A special metabolite constellation is found in lead poisoning, which imitates that in inherited PBG synthase deficiency porphyria. Their differential diagnosis is based on the impossibility of reactivating the enzyme in the porphyria condition in the absence of increased lead levels.

The key question between clinical medicine and the biochemical consultant focuses on the differentiation between porphyrias, the clinical symptoms of which are related to porphyrin metabolism, and secondary, non-inherited, acquired, clinically asymptomatic coproporphyrinurias, which generally do not have immediate clinical significance[4] (Table 7).

Clinical findings

Clinical findings include gastrointestinal, neurological and cardiovascular symptoms[40,41,42]. Colicky abdominal pain, associated with vomiting and constipation

Table 7 Secondary, clinically, asymptomatic coproporphyrinurias (acquired) related to various exposures and different aetiologies

Intoxications
Alcoholism (acute and/or chronic); foreign and environmental chemicals such as hexachlorobenzene, polyhalogenated biphenyls, dioxins (TCDD), vinyl chloride, carbon tetrachloride, benzene, chloroform; heavy metals such as lead, arsenic, mercury, etc.; drugs
Liver diseases
e.g., cirrhosis, active chronic hepatitis, toxic and infectious hepatitis, fatty liver, alcohol liver syndromes, drug injury, cholestasis, cholangitis, biliary cirrhosis
Adverse effect of drugs
Analgesics, sedatives, hypnotics, anaesthetics, etc. and sex hormones
Haematological diseases
e.g., haemolytic, sideroachrestic, sideroblastic, aplastic anaemias; ineffective erythropoiesis (intramedullary haemolysis); pernicious anaemia; thalassaemia; leukaemia; erythroblastosis; iron deficiency anaemia
Diabetes mellitus
Malignancies
e.g., hepatocellular tumours, hepatic metastases, pancreatic carcinoma, lymphomatosis and other systemic diseases
Disturbance of iron metabolism
e.g., haemosiderosis, idiopathic and secondary haemochromatosis
Hereditary hyperbilirubinaemias
e.g., Dubin–Johnson syndrome, Rotor's syndrome
Infectious diseases
Mononucleosis, acute poliomyelitis
Pregnancy
Fasting
Bronze baby syndrome
Myocardial infarction
Erythropoietic protoporphyria with liver involvement

or diarrhoea is very common and the initial sign of an acute clinical crisis in most cases. Tachycardia is observed in about one-third of patients. Tachycardia is a very sensitive sign of the clinical activity of the disease process. Neurological symptoms, which follow the abdominal manifestations, are highly variable. Peripheral neuropathy is very common and leads to paresis in arms and legs. In cases of severe course the cranial nerves are involved leading to a bulbar paralysis and respiratory impairment. In the acute porphyria syndrome seizures can occur, especially in patients with hyponatraemia due to the Schwartz–Bartter syndrome (inappropriate antidiuretic hormone release). Early regulatory treatment of the acute symptomatic expression of AIP is the treatment of choice to avoid a complicated course. There is no general rule for the appearance and the disappearance of clinical symptoms. The course of the acute hepatic porphyria syndrome is highly variable in the unknown (previously not diagnosed) and known porphyria patients.

The precipitating factors are of endogenous and exogenous origin. They can be differentiated into five classes[1,43].

1. Inducers of non-specific ALA synthase in the liver. An overproduction of ALA makes the partially deficient and the secondary controlling function of PBG deaminase now rate limiting[31].
2. Endocrine factors, including the cyclical premenstrual exacerbations. Oestrogens and progesterones are able to induce porphyria. On the other hand, a beneficial effect of hormonal oral contraceptives has been observed by different groups and is recommended as a therapeutic measure[44].
3. Caloric intake. Fasting, often in combination with alcohol intake, is a very important precipitating factor. The beneficial aspect of the early consideration of the glucose effect and nutritional management is recommended[33,45].
4. Certain drugs and foreign chemicals have the potential to induce cytochrome P450. Depletion of the regulatory haem leads to induction of hepatic ALA synthase and the initiation of the porphyria disease process resulting in an exacerbation of the acute hepatic porphyria.
5. Stress in all its variable forms can lead to a manifestation of acute hepatic porphyria. This may result from infections, alcohol excess and surgery, intercurrent illness or social problems (e.g. stress of relatives, examinations etc).

It should be noted that in some porphyria patients not one but several factors can act cumulatively to cause manifestation of symptomatic acute porphyria[41].

Therapy

Treatment of acute porphyrias includes the omission of precipitating factors, symptomatic measures according to the drug lists[34,38] and regulatory treatment by glucose and/or haem[1,2,46,47] (Table 8). Both glucose and haem effects on the porphyrin pathway have a proven experimental basis in vivo and in vitro studies[1–3]. In patients with acute porphyria of all four types, the glucose effect by itself causes a significant decrease of between 50 and 90% in urinary ALA, PBG and porphyrin excretion[33]. This biochemical response is associated with the

Table 8 Therapy of acute clinical porphyria crisis

Prerequisite	
1.	Confirmation of diagnosis by urinary ALA and PBG excess
2.	Elimination of all precipitating factors
Regulatory treatment	
3.	High dose glucose (400 g/day per os or i.v.)
4.	Haem arginate (3 mg/kg/day i.v. for 4 days)
Symptomatic treatment	
5.	Pain: opiates
6.	Hypertension, tachycardia: beta-blockers (e.g. propranolol)
7.	Nausea, vomiting: chlorpromazine or other phenothiazines
8.	Psychosis: chlorpromazine or other phenothiazine
9.	Epilepsy: diazepam, check for hyponatraemia
10.	Hyponatraemia: saline infusion, fluid restriction if signs of inappropriate secretion of antidiuretic hormone
11.	Motor neuropathy: physiotherapy

clinical response when intravenous glucose is administered in the ascending phase of the acute porphyria manifestation.

Instability of haematin was reported as one of the possible reasons for the variable clinical experience that has dampened the initial enthusiasm[48]. Haem arginate, however, is a stable and safe haem preparation[46,49]. Its clinical importance was reported in a Falk workshop years ago[50] and in current investigations[51].

Besides glucose and haem, another therapeutic approach should be mentioned: the application of long-acting synthetic luteinizing hormone releasing hormone agonistic analogues (LHRH) in porphyric women who have clinical manifestations of acute porphyria in relation to their menses[52,53]. Three females with repeated premenstrual clinical expression of acute hepatic porphyria (acute intermittent porphyria and hereditary coproporphyria) were treated successfully with a hormonal oral contraceptive or other exogenous hormones to stabilize the latent, subclinical phase of the disease[44]. LHRH analogues cause menopause: thus only those patients in whom the application of hormonal oral contraceptives does not improve the metabolic status of porphyrin parameters and the clinical symptoms should be treated with LHRH analogues[46]. We recommend that the application of LHRH analogues should be restricted to patients not responding to hormonal oral contraceptives. Research has also been undertaken into certain synthetic haem analogues in which the central iron is replaced by another element. Tin-protoporphyrin, a potent inhibitor of haem degradation by inhibition of haem oxygenase[54], suppresses chemically induced hepatic porphyria; unlike haem derivatives, tin-protoporphyrin is neither degraded nor does it induce the activity of haem oxygenase[54]. These studies may have potential clinical implications for the future.

Haem therapy

Haem and glucose administration are specific forms of treatment of the acute clinical manifestation of acute hepatic porphyrias. Both forms of treatment are considered as a regulatory therapy suppressing the induced ALA synthase in the liver which results in a decrease of porphyrin precursor and porphyrin excretion. In a consensus statement on the treatment of acute porphyrias by Mustajoki et al.[55] it was proposed that haem therapy is much more effective than high-dose glucose. Haem has been used increasingly often for the acute porphyria crisis during the last 20 years[32,46,50]. During the last 15 years, new haem compounds, such as haem arginate and a lyophilized form of haematin, were introduced[46,49,51].

The dose of haem is usually 3 mg/kg daily infused into a large peripheral vein for 4 consecutive days. The course may be shorter if the patient responds quickly or longer if the acute syndrome persists for more than 4 days. Of the available haem preparations, haem arginate (Normosang®) has been extensively studied, and it has proved to be stable and safe in clinical use[51]. The adverse effects, thrombophlebitis and coagulation abnormalities, associated with haematin, have been rare and mild when using haem arginate[55]. The choice of specific treatment depends on the severity of the acute symptoms[55]. In patients with severe manifestations haem therapy should be started immediately on admission[51].

Future aspects concerning treatment

A new aspect of therapy of acute porphyria syndromes includes the use of metalloporphyrins in combination with haem arginate. Although the activity of hepatic haem oxygenase, the rate-controlling enzyme for haem breakdown, has not been measured in patients with acute porphyria, it seems likely that activity of this enzyme is decreased, or at best is in the low normal range, due to the inborn defect in endogenous haem synthesis. Although never shown directly in humans, there is no reason to doubt that intravenously administered haem gains access to liver cells and induces haem oxygenase. Such induction probably contributes to the brevity of the biochemical effects of haem in acute porphyria, in which the liver is the main source of overproduced ALA, PBG, and porphyrins[56].

Tin-protoporphyrin prolongs the biochemical remission produced by haem arginate in acute hepatic porphyria. These findings suggest that inhibition of haem oxygenase by tin-protoporphyrin prolongs the biochemical remission induced by haem arginate in porphyric crises[57]. Furthermore, reduction of ALA synthase by zinc-mesoporphyrin and haem occurred after induction of ALA synthase by exposure of liver cells to several chemicals. These results suggest that low doses of zinc-mesoporphyrin and haem, in combination, may be a useful treatment for patients with acute porphyria[58].

The acute porphyrias in relapse are commonly treated with intravenous haem infusion to decrease the activity of ALA synthase, normally the rate-controlling enzyme in haem biosynthesis. The biochemical effects of haem treatment are short-lived, probably due in part to haem-mediated induction of haem oxygenase, the rate-controlling enzyme for haem degradation. The ability of zinc-mesoporphyrin to supplement the reduction of ALA synthase mRNA by haem, in a process similar to that observed with haem alone, provides a rationale for further investigation of this compound for eventual use as a supplement to haem therapy of the acute porphyrias and perhaps other conditions in which haem may be of benefit[59].

COMPOUND HETEROZYGOUS ACUTE PORPHYRIAS

δ-Aminolevulinic acid dehydratase deficiency porphyria (ADP)

A total of four patients with this seldom porphyria have been described up to date. First ADP (Doss porphyria) was reported in two young Germans, not related to each other, who have an intermittent severe acute hepatic porphyria syndrome and an activity of δ-aminolevulinic acid dehydratase (ALAD) of about 1% of controls[60]. Since 15 years of age, both patients suffered from repeated abdominal–neurological crises with cardiovascular symptoms, persistent paresis and transient respiratory paralysis. Despite marked ALAD deficiency, there was no anaemia in either patient. Family studies demonstrated that ALAD deficiency was inherited as an autosomal recessive trait[61]. Cloning and expression of the defective genes of one patient demonstrated that the patient was heteroallelic for ALAD deficiency with two separate point mutations, one producing an inactive enzyme and the other producing an unstable enzyme[62]. ALAD activity in the

Table 9 Molecular defects in hereditary ADP

Patient	*German B*	*German H*	*Swedish*	*Belgian*
CRIM(+)	20%	33%	28%	30%
Mutation				
Allele 1	A274T	V153M	G133R	G133R, K59N
Allele 2	R240W	delTC	V275M	F12L

two German patients was <10% from 1977 to 1997. An acute crisis in each patient was successfully treated by infusion of glucose and haem arginate[63].

Immunological and molecular investigations have been carried out in all four patients with ADP. In all cases the mutations were CRIM(+). The ALAD concentration ranges from 20 to 30%, whereas the enzyme activity is between 1 and 8% (Table 9). The different mutations on each allele cause a different amino acid exchange in nearly all cases[64]. This is the consequence of the heteroallelic or compound heterozygous molecular defect.

Compound heterozygous hereditary coproporphyria

A 10-year-old girl presented with skin symptoms of easy fragility, scars on hands and feet, and local reddening. Faecal coproporphyrin in the patient, the mother and the father were 76-, 7- and 5-fold higher, respectively, and more than 90% was present as isomer III. These three relatives were recognized as gene carriers of an hereditary coproporphyria by metabolite studies. Coproporphyrinogen oxidase activity in lymphocytes in the patient was 2% of normal. This extremely decreased enzyme activity confirms that the young patient represents a homozygous case of HCP. Molecular analysis in the family revealed that the child was compound heterozygous with the maternal mutation A to G at position 980 in exon 5 and the paternal single nucleotide exchange A to G at position 920 in exon 4. This is the first description of a compound heterozygous hereditary coproporphyria[65].

PORPHYRIA CUTANEA TARDA

Molecular genetics of porphyria cutanea tarda

PCT is due to a partial deficiency of uroporphyrinogen decarboxylase (EC 4.1.1.37) activity[66]. This enzyme's human gene sequence has been completely researched[67]. Judging by the decrease in uroporphyrinogen decarboxylase activity of about 50% compared to controls, half the cases seem to be genetically determined[68]. Familial or type II or III PCT may be inherited and sporadic or type I PCT may be more commonly acquired[1]. It has been shown that type I PCT is not due to mutations at the uroporphyrinogen decarboxylase locus. If inherited factors are involved, other loci must be affected[69]. A splice site mutation has been reported in patients with type II PCT. This mutation causes an exon 6 deletion from the corresponding mRNA. It seems to be common, since it was found in five of 22 unrelated pedigrees of type II PCT patients[70]. Seven new mutations of the uroporphyringen decarboxylase gene have been described in patients with type II PCT. Four were missense mutations, the others were an insertion, a deletion and a splicing defect. Screening of nine probands revealed that about half were gene carriers for haemochromatosis mutations[71]. In type III PCT[72] erythrocyte uroporphyrinogen decarboxylase activity and concentration is normal but hepatic uroporphyrinogen decarboxylase activity is decreased.

The homozygous type of PCT, hepatoerythropoietic porphyria, which can also occur as compound heterozygosity, results from a severe deficiency of uroporphyrinogen decarboxylase[66,73]. A zebrafish mutant with photosensitivity and a homozygous mutation in the uroporphyrinogen decarboxylase gene represents an animal model for this disease[74].

Pathogenesis

The pathogenesis of PCT is complex. Uroporphyrinogen decarboxylase catalyses the sequential removal of the four carboxylic groups of the carboxymethyl side chains in uroporphyrinogen resulting in coproporphyrinogen. This single enzyme can catalyze four successive decarboxylation reactions producing 7-, 6-, 5-, and 4-carboxylated porphyrinogens, and the occurrence of all these intermediates has been identified in urine, faeces and plasma. The enzyme activity in the liver can be inhibited by environmental chemicals such as polyhalogenated aromatic hydrocarbons.

PCT is the name of a heterogeneous group of porphyric diseases. Familial occurrence, termed type II, has been reported by Kushner, Nordmann, Elder[75–77] and our group[78]. At present, PCT is subdivided into type I, II and III[77]: type I with normal red cell uroporphyrinogen decarboxylase activity (sporadic), type II with reduced activity in all tissues (familial). In the inherited type uroporphyrinogen decarboxylase is about 50% of its normal value in all tissues, and the enzyme deficiency segregates as an autosomal dominant trait. Type III is a hereditary, familial form with normal erythrocyte uroporphyrinogen decarboxylase. The hallmark of all types of PCT is a cutaneous photosensitivity due to an increased accumulation of uro- and heptacarboxylic porphyrins. The most important precipitating environmental factors are alcohol and oestrogens, as has been observed for 40 years by different investigators[1]. In the aquired form type I hepatic uroporphyrinogen decarboxylase is also affected by hexachlorobenzene, dioxin and other chemicals foreign to the human body. The homozygous variant of PCT, hepatoerythropoietic porphyria, is accompanied by severe cutaneous complaints comparable to CEP.

The decarboxylase deficiency results in an accumulation of uro- and heptacarboxyporphyrin in the liver exhibiting red fluorescence of liver biopsy tissue under long-wave ultraviolet light. The highly carboxylated porphyrins are excreted in urine, and their chromatographic identification and quantification allows a rapid diagnosis. Partial fluorescence of liver tissue is characteristic for a latent subclinical PCT, whereas total fluorescence of the liver biopsy characterizes the clinically overt form of PCT with extrahepatic cutaneous manifestations.

PCT is associated with non-specific liver involvement. Iron seems to play an important role. The disease expression is triggered by alcohol and oestrogens[79] in the majority of cases, and in a minority through haemodialysis, AIDS and hepatitis C virus infection (HCV). Recent studies in New Zealand[80] and Germany[81] have shown that PCT seems to have strong associations with an excessive use of alcohol and oestrogens but not with HCV infections. These results are in contrast to those published by authors from France, Spain, Italy and Poland[82–86].

Diagnosis of porphyria cutanea tarda

An extreme porphyrinuria (> 50-fold above normal levels) with dominance of uro- and heptacarboxyporphyrin is characteristic for the clinically manifest cutaneous phase of chronic hepatic porphyria. The excretion of porphyrin precursors is normal, although a slight elevation of ALA excretion may be found in alcohol-induced forms of the disease. In contrast to the acute hepatic porphyrias, the disease process of chronic hepatic porphyria develops slowly over months to years. In this time it passes through different subclinical stages, each of which is characterized by a continuous, gradual elevation of porphyrin excretion with a reversal of the copro-uroporphyrin ratio in their course. Under physiological circumstances, the copro-uroporphyrin ratio is about 4:1, by its reversal the chronic hepatic porphyria process is initiated[4]. When porphyrinuria rises to more than 2 μmol/24 h, an extensive porphyrin accumulation in the liver is indicated. The typical cutaneous symptoms depend on the level of porphyrinuria, which in turn is determined by the extent of hepatic porphyrin accumulation. A decline of porphyrinuria and porphyrinemia corresponds with the elimination of porphyrins from the liver and a remission of cutaneous symptoms. A dermatological remanifestation can be predicted by the preceding porphyrinuria. This allows for the institution of preventive and therapeutic measures.

Monitoring treatment

PCT is understood to be a cutaneous chronic hepatic porphyria because the centre of the disease process is the liver. The extent of hepatic accumulation of uro- and heptacarboxyporphyrin determines the onset and severity of the cutaneous manifestations. The decisive aim in therapy is the elimination of porphyrin from the liver via blood into urine. Venesection and chloroquine are effective[1]. Urinary porphyrin excretion patterns clearly reflect the hepatic porphyrin content, and monitoring of treatment by analysing urinary porphyrins is highly reliable. Alternatively, plasma porphyrins may be studied. Methodologically, however, when using high-performance thin-layer chromatography or high-performance liquid chromatography, sample preparation for chromatography is much easier when urine specimens are used.

The rate of urinary uro- and heptacarboxyporphyrin excretion correlates quantitatively with the porphyrin storage in the liver which is, in turn, directly related to the expression of cutaneous symptoms. This means that high-grade porphyrinuria (> 6 μmol/24 h) is associated with cutaneous lesions, whereas cutaneous symptoms are not found with low-grade porphyrinuria (< 1 μmol/24 h; normal limit < 0.2 μmol/24 h) in spite of the dominance of uro- and heptacarboxyporphyrin. Low-grade porphyrinuria has characteristic constellations of porphyrins that reflect the different subclinical stages of chronic hepatic porphyria leading to PCT[68]. During treatment, these stages are passed in the reverse direction, with the only difference that under chloroquine treatment uroporphyrin may stay dominant even in low-grade pathological porphyrinuria (< 0.3 μmol/ 24 h). After the omission of alcohol or oestrogens, porphyrinuria may decline by 30–50% with a disappearance of the cutaneous symptoms[87]. Under low-dose chloroquine treatment, porphyrinuria may rise temporarily because of a drug-induced elimination of porphyrins from the liver. Thereafter, porphyrinuria decreases, and the cutaneous manifestations disappear; no new dermal lesions appear while the old ones heal. The intensity of chloroquine treatment can be controlled precisely by using the decrease in porphyrinuria as the measure of treatment effectiveness. When porphyrinuria drops below 0.5 μmol/24 h, a relatively stable phase of latency is achieved. If the chloroquine treatment is continued for 3–6 months beyond this improvement, porphyrinuria may decline to normal values (< 0.2 μmol/24 h) under the condition that alcohol and oestrogens (including oral contraceptives) for women are avoided.

The study of urine porphyrins is recommended every 3 months to recognize reactivation of the chronic hepatic porphyria process before cutaneous symptoms occur, especially in patients with the genetically predisposing form (type II). In contrast to the pharmacogenetic acute hepatic porphyrias with their intermittent acute development of the clinical syndrome, in PCT the biochemical and clinical manifestations develop slowly over months and, in many cases, even over years.

In conclusion, the study of urinary porphyrins may be the optimal method for laboratory monitoring of PCT treatment. As in AIP, enzyme studies are not of importance and may even be misleading, because the uroporphyrinogen decarboxylase as well as the PBG deaminase activity in red cells remains constant throughout life and does not provide any information about the biochemical and clinical activity of the porphyria disease process. Furthermore these activities may even be normal in several cases of this disease.

ERYTHROPOIETIC PROTOPORPHYRIA

Photosensitivity, hepatic manifestations, pathological mechanisms and treatment of erythropoietic protoporphyria (EPP) have been reviewed by Cox[88].

Molecular genetics of erythropoietic protoporphyria

EPP is associated with a partial deficiency of ferrochelatase activity and is inherited in an autosomal dominant fashion with a variable degree of penetrance, although recessive inheritance patterns have also been demonstrated[89,90]. Patients with clinical manifestations of EPP have lower ferrochelatase activities than the expected 50%. Magness and Brenner[91] have shown that an exon 10 deletion alone in mouse embryonic stem cells is insufficient to decrease ferrochelatase activity to the levels in protoporphyric patients. Furthermore, it has been shown that co-inheritance of a ferrochelatase gene defect and a wild-type low-expressed allele is generally involved in the clinical expression of EPP[92]. The first de novo mutation, two deletions and two point mutations, were detected in Finnish EPP families[93]. Other large and small deletions occur in the ferrochelatase gene in patients with EPP. A five base-pair deletion was found in the ferrochelatase gene of a Swiss family with EPP[94]. Mutation analysis was performed in four Spanish EPP families resulting in the identification of four different mutations in the ferrochelatase gene. Two of them were a missense and a frameshift mutation. The third and the fourth Spanish patients carried a nonsense and a missense mutation. The frameshift mutation predicted formation of an abrupt mRNA. One of the missense mutations was expressed in *Escherichia coli*. The mutant ferrochelatase exhibited only 0.8% of the wild-type ferrochelatase activity[95]. Twenty different mutations, 15 of which were new, have been characterized in 26 of 29 EPP patients of Swiss and French origin. All the patients, including those with liver complications, were heterozygous for the mutations. Among the pedigrees with liver complication, mutations were common, which lead to a null allele after bacterial expression of the cDNA[96].

The human ferrochelatase promotor has been analysed in transgenic mice. It has been shown that the 5 flanking region of the ferrochelatase gene is necessary and sufficient to confer high levels of transgene expression in erythroid tissue[97].

Two patients with a compound heterozygous, autosomal recessive form of EPP have been reported[89,98]. Only one of them developed hepatic failure[99].

Bovine protoporphyria may be a useful animal model for the human disease. A novel stop codon mutation (X417L) of the ferrochelatase sequence from cattle has been identified and is probably responsible for EPP in these animals[100].

Ferrochelatase deficiency, protoporphyrinaemia, photosensitivity and liver involvement

EPP is associated with a partial deficiency of ferrochelatase activity and is inherited in an autosomal dominant fashion with a variable degree of penetrance[4,101,102]. Also recessive patterns of inheritance have been demonstrated[89,103,104]. Biochemically, the deficient ferrochelatase results in massive accumulations of protoporphyrin in erythrocytes, plasma, and faeces. Clinically, the disease is characterized by the childhood onset of cutaneous photosensitivity in light-exposed areas, but skin lesions are milder and less disfiguring than those seen in congenital erythropoietic porphyria and porphyria cutanea tarda[4]. The most important clinical complication is liver involvement[105–107]. In this context EPP was also designated as erythrohepatic protoporphyria[105,108]. Porphyrin and clinical studies in patients after liver transplantation reveal the immanent protoporphyrinaemia due to the ferrochelatase deficiency and justify the terminus EPP[108].

EPP is the most common form of erythropoietic porphyria. Three hundred case reports were published as of 1976. There is no racial or sexual predilection.

Clinical expression

EPP appears in early childhood often with season-dependent light dermatosis. The photosensitivity leads to burning, itching, pain, oedema, erythema, blisters and scars as well as petechiae. A slight anaemia occurs in about 25% of all cases. One-third of the patients develop an hepatobiliary disease. Serious forms lead to liver cirrhosis with cholestasis. The liver complication is the most important clinical aspect of the progressing EPP. The clinical suspicion of an EPP will be proved by the demonstration of enhanced concentrations of free protoporphyrin in erythrocytes and plasma.

Diagnosis and monitoring of treatment of erythropoietic protoporphyria

As in the acute and chronic hepatic porphyrias, the excess of porphyrin metabolites determines the disease process in EPP. Protoporphyrin, which is lipophilic, is cleared by hepatobiliary elimination, so protoporphyrinaemia (> 10 μmol/l erythrocytes) is accompanied by an increased faecal protoporphyrin excretion. Protoporphyrin has a concentration-dependent hepatotoxic effect. In about one-quarter of the patients with EPP hepatobiliary involvement occurs, resulting from the accumulation of protoporphyrin in the liver[107,109]. In the final stage of protoporphyric liver disease, fatal hepatic failure can be the consequence[110,111].

An early and most sensitive indicator of hepatic involvement in EPP is an increase of urinary coproporphyrin excretion. The specific diagnostic feature of the coproporphyrinuria is a change of the isomer I/III composition with an elevation and dominance of coproporphyrin isomer I (40–80% of total coproporphyrin). Therefore, monitoring urinary porphyrins is of decisive importance for early recognition of the erythrohepatic phase of EPP and for initiating therapeutic measures in order to eliminate protoporphyrin from the liver, to reduce hepatic protoporphyrin synthesis, and to interrupt enterohepatic circulation of protoporphyrin[102,107,112]. Severe hepatic protoporphyrin-induced disease (cholestatic cirrhosis) is associated with excessive protoporphyrinaemia (> 20 μmol/l erythrocytes), moderate coproporphyrinuria (> 0.2 μmol/24 h; normal < 0.1 μmol/24 h), and variable faecal protoporphyrin excretion. A decrease in faecal protoporphyrin excretion in patients with severe cirrhosis is a prognostically disadvantageous sign.

Rüfenacht et al.[113] have developed a molecular diagnostic procedure for screening of five known mutations in the ferrochelatase gene among Swiss EPP patients by single denaturing gradient gel electrophoresis. However, DNA-based testing is not usually needed for rapid diagnosis or management of symptomatic subjects, but it is useful for kindred evaluation and genetic counseling[114].

Treatment: cholic acids and liver transplantation

Therapy with ursodeoxycholic acid is indicated in EPP patients with incipient liver involvement. In some patients, treatment with ursodeoxycholic acid has stabilized liver functions for up to 2 years[115]. In EPP ursodeoxycholic acid is used to prevent hepatic accumulation of protoporphyrin in the liver and to facilitate its hepatic transport and secretion into bile[102].

The excretory function of the liver for protoporphyrin is impaired by advanced cirrhosis with cholestasis. In such cases, transplantation of the liver is the only therapeutic option[115–120]. After liver transplantation erythrocyte protoporphyrin levels fall rapidly and faecal protoporphyrin increases, indicating hepatic clearance of protoporphyrin by the transplanted liver. The total urinary coproporphyrin excretion tends to move to near normal rates. The coproporphyrin isomers remain shifted towards isomer I, reflecting low-grade cholestasis of the transplanted liver[121].

Orthotopic liver transplantations were performed on five patients with persistent jaundice due to protoporphyrin-induced biliary liver cirrhosis[115,118–120,122]. The liver explants from protoporphyria patients exhibit a brownish-black pigmentation due to the deposition of protoporphyrin and bile pigments. A summary of 10 other cases of EPP treated by liver transplantation was presented[123]. Some patients illustrate the point that continued reflux of protoporphyrin from extrahepatic sites can potentially cause recurrent protoporphyric injury to the liver allograft[123]. Two EPP patients were followed for 7 years after liver transplantation. In one patient, long periods with normal liver tests, low protoporphyrin levels and the absence of photosensitivity were followed by episodes of cholestasis and elevated protoporphyrin levels in blood, faeces and liver tissue. Sequential liver biopsies of both patients showed various degrees of liver injury related to variations of the hepatic protoporphyrin concentrations. Eight and six months respectively after liver transplantation the livers of both patients showed fibrosis and hepatocellular protoporphyrin accumulation[124]. Liver protoporphyrin levels in EPP patients with advanced protoporphyric liver disease are much higher than levels in blood and bile, in part because protoporphyrin forms crystalline deposits in liver tissue[125].

In conclusion, urinary coproporphyrin monitoring, including its isomer composition, is an important parameter for diagnosis and for assessing the course of the hepatobiliary phase and complications of EPP.

Autosomal recessive variant of protoporphyria

Studies by Sarkany and Cox[89] suggest that hepatic failure in protoporphyria may represent an autosomal recessive type of ferrochelatase deficiency. The authors describe a family in which two siblings with protoporphyria suffered from severe photosensitivity and developed hepatic failure requiring liver transplantation. A micronodular cirrhosis was seen on light microscopy of a liver biopsy specimen with deposition of a brown pigment which exhibits positive birefringence under polarized light. Two different mutations were found in the ferrochelatase gene. The asymptomatic parents of the two siblings were heterozygous for the two distinct ferrochelatase mutations. Both mutations cause severe ferrochelatase deficiency. The affected offspring were compound heterozygotes for these mutations. In conclusion, these patients suffered from an autosomal recessive form of protoporphyria with protoporphyrin-induced photosensitivity and cholestatic liver disease[103].

CONGENITAL ERYTHROPOIETIC PORPHYRIA

Molecular genetics of congenital erythropoietic porphyria

CEP is a rare, recessively inherited disorder, and mutations in the uroporphyrinogen-III synthase (EC 4.2.1.75) gene detected in CEP patients are heterogeneous. The exception to this rule is a single missense mutation, designated

C73R, which represents more than 40% of all uroporphyrinogen-III synthase alleles. Thus, C73R is a hotspot mutation for CEP[126].

Clinical expression and diagnosis

Patients with CEP pass reddish coloured urine, which is an early sign of this porphyria. Skin photosensitivity is manifested by vesiculobullous lesions which arise on the face, hands and other sun-exposed areas of skin. Cutaneous symptoms worsen during strong sunlight. Healing is followed by scarring, hyperpigmentation and hypertrichosis. Furthermore erythrodontia occurs in patients with CEP.

Urine of CEP patients contains large amounts of uroporphyrin and to a lesser extent of coproporphyrin. Hepta-, hexa- and pentacarboxylic porphyrins are also increased. Urinary excretion of the porphyrin precursors ALA and PBG is within the normal range. Excessive quantities of porphyrins are also excreted with the faeces. Urinary and faecal coproporphyrin isomers I and III reveal an excessive elevation of isomer I to about 90%[127].

Therapy

Allogenic bone marrow transplantation is the only curative treatment available for severe cases. A successful stem cell transplantation using blood from an HLA-identical brother in patients suffering from CEP has been reported by Zix-Kieffer et al.[128] and Freesemann et al.[129].

Gene therapy may play an important role in the healing of this erythropoietic porphyria for the future. A retroviral transfer in deficient human fibroblasts, immortalized lymphoblasts as well as bone marrow cells has been investigated: a complete restoration of the enzymatic activity and full metabolic correction has been obtained[130]. Another group transduced CEP fibroblasts by retroviral vectors with the wild-type and an optimized uroporphyrinogen-III synthase sequence. The endogenous enzyme activity of the cells could be enhanced up to nearly 20-fold without selection by this treatment[131].

DUAL PORPHYRIAS

Simultaneous presence of the enzyme deficiencies of two types of hereditary porphyria in one individual or in the same family is characteristic of dual porphyrias. These conditions are rare, and have been reported as a combination of two acute hepatic porphyrias, AIP and VP, known as the Chester type[10]. Coexistence of an acute and a non-acute hepatic porphyria (AIP and PCT or VP and PCT) is also described by literature[12,13,132], and two non-acute porphyrias may exist in the same person[133].

SECONDARY COPROPORPHYRINURIA

The secondary coproporphyrinurias, which are characterized by a mild-to-moderate coproporphyrinuria without uroporphyrinuria, δ-aminolevulinic aciduria, or PBGuria are the most frequent disturbances of haem biosynthesis. They arise as a result of the variable and complex effects many disorders and conditions have on normal porphyrin biosynthesis (Table 7). These secondary asymptomatic coproporphyrinurias do not develop clinical symptoms by themselves. Therefore, secondary porphyrinurias cannot explain clinical symptoms, even acute porphyria like symptoms. Thus, porphyrinuria does not necessarily mean porphyria. Treatment of these subclinical disturbances of porphyrin metabolism is not indicated (with the exception of subclinical lead poisoning); instead, the underlying associated disease has to be diagnosed and treated. From the clinical point of view the overinterpretation of secondary coproporphyrinuria as being hepatic porphyrias is the most frequent reason for errors in diagnosis and therapy in this field[134].

CONCLUSION

Elevated levels of urinary ALA and PBG are the conditio sine qua non for diagnosing clinical symptoms as AIP. In contrast, in PCT normal porphyrin precursors and excessive excretion of high-carboxylated porphyrins (uroporphyrin and heptacarboxyporphyrin) are of diagnostic significance.

The acute clinical crisis in AIP is treated by intravenous high-dose glucose and haem arginate, including avoidance of harmful drugs. PCT is treated by phlebotomy and low-dose chloroquine as well as by avoidance of alcohol and oestrogens. The hepatobiliary complication in EPP is treated by ursodeoxycholic acid and liver transplantation.

ACKNOWLEDGEMENT

This article contains results which were supported by the Hans-Fischer-Gesellschaft, Munich and the German Research Association (grant GR 1363/2-2).

REFERENCES

1. Kappas A, Sassa S, Galbraith RA, Nordmann Y. The porphyrias. In: Scriver CR, Beaudet AL, Sly WS, Vale D, eds. The Metabolic and Molecular Bases of Inherited Disease, 7th edn. New York: McGraw-Hill, Inc., 1995: pp. 2103–51.
2. Doss M. Hepatic porphyrias: Pathobiochemical, diagnostic, and therapeutic implications. In: Popper H, Schaffner F, eds. Progress in Liver Diseases. Vol. VII. New York: Grune & Stratton, 1982: pp. 573–97.
3. Meyer UA. Hepatic porphyrias. In: Bianchi L, Gerok W, Landmann L, Sickinger K, Stalder GA, eds. Liver in Metabolic Diseases. Boston: MTP Press Limited, 1983: pp. 379–84.
4. Doss MO, Sassa S. The porphyrias. In: Noe DA, Rock RC, eds. Laboratory Medicine. The Selection and Interpretation of Clinical Laboratory Studies, Chapter 26. Baltimore, MD: Williams & Wilkins, 1994: pp. 535–53; 902–3.
5. Grandchamp B, Phung N, Nordmann Y. Homozygous case of inheritary coproporphyria. Lancet. 1977;2:1348–9.
6. Nordmann Y, Grandchamp B, de Verneuil H, Phung L, Cartigny B, Fontaine G. Harderoporphyria: a variant hereditary coproporphyria. J Clin Invest. 1983;72:1139–49.
7. Doss M, v Tiepermann R, Köpp W. Harderoporphyrin coproporphyria. Lancet. 1984;1:292.

8. Kordac V, Deybach JCh, Martasek P et al. Homozygous variegate porphyria. Lancet. 1984;1:851.
9. Murphy GM, Hawk JLM, Magnus IA, Barrett DF, Elder GH, Smith SG. Homozygous variegate porphyria: two similar cases in unrelated families. J R Soc Med. 1966;79:361.
10. McColl KEL, Tompson GG, Moore MR, Goldberg A, Church SE, Quadiri MR, Youngs GR. Chester porphyria: biochemical studies of a new form of acute porphyria. Lancet. 1985;2:796–9.
11. Day RS, Eales L, Meissner D. Coexistent variegate porphyria and porphyria cutanea tarda. N Engl J Med. 1982;307:36–41.
12. Sieg I, Bhutani LK, Doss MO. Dual porphyria of coexisting variegata and cutanea tarda. Eur J Clin Chem Clin Biochem. 1995;33:405–10.
13. Doss M. New dual form of porphyria. Lancet. 1988;1:945–6.
14. Grandchamp B, Puy H, Lamoril J, Deybach JC, Nordmann Y. Molecular pathogenesis of hepatic acute porphyrias. In: Schmid R, Blum HE, Maier P, Bianchi L, Gerok W, Stalder GA, eds. Acute and Chronic Liver Diseases: Molecular Biology and Clinics. Dordrecht: Kluwer, 1996: pp. 192.
15. Mustajoki S, Pihlaja H, Ahola H, Peterson NE, Mustajoki P, Kauppinen R. Three splicing defects, an insertion, and two missense mutations responding for acute intermittent porphyria. Hum Genet. 1998;102:541–8.
16. Grandchamp B. Acute intermittent porphyria. Semin Liver Dis. 1998;18:17–24.
17. Schreiber WE, Jamani A, Armstrong A, Armstrong JG. AIP in a native North American family. Am J Clin Pathol. 1995;103:730–4.
18. Greene-Davis ST, Neumann PE, Mann OE et al. Detection of a R173W mutation in the porphobilinogen deaminase gene in the Nova Scotian foreign protestant population with acute intermittent porphyria: a founder effect. Clin Biochem. 1997;30:607–12.
19. Lee JS, Anvret M. Identification of the most common mutation within the porphobilinogen deaminase gene in Swedish patients with acute intermittent porphyria. Proc Natl Acad Sci USA. 1991;88:10912–15.
20. Gu XF, de Rooij F, Lee JS et al. High prevalence of a point mutation in the porphobilinogen deaminase gene in Dutch patients with acute intermittent porphyria. Hum Genet. 1993;91:128–30.
21. Mustajoki S, Kauppinen R, Mustajoki P, Suomalainen A, Peltonen L. Steady-state transcript levels of the porphobilinogen deaminase gene in patients with acute intermittent porphyria. Genome Res. 1997;7:1054–60.
22. Petersen NE, Nissen H, Hørder M, Senz J, Jamani A, Schreiber WE. Mutation screening by denaturing gradient gel electrophoresis in North American patients with acute intermittent porphyria. Clin Chem. 1998;44:1766–8.
23. Bjersing L, Andersson C, Lithner F. Hepatocellular carcinoma in patients from northern Sweden with AIP: morphology and mutations. Cancer Epidemiol Biomark Prevent. 1996;5:393–7.
24. Chretien S, Dubart A, Beaupain D et al. Alternative transcription and splicing of the human PBG deaminase gene result either in tissue specific or in housekeeping expression. Proc Natl Acad Sci USA. 1988;85:6–10.
25. Gross U, Honcamp M, Doss MO. Heterogeneity of AIP: a subtype with normal PBG deaminase activity in erythrocytes in Germany. Eur J Clin Chem Clin Biochem. 1996;34:613–18.
26. Mustajoki P, Kauppinen R, Lannfelt L, Koistinen J. Frequency of low PBG deaminase activity in Finland. J Intern Med. 1992;231:389–95.
27. Puy H, Gross U, Deybach JCh, Robréau AM, Frank M, Nordmann Y, Doss M. Exon 1 donor splice site mutations in the porphobilinogen deaminase gene in the non-erythroid variant form of acute intermittent porphyria. Hum Genet. 1998;103:570–5.
28. Lindberg RLP, Martini R, Baumgartner M, Erne B, Borg J, Zielasek J et al. Motor neuropathy in porphobilinogen deaminase-deficient mice imitates the peripheral neuropathy of human acute porphyria. J Clin Invest. 1999;103:1127–34.
29. Meyer UA, Schuurmans MM, Lindberg RLP. Acute porphyrias: Pathogenesis of neurologic manifestations. Semin Liv Dis. 1998;18:43–52:
30. Elder GH. Metabolic abnormalities in the porphyrias. Semin Dermatol. 1986;5:88–98.
31. Doss M. Relationships between acute hepatic porphyrias due to genetic variability of primary enzyme defects and limiting function of uroporphyrinogen synthase. Int J Biochem. 1978;9:911–16.

32. Bonkowsky HL, Tschudy DP, Collins A, Doherty J, Bossenmaier I, Cardinal R, Watson CJ. Repression of the overproduction of porphyrin precursors in acute intermittent porphyria by intravenous infusions of hematin. Proc Natl Acad Sci USA. 1971;68:2725–9.
33. Doss M, Sixel-Dietrich F, Verspohl F. 'Glucose effect' and rate limiting function of uroporphyrinogen synthase on porphyrin metabolism in hepatocyte culture: relationship with human acute hepatic porphyrias. J Clin Chem Clin Biochem. 1985;23:505–13.
34. Bonkowsky HL, Schady W. Neurologic manifestations of acute porphyria. Semin Liver Dis. 1982;2:108–24.
35. Litman DA, Correia MA. L-Tryptophan a common denominator of biochemical and neurological events of acute porphyrias? Science. 1983;22:1031–3.
36. Thunell S, Anderson C, Carlmark B, Floderus Y, Grönqvist SO, Harper P et al. Markers for vulnerability in acute porphyria. A hypothesis paper. Eur J Clin Chem Clin Biochem. 1995;33:179–94.
37. Demasi M, Penatti CAA, deLucia R, Bechara EJH. The prooxidant effect of δ-aminolevulinic acid in the brain tissue of rats: implications in neuropsychiatric manifestations in porphyrias. Free Rad Biol Med. 1996;20:2919.
38. Moore MR. International review of drugs in acute porphyria – 1980. Int J Biochem. 1980;12:1089–97.
39. Mustajoki P, Desnick RJ. Genetic heterogeneity in acute intermittent porphyria: characterisation and frequency of porphobilinogen deaminase mutations in Finland. Br Med J. 1985;291:505–9.
40. Stölzel U, Doss MO, Dissmann T, Cervós-Navarro J, Riecken EO. Gastroenterologische und neurologische Manifestation bei akuter intermittierender Porphyrie. Med Klin. 1987;82:520–5.
41. Sieg I, Rohrbacher C, Bavastro P, Doss MO. Kumulative Manifestationsfaktoren bei akuter intermittierender Porphyrie. Med Klin. 1992;87:318–22.
42. Hift RJ, Meissner PN, Kirsch RE. Clinical diagnosis, prevention and management of the hepatic porphyrias. In: Schmid R, Blum HE, Maier KP, Bianchi L, Gerok W, Stalder GA, editors. Acute and Chronic Liver Diseases: Molecular Biology and Clinics. Dordrecht: Kluwer Academic Publishers, 1996: pp. 201–15.
43. Kauppinen R, Mustajoki P. Prognosis of acute porphyria: occurrence of acute attacks, precipitating factors, and associated disease. Medicine. 1992;71:1–13.
44. Gross U, Honcamp M, Daume E, Frank M, Düsterberg B, Doss MO. Hormonal oral contraceptives, urinary porphyrin excretion and porphyrias. Horm Metab Res. 1995;27: 379–83.
45. Robert TL, Varella L, Meguid MM. Nutrition management of acute intermittent porphyria. Nutrition. 1994;10:551–5.
46. Kauppinen R, Timonen K, Mustajoki P. Treatment of the porphyrias. Ann Med. 1994;26:31–8.
47. Doss MO. Diagnosis and therapy of acute porphyrias: state of the art. In: Mustajoki P, ed. New Therapeutic Approach to Hepatic Porphyrias. Basel, Switzerland: Falk Foundation, 1987: pp. 19–29.
48. Goetsch CA, Montgomery Bissell D. Instability of hematin used in the treatment of acute hepatic porphyria. N Engl J Med. 1986;315:235–8.
49. Mustajoki P. Prevention and treatment of acute porphyric attacks. Ann Clin Res. 1985;17:289–91.
50. Mustajoki P (ed). New therapeutic approach to hepatic porphyrias. Workshop Short Report. Freiburg: Falk Foundation, 1987.
51. Mustajoki P, Nordmann Y. Early administration of heme arginate for acute porphyric attacks. Arch Intern Med. 1993;153:2004–8.
52. Anderson KE. LHRH analogues for hormonal manipulation in acute intermittent porphyria. Semin Hepatol. 1989;26:10–15.
53. Anderson KE, Spitz IM, Bardin CW, Kappas A. A gonadotropin releasing hormone analogue prevents cyclical attacks of porphyria. Arch Intern Med. 1990;150:1469–74.
54. Galbraith RA, Drummond GS, Kappas A. Sn-protoporphyrin suppresses chemically induced experimental hepatic porphyria. Potential clinical implications. J Clin Invest. 1985;76:2436–9.
55. Mustajoki P, Anderson KE, Bloomer J, Doss MO, Moore MR, Nordmann Y et al. Treatment of acute porphyrias. Consensus Statement 1994. P. Mustajoki, Third Department of Medicine, University Central Hospital, University of Helsinki, Finland.

56. Bonkovsky HL. Advances in understanding and treating 'the little imitator,' acute porphyria. Gastroenterology. 1993;105:590–4.
57. Dover SB, Moore MR, Fitzsimmons EJ, Graham A, McColl KEL. Tin protoporphyrin prolongs the biochemical remission produced by heme arginate in acute hepatic porphyria. Gastroenterology. 1993;105:500–6.
58. Cable EE, Cable JW, Bonkovsky HL. Repression of hepatic δ-aminolevulinate synthase by heme and metalloporphyrins: relationship to inhibition of heme oxygenase. Hepatology. 1993;18:119–27.
59. Cable EE, Pepe JA, Karamitsios NC, Lambrecht RW, Bonkovsky HL. Differential effects of metalloporphyrins on messenger RNA levels of δ-aminolevulinate synthase and haem oxygenase. J Clin Invest. 1994;94:649–54.
60. Doss M, v Tiepermann R, Schneider J, Schmid H. New type of hepatic porphyria and porphobilinogen synthase defect and intermittent acute clinical manifestation. Klin Wochenschr. 1979;57:1123–7.
61. Doss M, Benkmann HG, Goedde HW. δ-Aminolevulinic acid dehydratase (porphobilinogen synthase) in two families with inherited enzyme deficiency. Clin Genet. 1986;30:191–8.
62. Ishida N, Fujita H, Fukuda Y, Noguchi T, Doss M, Kappas A, Sassa S. Cloning and expression of the defective genes from a patient with (δ-aminolevulinate dehydratase porphyria. J Clin Invest. 1992;89:1431–7.
63. Gross U, Sassa S, Jacob K, Deybach JCh, Nordmann Y, Frank M, Doss MO. 5-Aminolevulinic acid dehydratase deficiency porphyria: a twenty-year clinical and biochemical follow up. Clin Chem. 1998;44:1892–6.
64. Sassa S. ALAD porphyria. Semin Liv Dis. 1998;18:95–101.
65. Doss MO, Gross U, Lamoril J, Kranl Ch, Jacob K, Doss M et al. Compound heterozygous hereditary coprophyria with fluorescing teeth. Ann Clin Biochem. 1999;36:680–2.
66. Elder GH, Roberts AG. Uroporphyrinogen decarboxylase. J Bioenerg Biomembr. 1995;27: 207–13.
67. Moran-Jimenez MJ, Ged C, Romana M et al. Uroporphyrinogen decarboxylase: complete human gene sequence and molecular study of three families with hepatoerythropoietic porphyria. Am J Hum Genet. 1996;58:712–21.
68. Doss MO, Frank M, Braun-Falco O. Porphyria cutanea tarda: erythrocyte decarboxylase activity in 471 consecutive patients. Curr Prob Dermatol. 1991;20:97–105.
69. Garey JR, Franklin KF, Brown DA, Harrison LM, Metcalf KM, Kushner JP. Analysis of uroporphyrinogen decarboxylase complementary DNAs in sporadic porphyria cutanea tarda. Gastroenterology. 1993;105:165–9.
70. Garey R, Harrison LM, Franklin KF, Metcalf KM, Radisky ES, Kushner JP. Uroporphyrinogen decarboxylase: a splice site mutation causes the deletion of exon 6 in multiple families with porphyria cutanea tarda. J Clin Invest. 1990;86:1416–22.
71. Mendez M, Sorkin L, Rossetti MV et al. Familial porphyria cutanea tarda: Characterization of seven novel uroporphyrinogen decarboxylase mutations and frequency of common hemochromatosis alleles. Am J Hum Genet. 1998;63:1363–75.
72. Held JL, Sassa S, Kappas A, Harber LC. Erythrocyte uroporphyrinogen decarboxylase activity in porphyria cutanea tarda: a study of 40 consecutive patients. J Invest Dermatol. 1989;93:332–4.
73. de Verneuil H, Bourgeois F, de Rooij F et al. Characterization of a new mutation (R292G) and a deletion at the human urporphyrinogen decarboxylase locus in two patients with hepatoerythropoietic porphyria. Hum Genet. 1992;89:548–52.
74. Wang H, Long Q, Marty SD, Sassa S, Lin S. A zebrafish model for hepatoerythropoietic porphyria. Nature Genet. 1998;20:239–43.
75. Kushner JP, Barbuto AJ, Lee GR. An inherited enzymatic defect in porphyria cutanea tarda. J Clin Invest. 1976;58:1089–97.
76. de Verneuil H, Atiken G, Nordmann Y. Familial and sporadic porphyria cutanea. Two different diseases. Hum Genet. 1978;42:145–51.
77. Elder GH, Roberts AG, de Salamanca RE. Genetics and pathogenesis of human uroporphyrinogen decarboxylase defects. Clin Biochem. 1989;22:163–8.
78. Doss M, v Tiepermann R, Look D. Hereditäre und nicht-hereditäre Form der chronischen hepatischen Porphyrie: Unterschiedliches Verhalten der Uroporphyrinogen-Decarboxylase in Leber und Erythrozyten. Klin Wochenschr. 1980;58:1347–56.

79. Sixel-Dietrich F, Doss M. Hereditary uroporphyrinogen decarboxylase deficiency predisposing porphyria cutanea tarda (chronic hepatic porphyria) in females after oral contraceptive medication. Arch Dermatol Res. 1985;278:13–16.
80. Salmon P, Oakley A, Rademaker M, Duffill M. Hepatitis C virus infection and porphyria cutanea tarda in Australasia. Arch Dermatol. 1996;132:91.
81. Stölzel U, Köstler E, Koszka C et al. Low prevalence of hepatitis C virus infection in porphyria cutanea tarda in Germany. Hepatology. 1995;21:1500–3.
82. Lacour JPH, Bodokh I, Castanet J, Bekri S, Ortonne JP. Porphyria cutanea tarda and antibodies to hepatitis C virus. Br J Dermatol. 1993;128:121–3.
83. deCastro M, Sanchez J, Herrera JF et al. Hepatitis C virus antibodies and liver disease in patients with porphyria cutanea tarda. Hepatology. 1993;17:551–7.
84. Ferri C, Baicchi U, LaCivita L et al. Hepatitis C virus-related autoimmunity in patients with porphyria cutanea tarda. Eur J Clin Invest. 1993;23:851–5.
85. Fargion S, Piperno A, Cappellini MD. Hepatitis C virus and porphyria cutanea tarda: evidence of a strong association. Hepatology. 1992;16:1322–6.
86. Dabrowska E, Jablonska-Kaszewska I, Falkiewicz B. High prevalence of hepatitis C virus infection in patients with porphyria cutanea tarda in Poland. Clin Exp Dermatol. 1998;23:95–6.
87. Topi GC, Amantea AA, Griso D. Recovery from porphyria cutanea tarda with no specific therapy other than avoidance of hepatic toxins. Br J Dermatol. 1984;111:75–82.
88. Cox TM. Erythropoietic protoporphyria. J Inher Metab Dis. 1997;20:258–69.
89. Sarkany RPE, Alexander GJMA, Cox TM. Recessive inheritance of erythropoietic protoporphyria with liver failure. Lancet. 1994;343:1394–6.
90. Deybach JC, DaSilva V, Pasquier Y, Nordmann Y. Ferrochelatase in human erythropoietic protoporphyria: the first case of a homozygous form of the enzyme deficiency. In: Nordmann Y, ed. Porphyrins and Porphyrias. Colloque INSERM/John Libbey Eurotext Ltd. 1986;134:163–73.
91. Magness ST, Brenner DA. Targeted disruption of the mouse ferrochelatase gene producing an exon 10 deletion. Biochim Biophys Acta. 1986;1453:161–74.
92. Gouya L, Puy H, Lamoril J et al. Inheritance in erythropoietic protoporphyria: A common wild type ferrochelatase allelic variant with low expression accounts for clinical manifestation. Blood. 1999;93:2105–10.
93. Henriksson M, Timonen K, Mustajoki P. Four novel mutations in the ferrochelatase gene among erythropoietic protoporphyria patients. J Invest Dermatol. 1996;106:346–50.
94. Schneider-Yin X, Schäfer BW, Tönz O, Minder EI. Human ferrochelatase: a novel mutation in patients with erythropoietic protoporphyria and an isoform caused by alternative splicing. Hum Genet. 1995;95:391–6.
95. Gouya L, Schneider-Yin X, Rüfenacht U, Herrero C, Lecha M, Mascaro JM et al. Mutations in the ferrochelatase gene of four Spanish patients with erythropoietic protoporphyria. J Invest Dermatol. 1998;111:406–9.
96. Rüfenacht UB, Gouya L, Schneider-Yin X et al. Systematic analysis of molecular defects in the ferrochelatase gene from patients with erythropoietic protoporphyria. Am J Hum Genet. 1998;62:1341–52.
97. Magness ST, Tugores A, Diala ES, Brenner DA. Analysis of the human ferrochelatase promotor in transgenic mice. Blood. 1998;92:320–8.
98. Lamoril J, Boulechfar S, Verneuil H de, Grandchamp B, Nordmann Y, Deybach J-C. Human erythropoietic protoporphyria: two point mutations in the ferrochelatase gene. Biochem Biophys Res Commun. 1991;181:594–9.
99. Todd DJ. Molecular genetics of erythropoietic protoporphyria. Photodermatol Photoimmunol Photomed. 1998;14:70–3.
100. Jenkins MM, LeBoef RD, Ruth GR, Bloomer JR. A novel stop codon mutation (X417L) of the ferrochelatase gene in bovine protoporphyria, a natural animal model of the human disease. Biochim Biophys Acta. 1998;1408:18–24.
101. Poh-Fitzpatrick MB. Erythropoietic protoporphyria. Semin Dermatol. 1986;5:99–105.
102. Todd DJ. Erythropoietic protoporphyria. Br J Dermatol. 1994;131:751–66.
103. Sarkany RPE, Cox TM. Autosomal recessive erythropoietic protoporphyria: a syndrome of severe photosensitivity and liver failure. Q J Med. 1995;88:541–9.
104. Deybach JC, DaSilva V, Pasquier Y, Nordmann Y. Ferrochelatase in human erythropoietic protoporphyria: the first case of a homozygous form of the enzyme deficiency. In:

Nordmann Y, ed. Porphyrins and Porphyrias. Colloque INSERM/John Libbey Eurotext Ltd. 1986;134:163–73.
105. Eales L. Liver involvement in erythropoietic protoporphyria. Int J Biochem. 1980;12:915–23.
106. Bloomer JR. The liver in protoporphyria. Hepatology (Balt.). 1988;8:402–7.
107. Doss MO, Frank M. Hepatobiliary implications and complications in protoporphyria. A 20-year study. Clin Biochem. 1989;22:223–9.
108. Johnson JA, Fusaro RM. Prognosis of liver transplantation in patients with erythropoietic protoporphyria. Transplantation. 1989;48:175–6.
109. Bloomer JR. The liver in protoporphyria. Hepatology. 1988;8:402–7.
110. Mercurio MG, Prince G, Weber FL Jr, Jacobs G, Zaim MT, Bickers DR. Terminal hepatic failure in erythropoietic protoporphyria. J Am Acad Dermatol. 1993;29:829–33.
111. Rank JM, Carithers R, Bloomer J. Evidence for neurological dysfunction in end-stage protoporphyric liver disease. Hepatology. 1993;18:1404–9.
112. Nordmann Y. Erythropoietic protoporphyria and hepatic complications. Hepatology. 1992;16:4–6.
113. Rüfenacht UB, Schneider-Yin X, Schäfer BW, Taketani S, Deybach JCh, Minder E. Rapid molecular diagnosis of erythropoietic protoporphyria among Swiss patients. Clin Chem Lab Med. 1998;36:763–5.
114. Bonkovsky HL, Barnard GF. Diagnosis of porphyric syndromes: a practical approach in the era of molecular biology. Semin Liver Dis. 1998;18:57–65.
115. Frank M, Doss MO. Leberzirrhose bei Protoporphyrie: Gallensäurentherapie und Lebertransplantation. Z Gastroenterol. 1995;33:399–403.
116. Polson RJ, Lim CK, Rolles K, Calne Y, Williams R. The effect of liver transplantation in a 13 year old boy with erythropoietic protoporphyria. Transplantation. 1988;46:386–9.
117. Samuel D, Boboc B, Bernuau J, Bismuth H, Benhamou JP. Liver transplantation for protoporphyria. Evidence for the predominant role of the erythropoietic tissue in protoporphyrin overproduction. Gastroenterology. 1988;95:816–19.
118. Steinmüller T, Doss MO, Steffen R et al. Lebertransplantation bei erythrohepatischer Protoporphyrie. Dtsch Med Wschr. 1992;117:1097–102.
119. Gauer EB, Doss MO, Riemann FJ. Erythrohepatische Protoporphyrie. Eine seltene Differentialdiagnose des parenchymatösen Ikterus. Dtsch Med Wschr. 1995;120:713–17.
120. Lock G, Holstege A, Mueller AR et al. Liver failure in erythropoietic protoporphyria associated with choledocholithiasis and severe post-transplantation polyneuropathy. Liver. 1996;16:211–17.
121. Gross U, Frank M, Doss MO. Hepatic complications of erythropoietic protoporphyria. Photodermatol Photoimmunol Photomed. 1998;14:52–7.
122. Wagner S, Doss MO, Wittekind C, Bäcker U, Meesen D, Schmidt FW. Erythrohepatische Protoporphyrie mit rasch progredienter Leberzirrhose. Dtsch Med Wschr. 1989;114:1837–41.
123. de Torres I, Demetris AJ, Randhawa PS. Recurrent hepatic allograft injury in erythropoietic protoporphyria. Transplantation. 1996;61:1412–33.
124. Meermann L, Haagsma EB, Gouw ASH, Slooff MJH, Jansen PLM. Long-term follow-up after liver transplantation for erythropoietic protoporphyria. Eur J Gastroenterol Hepatol. 1999;11:431–8.
125. Bloomer JR. Hepatic protoporphyrin metabolism in patients with advanced protoporphyric liver disease. Yale J Biol Med. 1997;70:323–30.
126. Frank J, Wang X, Lam HM, Aita VM, Jugert FK, Goerz G et al. C73R is a hotspot mutation in the uroporphyrinogen III synthase gene in congenital erythropoietic porphyria. Am Hum Genet. 1998;62:225–30.
127. Freesemann AG, Bhutani LK, Jacob K, Doss MO. Interdependence between degree of porphyrin excess and disease severity in congenital erythropoietic porphyria (Günther's disease). Arch Dermatol Res. 1997;289:272–6.
128. Zix-Kieffer I, Langer B, Eyer D et al. Successful cord blood stem cell transplantation for congenital erythropoietic porphyria (Günther's disease). Bone Marrow Transplant. 1996;18:217–20.
129. Freesemann AG, Greil J, Beck JD, Doss MO. Porphyrinstoffwechsel vor und nach allogener Knochenmarkstransplantation bei kongenitaler erythropoetischer Porphyrie. Med Klin. 1999;94:145.
130. Mazurier F, Moreau-Gaudry F, Salesse S et al. Gene transfer of the uroporphyrinogen III synthase cDNA into haematopoietic progenitor cells in view of a future gene therapy in congenital erythropoietic porphyria. J Inher Metab Dis. 1997;20:247–57.

131. Kauppinen R, Glass IA, Aizencang G, Astrin KH, Atweh GF, Desnick RJ. Congenital erythropoietic porphyria: Prolonged high-level expression and correction of the heme biosynthetic defect by retroviral-mediated gene transfer into porphyric and erythroid cells. Mol Gen Metab. 1998;65:10–17.
132. Doss MO. Dual porphyria in double heterozgotes with porphobilinogen deaminase and uroporphyrinogen decarboxylase deficiencies. Clin Genet. 1989;35:146–51.
133. Freesemann AG, Hofweber K, Doss MO. Coexistence of deficiencies of uroporphrinogen III synthase and decarboxylase in a patient with congenital erythropoietic porphyria and his family. Eur J Clin Chem Clin Biochem. 1997;35:35–9.
134. Doss MO. Porphyrinurias and occupational disease. Ann NY Acad Sci. 1987;514:204–18.

27
Presentation of the Hans Popper Award

J. L. BOYER

A major highlight of this Congress is the presentation of the Hans Popper Award. This award was created by the Falk Foundation and is presented for the 4th time. The prize is endowed with a check for $25 000 and is awarded to a scientist under 50 years of age for outstanding publications in the field of clinical and experimental hepatology.

Hans Popper, for whom the Award is named, is widely considered to be the father of modern hepatology. Hans Popper was born in 1903 in Vienna where he entered medical school and pursued biochemical research and training in pathology. His interest in liver diseases began in the First Department of Medicine at the University of Vienna but when Austria was occupied in 1938 he continued his work in the United States at the Hektoen Institute in Chicago. There he organized the first informal meetings of clinical scientists interested in liver disease which led in 1950 to the establishment of the first organized liver society, the American Association for the Study of the Liver. In 1956 he became pathologist-in-chief at the Mt Sinai Hospital in New York, and later the first Dean of the new Mount Sinai Medical School. This award memorializes the seminal influence that he has made on the field of Hepatology as reflected not only in his prolific writings, his many lectures and unending research, but also for the extraordinary enthusiasm that he projected for all things hepatological and for the encouragement that he consistently gave to all within his influence.

This year the Falk Foundation presents the Hans Popper Award to a research team, whose leader, Dr. Michael Houghton, accepts the award and provides the Hans Popper Award presentation.

Following the discovery of the Hepatitis B virus in 1976 and hepatitis A in 1973, diagnostic tests were developed to detect these viruses in serum. This work confirmed the existence of a third type of virus, long suspected on clinical grounds. This virus came to be known as the non-A, non-B virus. Clinical studies of non-A, non-B hepatitis revealed much of its natural history including development of chronic hepatitis, its progression to cirrhosis in some patients, and histological features that were characteristic. However efforts to isolate this virus failed despite the work of many investigators and the testing of numerous candidate viruses against a panel of known infectious sera at the National Institutes of Health, using classic virological and immunological approaches.

The landmark discovery came in 1989 when Michael Houghton and his colleagues Qui-Lim Choo and George C. Kuo at Chiron Corporation in Emeryville, California and Daniel W. Bradley at the Center for Disease Control in Atlanta, Georgia used molecular biology techniques and succeeded in cloning parts of the hepatitis C virus, which then led to the development of diagnostic antibody tests for this disease. This discovery, one of the most important in the field of hepatology in this century, has had an enormous worldwide impact. The hepatitis C virus has now been identified as the cause of both acute and chronic hepatitis, cirrhosis and hepatocellular carcinoma, as well as the agent responsible for several extrahepatic disorders, including mixed essential cryoglobulinaemia and glomerulonephritis. More then 200 million patients are infected with this virus throughout the world and cirrhosis secondary to chronic hepatitis C is now the leading cause of liver failure leading to transplantation. This discovery not only led to major improvements in diagnosis but also to rational antiviral therapy and attempts to irradiate this chronic virus infection.

Michael Houghton is Director of non-A, non-B hepatitis research at Chiron Corporation. He received his education in England, graduating with honors in the biological sciences from the University of East Anglia in 1972. He received a PhD in biochemistry from King's College, University of London in 1977 and then began his professional career as Senior Research Investigator at the Searle Research Laboratories in Buckinghamshire, England before moving to his present position at Chrion Corporation in 1982.

Dr. Qui-Lim Choo is a Senior Scientist at Chiron Corporation. He received his undergraduate training at Queen Elizabeth College, University of London in 1973 and his PhD in Biochemistry at King's College, University of London in 1980. After two years of postdoctoral training with Dr. William Rutter at the University of California, San Francisco, he joined the Chiron Corporation.

George C. Kuo is Director of immunochemistry at Chiron Corporation. He received his undergraduate training at the National Taiwan University in 1961 and his PhD degree from Albert Einstein College of Medicine in molecular biology in 1972. He joined the Chiron Corporation in 1981.

Daniel W. Bradley is Chief of Hepatitis at the Centers for Disease Control in Atlanta, Georgia. His undergraduate training was at San Jose State College in California, graduating in 1964. In 1970 he received a PhD degree from the University of Arizona in Tucson, before joining the Centers for Disease Control in Phoenix, Arizona in 1971.

Dr. Houghton and his three colleagues are co-recipients of many honours for their work on hepatitis C, including the Karl Landsteiner Award from the American Association of Blood Banks in 1992; the Robert Koch Award from Germany in 1993; and the William Beaumont Prize from the American Gastroenterology Association in 1994.

Index

Falk Symposium Series

99. Goebell H, Holtmann G, Talley NJ, eds. *Functional Dyspepsia and Irritable Bowel Syndrome: Concepts and Controversies.* Falk Symposium 99. 1998 ISBN 0-7923-8735-X
100. Blum HE, Bode Ch, Bode JCh, Sartor RB, eds. *Gut and the Liver.* Falk Symposium 100. 1998 ISBN 0-7923-8736-8
101. Rachmilewitz D, ed. *V International Symposium on Inflammatory Bowel Diseases.* Falk Symposium 101. 1998 ISBN 0-7923-8743-0
102. Manns MP, Boyer JL, Jansen PLM, Reichen J, eds. *Cholestatic Liver Diseases.* Falk Symposium 102. 1998 ISBN 0-7923-8746-5

102B. Manns MP, Chapman RW, Stiehl A, Wiesner R, eds. *Primary Sclerosing Cholangitis.* International Falk Workshop. 1998. ISBN 0-7923-8745-7

103. Häussinger D, Jungermann K, eds. *Liver and Nervous System.* Falk Symposium 102. 1998 ISBN 0-7924-8742-2

103B. Häussinger D, Heinrich PC, eds. *Signalling in the Liver.* International Falk Workshop. 1998 ISBN 0-7923-8744-9

103C. Fleig W, ed. *Normal and Malignant Liver Cell Growth.* International Falk Workshop. 1998 ISBN 0-7923-8748-1

104. Stallmach A, Zeitz M, Strober W, MacDonald TT, Lochs H, eds. *Induction and Modulation of Gastrointestinal Inflammation.* Falk Symposium 104. 1998 ISBN 0-7923-8747-3
105. Emmrich J, Liebe S, Stange EF, eds. *Innovative Concepts in Inflammatory Bowel Diseases.* Falk Symposium 105. 1999 ISBN 0-7923-8749-X
106. Rutgeerts P, Colombel J-F, Hanauer SB, Schölmerich J, Tytgat GNJ, van Gossum A, eds. *Advances in Inflammatory Bowel Diseases.* Falk Symposium 106. 1999 ISBN 0-7923-8750-3
107. Špičák J, Boyer J, Gilat T, Kotrlik K, Mareček Z, Paumgartner G, eds. *Diseases of the Liver and the Bile Ducts – New Aspects and Clinical Implications.* Falk Symposium 107. 1999 ISBN 0-7923-8751-1
108. Paumgartner G, Stiehl A, Gerok W, Keppler D, Leuschner U, eds. *Bile Acids and Cholestasis.* Falk Symposium 108. 1999 ISBN 0-7923-8752-X
109. Schmiegel W, Schölmerich J, eds. *Colorectal Cancer – Molecular Mechanisms, Premalignant State and its Prevention.* Falk Symposium 109. 1999 ISBN 0-7923-8753-8
110. Domschke W, Stoll R, Brasitus TA, Kagnoff MF, eds. *Intestinal Mucosa and its Diseases – Pathophysiology and Clinics.* Falk Symposium 110. 1999 ISBN 0-7923-8754-6

110B. Northfield TC, Ahmed HA, Jazwari RP, Zentler-Munro PL, eds. *Bile Acids in Hepatobiliary Disease.* Falk Workshop. 2000 ISBN 0-7923-8755-4

111. Rogler G, Kullmann F, Rutgeerts P, Sartor RB, Schölmerich J, eds. *IBD at the End of its First Century.* Falk Symposium 111. 2000 ISBN 0-7923-8756-2
112. Krammer HJ, Singer MV, eds. *Neurogastroenterology: From the Basics to the Clinics.* Falk Symposium 112. 2000 ISBN 0-7923-8757-0
113. Andus T, Rogler G, Schlottmann K, Frick E, Adler G, Schmiegel W, Zeitz M, Schölmerich J, eds. *Cytokines and Cell Homeostasis in the Gastrointestinal Tract.* Falk Symposium 113. 2000 ISBN 0-7923-8758-9
114. Manns MP, Paumgartner G, Leuschner U, eds. *Immunology and Liver.* Falk Symposium 114. 2000 ISBN 0-7923-8759-7

Falk Symposium Series

115. Boyer JL, Blum HE, Maier K-P, Sauerbruch T, Stalder GA, eds. *Liver Cirrhosis and its Development.* Falk Symposium 115. 2000 ISBN 0-7923-8760-0
116. Riemann JF, Neuhaus H, eds. *Interventional Endoscopy in Hepatology.* Falk Symposium 116. 2000 ISBN 0-7923-8761-9

116A. Dienes HP, Schirmacher P, Brechot C, Okuda K, eds. *Chronic Hepatitis: New Concepts of Pathogenesis, Diagnosis and Treatment.* Falk Workshop. 2000 ISBN 0-7923-8763-5

www.ingramcontent.com/pod-product-compliance
Ingram Content Group UK Ltd.
Pitfield, Milton Keynes, MK11 3LW, UK
UKHW020234290926
15470UKWH00002B/538
* 9 7 8 0 7 9 2 3 8 7 6 0 2 *